2006
YEAR BOOK OF
HAND AND UPPER
LIMB SURGERY®

The 2006 Year Book Series

Year Book of Allergy, Asthma, and Clinical Immunology™: Drs Rosenwasser, Boguniewicz, Milgrom, Routes, and Weber

Year Book of Anesthesiology and Pain Management™: Drs Chestnut, Abram, Black, Gravlee, Lee, Mathru, and Roizen

Year Book of Cardiology®: Drs Gersh, Cheitlin, Elliott, Graham, Sundt, and Waldo

Year Book of Critical Care Medicine®: Drs Dellinger, Parrillo, Balk, Bekes, Dorman, and Dries

Year Book of Dentistry®: Drs McIntyre, Belvedere, Buhite, Davis, Henderson, Johnson, Jureyda, Ohrbach, Olin, Scott, Spencer, and Zakariasen

Year Book of Dermatology and Dermatologic Surgery™: Drs Thiers and Lang

Year Book of Diagnostic Radiology®: Drs Osborn, Birdwell, Dalinka, Gardiner, Levy, Maynard, Oestreich, and Rosado de Christenson

Year Book of Emergency Medicine®: Drs Burdick, Hamilton, Handly, Quintana, and Werner

Year Book of Endocrinology®: Drs Mazzaferri, Bessesen, Clarke, Howard, Kennedy, Leahy, Meikle, Molitch, Rogol, and Schteingart

Year Book of Family Practice®: Drs Bowman, Apgar, Dexter, Miser, Neill, and Scherger

Year Book of Gastroenterology™: Drs Lichtenstein, Burke, Campbell, Dempsey, Drebin, Ginsberg, Katzka, Kochman, Morris, Rombeau, Shah, and Stein

Year Book of Hand Surgery and Upper Limb Surgery®: Drs Chang and Steinmann

Year Book of Medicine®: Drs Barkin, Frishman, Garrick, Loehrer, Phillips, Pillinger, and Snydman

Year Book of Neonatal and Perinatal Medicine®: Drs Fanaroff, Maisels, and Stevenson

Year Book of Neurology and Neurosurgery®: Drs Gibbs and Verma

Year Book of Nuclear Medicine®: Drs Coleman, Blaufox, Royal, Strauss, and Zubal

Year Book of Obstetrics, Gynecology, and Women's Health®: Dr Shulman

Year Book of Oncology®: Drs Loehrer, Arceci, Glatstein, Gordon, Hanna, Morrow, and Thigpen

Year Book of Ophthalmology®: Drs Rapuano, Cohen, Eagle, Flanders, Hammersmith, Myers, Nelson, Penne, Sergott, Shields, Tipperman, and Vander

Year Book of Orthopedics®: Drs Morrey, Beauchamp, Peterson, Swiontkowski, Trigg, and Yaszemski

Year Book of Otolaryngology-Head and Neck Surgery®: Drs Paparella, Gapany, and Keefe

2006

The Year Book of HAND AND UPPER LIMB SURGERY®

Editors

James Chang, MD
Associate Professor of Surgery and Orthopedic Surgery, Residency Program Director, Plastic Surgery, Stanford University Medical Center, Stanford, California; Chief, Plastic Surgery, Palo Alto Veterans Administration Health Care System, Palo Alto, California

Scott P. Steinmann, MD
Associate Professor of Orthopedic Surgery, Mayo Clinic, Rochester, Minnesota

Editors Emeritus

Peter C. Amadio, MD
Professor of Orthopedic Surgery, Mayo Clinic, Rochester, Minnesota

Richard A. Berger, MD, PhD
Professor of Orthopedic Surgery and Anatomy, Mayo Clinic, Rochester, Minnesota

Robert A. Chase, MD
Emile Holman Professor of Surgery (Emeritus), Stanford University School of Medicine, Stanford, California

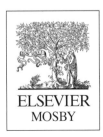

ELSEVIER
MOSBY

James H. Dobyns, MD
Emeritus Professor of Orthopedic Surgery, Mayo Foundation, Rochester, Minnesota; Clinical Professor, University of Texas Science Center, San Antonio, Texas

Vincent R. Hentz, MD
Professor of Surgery, Robert A. Chase Hand and Upper Limb Center, Department of Orthopaedic Surgery, Stanford University School of Medicine, Stanford, California

Amy L. Ladd MD
Professor of Orthopedic Surgery, Robert A. Chase Hand and Upper Limb Center, Department of Orthopaedic Surgery, Stanford University School of Medicine; Chief, Pediatric Hand Clinic, Lucile Packard Children's Hospital, Stanford University Medical Center, Stanford, California

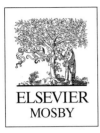

Vice President, Continuity Publishing: John A. Schrefer
Developmental Editor: Timothy Maxwell
Senior Manager, Continuity Production: Idelle L. Winer
Senior Issue Manager: Donna M. Adamson
Illustrations and Permissions Coordinator: Dawn Vohsen

Printed in the United States of America
Composition by Thomas Technology Solutions, Inc.
Printing/binding by Sheridan Books, Inc.

Editorial Office:
Elsevier
Suite 1800
1600 John F. Kennedy Blvd.
Philadelphia, PA 19103-2899

International Standard Serial Number: 1551-7977
International Standard Book Number: 1-4160-3313-0
                                    978-1-4160-3313-4

Contributing Editors

Kimberly K. Amrami, MD
Consultant in Diagnostic Radiology; Assistant Professor of Radiology; Chair, Division of Body MRI, Mayo Clinic, Rochester, Minnesota

Kodi Azari, MD
Assistant Professor of Surgery, Division of Plastic Surgery, Department of Surgery, University of Pittsburgh Medical Center, Pittsburgh, Pennsylvania

Keith Bengtson, MD
Assistant Professor of Physical Medicine and Rehabilitation, Mayo Clinic, Rochester, Minnesota

Stacey H. Berner, MD
Chief, Division of Hand Surgery, Northwestern Hospital Center, Owings Mills, Maryland

Rudy Buntic, MD
Attending Microsurgeon, Division of Microsurgery, Department of Plastic Sugery, The Buncke Clinic, California Pacific Medical Center, San Francisco, California

Charles Carroll IV, MD
Associate Professor of Clinical Orthopedic Surgery, Feinberg School of Medicine, Northwestern University, Chicago, Illinois

Alphonsus Chong, MD
Associate Consultant, Department of Hand and Reconstructive Microsurgery, National University Hospital, Singapore

Kevin C. Chung, MD, MS
Associate Professor, Plastic Surgery, University of Michigan Health Center, Ann Arbor, Michigan

Matthew Concannon, MD
Associate Professor of Surgery, Director, Hand & Microsurgery, Division of Plastic & Reconstructive Surgery, University of Missouri Health Sciences Center, Columbia, Missouri

William P. Cooney, MD
Professor of Orthopaedic Surgery, Mayo Clinic, Rochester, Minnesota

David G. Dennison, MD
Assistant Professor of Orthopedic Surgery, Mayo Clinic, Rochester, Minnesota

Scott F. M. Duncan, MD, MPH
Assistant Professor of Orthopedic Surgery, Mayo Clinic, Scottsdale, Arizona

Marybeth Ezaki, MD
Professor, Orthopaedic Surgery, University of Texas Southwestern Medical School; Director of Hand Surgery, Texas Scottish Rite Hospital for Children, Dallas, Texas

Leesa M. Galatz, MD
Assistant Professor, Shoulder and Elbow Service, Washington University School of Medicine, St. Louis, Missouri

Robert Goitz, MD
Assistant Professor of Orthopaedic Surgery, Division of Hand and Upper Extremity Surgery, Department of Orthopedic Surgery, University of Pittsburgh Medical Center, Pittsburgh, Pennsylvania

Ranjan Gupta, MD
Associate Professor of Orthopaedic Surgery, Department of Orthopedic Surgery, University of California, Irvine Medical Center, Orange, California

Doron I. Ilan, MD
Attending Orthopaedic Surgeon, Hand and Upper Extremity, Rivertown Orthopaedics, Ardsley, New York

Julie A. Katarincic, MD
Assistant Professor of Orthopedics, Brown Medical School, Providence, Rhode Island

Charles Lee, MD
Attending Surgeon, Buncke Microsurgery Clinic, California Pacific Medical Center, San Francisco, California

Sven Lichtenberg, MD
Orthopaedic Surgeon, Sports Medicine, Department of Shoulder and Elbow Surgery, ATOS-Clinic Heidelberg, Heidelberg, Germany

Timothy R. McAdams, MD
Assistant Professor, Robert A. Chase Hand and Upper Limb Center, Department of Orthopaedic Surgery, Stanford University School of Medicine, Stanford, California

Steven L. Moran, MD
Assistant Professor of Orthopedic Surgery, Mayo Clinic, Rochester, Minnesota

Peter M. Murray, MD
Associate Professor of Orthopedic Surgery, Mayo Clinic, Jacksonville, Florida

Toshihiko Ogino, MD, PhD
Professor and Chair, Department of Orthopaedics, Yamagata University School of Medicine, Yamagata, Japan

Marianne Outzen, MS, OTR/L
Occupational Therapist, Stanford Hand Rehabilitation Clinic, Palo Alto, California

Kevin J. Renfree, MD
Assistant Professor of Orthopedic Surgery, Mayo Clinic, Scottsdale, Arizona

Marco Rizzo, MD
Assistant Professor of Orthopedic Surgery, Mayo Clinic, Rochester, Minnesota

Alberto G. Schneeberger
Shoulder and Elbow Surgery, Seefeldstr. 27, 8008 Zurich, Switzerland

Alexander Y. Shin, MD
Associate Professor of Orthopedic Surgery, Mayo Clinic, Rochester, Minnesota

Walter Short, MD
Professor of Orthopedic Surgery, State University of New York, Upstate Medical, University Hospital, Syracuse, New York

Robert R. Slater, Jr, MD
Department of Orthopedic Surgery, The Permanente Medical Group, Roseville, California

John W. Sperling, MD
Associate Professor of Orthopedic Surgery, Mayo Clinic, Rochester, Minnesota

Matthew Tomaino, MD
Professor of Orthopaedics, University of Rochester Medical Center; Chief, Division of Hand, Shoulder, and Elbow Surgery, Strong Memorial Hospital, Rochester, New York

Brad Wilhelmi, MD
Associate Professor, Division of Plastic Surgery, Southern Illinois University School of Medicine, Springfield, Illinois

Jeffrey Yao, MD
Assistant Professor, Robert A. Chase Hand and Upper Limb Center, Department of Orthopaedic Surgery, Stanford University School of Medicine, Stanford, California

Table of Contents

Journals Represented

Journals represented in this YEAR BOOK are listed below.

Acta Orthopaedica Scandinavica
Acta Radiologica
American Journal of Roentgenology
American Journal of Sports Medicine
Anesthesia and Analgesia
Annals of Internal Medicine
Annals of Plastic Surgery
Annals of Rheumatic Diseases
Archives of Physical Medicine and Rehabilitation
Arthritis and Rheumatism
Arthroscopy
British Association of Plastic Surgeons
British Journal of Plastic Surgery
Canadian Journal of Surgery
Clinical Biomechanics
Clinical Orthopaedics and Related Research
Injury
Journal of Bone and Joint Surgery (American Volume)
Journal of Bone and Joint Surgery (British Volume)
Journal of Computer Assisted Tomography
Journal of Hand Surgery (American)
Journal of Hand Surgery (British)
Journal of Orthopaedic Trauma
Journal of Orthopaedic and Sports Physical Therapy
Journal of Pathology
Journal of Pediatric Orthopaedics
Journal of Reconstructive Microsurgery
Journal of Rheumatology
Journal of Surgical Research
Microsurgery
Neurology
Neurosurgery
Orthopedics
Plastic and Reconstructive Surgery
Radiographics
Radiology
Transplantation

STANDARD ABBREVIATIONS

The following terms are abbreviated in this edition: acquired immunodeficiency syndrome (AIDS), cardiopulmonary resuscitation (CPR), central nervous system (CNS), cerebrospinal fluid (CSF), computed tomography (CT), deoxyribonucleic acid (DNA), electrocardiography (ECG), health maintenance organization (HMO), human immunodeficiency virus (HIV), intensive care unit (ICU), intramuscular (IM), intravenous (IV), magnetic resonance (MR) imaging (MRI), ribonucleic acid (RNA), and ultrasound (US).

NOTE

The YEAR BOOK OF HAND AND UPPER LIMB SURGERY® is a literature survey service providing abstracts of articles published in the professional literature. Every effort is made to assure the accuracy of the information presented in these pages. Neither the editors nor the publisher of the YEAR BOOK OF HAND AND UPPER LIMB SURGERY® can be responsible for errors in the original materials. The editors' comments are their own opinions. Mention of specific products within this publication does not constitute endorsement.

To facilitate the use of the YEAR BOOK OF HAND AND UPPER LIMB SURGERY® as a reference tool, all illustrations and tables included in this publication are now identified as they appear in the original article. This change is meant to help the reader recognize that any illustration or table appearing in the YEAR BOOK OF HAND AND UPPER LIMB SURGERY® may be only one of many in the original article. For this reason, figure and table numbers will often appear to be out of sequence within the YEAR BOOK OF HAND AND UPPER LIMB SURGERY®.

Introduction

We are honored to continue the tradition of co-editing the YEAR BOOK OF HAND AND UPPER LIMB SURGERY. This is the 22nd consecutive edition of the YEAR BOOK series dedicated to the hand. The founding editors of this series were Drs James Dobyns and Robert Chase. They were succeeded by Drs Peter Amadio and Vincent Rod Hentz, and, more recently, by Drs Richard Berger and Amy Ladd.

Over the past 22 years, there have been tremendous changes in the way advances in hand surgery are disseminated. Numerous international journals have replaced the few specialty journals; online searches have replaced card catalogs; and PDF files have replaced reprints.

With greater access to primary literature, there is even greater need for an annual compendium of the best and most innovative articles pertaining to hand surgery. Today, the typical reader performs an online literature search and downloads the appropriate articles. "Collateral reading," where one flips through a journal and happens across another topic of interest, has therefore decreased. This YEAR BOOK allows the hand surgeon to draw upon the wide spectrum of journals publishing articles in hand surgery.

You will notice that we have expanded the pool of contributing editors. These contributing editors are truly the experts in their areas of hand surgery. We have asked them to focus on their own clinical and research experience to provide the reader with the proper perspective for each article. Also, critical figures are reproduced to help orient the reader.

We would like to thank our assistants, Ms Natalie Sobotta (for Dr Steinmann) and Ms Pam Rawls (for Dr Chang) for their efforts in managing the abstracts and manuscripts. We would also like to acknowledge the excellent guidance of Mr Timothy Maxwell, the development editor of the YEAR BOOK for Elsevier.

We hope you find this year's edition worthy of our predecessors and of great educational benefit to you!

James Chang, MD
Scott P. Steinmann, MD

1 Shoulder: Trauma

Internal Fixation of Proximal Humeral Fractures With a Locking Compression Plate: A Retrospective Evaluation of 72 Patients Followed for a Minimum of 1 Year
Björkenheim J-M, Pajarinen J, Savolainen V (Helsinki Univ Central Hosp)
Acta Orthop Scand 75:741-745, 2004   1–1

Background.—About 80% of proximal humeral fractures involve only slight displacement and can be managed nonoperatively. Fractures that are more complex often are liable to a failure of osteosynthesis, avascular necrosis of the humeral head, or a nonunion or malunion of the fracture, producing a painful shoulder that functions poorly. Prosthetic replacement of the humeral head has not proved satisfactory functionally. A new technique (Philo) was developed to preserve the humeral head's biologic integrity and yield an anatomic reduction by using multiple screws with angular stability. Outcomes with the new locking compression plate method were reported.

Methods.—Seventy-two patients (72 fractures) underwent treatment with the new plate and were followed up for a minimum of 1 year. Patients ranged in age from 27 to 89 years (mean age, 67 years). The complications and functional outcomes were documented.

Results.—Forty-eight fractures healed in good anatomic position and had no associated complications. Nineteen healed in slight varus position, and 2 failed to unite and required reoperation. Avascular necrosis developed in 3 fractures that were AO/ASIF type C. Loss of fixation at the humeral shaft required reoperation in 2 patients; in these cases, the drill holes in the shaft had been made with an oversized drill bit. After refixation of the plate to the shaft, these fractures healed in good position. According to the Constant score for functional outcome, 4 patients scored excellent, 32 good, 31 moderate, and 5 poor. Patients with a 2- or 3-fragment fracture had better results than those with a 4-part fracture. Of 23 patients who were working before their injury, 18 returned to their previous vocation. All patients reported a return to their preinjury level of activity. Even elderly patients were satisfied with their functional level.

Conclusions.—The Philos plate produced a high level of satisfaction with the functional capacity achieved. Thirty-six of the 72 patients had Constant scores of excellent or good. Only 5 patients had a poor result. The number of complications associated with the plate was minimal, and all were handled within the 1-year follow-up period.

▶ This is an early report on a new device for fixation of proximal humerus fractures. Seventy-two patients with Neer type 2-, 3-, and 4-part fractures were stabilized with the use of this precontoured plate with locking screw fixation. The authors used a standard deltopectoral approach with attachment of the plate to the shaft. Reduction and assembly of the fractured proximal humerus to the plate were achieved with K-wire fixation. Six to 9 locking screws were placed into the fixed angle locking screw holes to provide final stability to the fracture. Only 2 fractures failed to unite, and there were 3 cases of avascular necrosis. There were no cases of subacromial impingement of the plate. This new device is similar in function to the new volar locking plate used for distal radius fractures. This device shows excellent promise, although plate breakage has been reported by others. Newer second-generation implants will hopefully build upon this early successful implant.

S. P. Steinmann, MD

The Impacted Varus (A2.2) Proximal Humeral Fracture: Prediction of Outcome and Results of Nonoperative Treatment in 99 Patients
Court-Brown CM, McQueen MM (Royal Infirmary of Edinburgh, Scotland)
Acta Orthop Scand 75:736-740, 2004   1–2

Background.—Impacted varus fracture has been viewed as predisposing to an increased incidence of impingement syndrome and shoulder pain if not treated operatively. The outcome of impacted varus fractures handled nonoperatively was evaluated, noting in particular factors influencing results.

Methods.—Ninety-nine impacted varus proximal humeral fractures were treated and analyzed prospectively. Ninety-one percent of the patients had been injured in a simple fall. They ranged in age from 23 to 94 years (mean age, 68 years). Nonoperative treatment included immobilization in a sling for 2 weeks, followed by a course of physiotherapy based on the program of Neer, with the duration determined by the physiotherapist. Evaluations were conducted after 6, 13, 26, and 52 weeks, noting the time to return to routine activities appropriate for an elderly population, the power of abduction and flexion, and radiographic results.

Results.—Union was present in all the fractures treated. After 1 year of continuously improving Neer scores, 79% of the patients had good or excellent results. Subjective scores (strength, reach, and mobility) showed greater improvement than more objective scores (glenohumeral movement and power). Increased varus angulation on radiographs did not translate to increased pain or significantly decreased function. Age correlated with outcome, with patients younger than 40 years having nearly normal shoulder strength after 1 year, but 80- to 99-year-old patients having significantly reduced glenohumeral movement and power. However, even the oldest patients assessed their strength, reach, and stability at 90% of normal levels.

Increasing age also correlated with decreasing reach, flexion, abduction, and internal rotation but did not correlate with pain. Seventeen patients had no physiotherapy. At 1 year, the Neer score was 88 for patients having physiotherapy and 74 for those not having physiotherapy. Multivariate analysis revealed the difference in outcome was a function of age rather physiotherapy.

Conclusions.—The outcome for these patients was good after nonoperative therapy. Their subjective ratings exceeded objective findings. The degree of varus angulation was not an indication of outcome, but age was. Physiotherapy did not improve the results achieved.

▶ This study examined the nonoperative outcome of the impacted varus proximal humerus fracture, which is the second most common fracture type after the impacted valgus type. It has been presumed that this fracture might lead to an increased incidence of impingement syndrome if not surgically treated. A total of 131 patients with impacted varus fractures were treated over a 4-year period. A single fall was the cause of injury in 91%. Patients were placed in a sling for 2 weeks and then placed in a physiotherapy regimen of Neer. All fractures united. A higher varus angle was associated with increasing age. Increasing varus angle, however, was not associated with decreased function. There was also no association between pain and increasing varus angle, suggesting that an impingement syndrome is not a significant problem in these patients. Interestingly, physiotherapy was not demonstrated to be useful in the treatment of this fracture. This is another article from a group that has previously reported about the benefit of a nonoperative approach to many humeral fractures. The old adage "they all do well" might be true after all.

S. P. Steinmann, MD

Internal Fixation of Complex Fractures of the Proximal Humerus
Gerber C, Werner CML, Vienne P (Univ of Zürich, Switzerland)
J Bone Joint Surg Br 86-B:848-855, 2004   1–3

Background.—Approximately 20% of fractures of the proximal humerus are associated with displaced fracture fragments. These displaced fragments are unstable and may have disruption of their blood supply. Their treatment is controversial. Displaced and unstable extra-articular fractures are more commonly treated by operative reduction and fixation with a variety of techniques. However, treatment is more controversial for articular fractures, which carry a high risk of avascular necrosis and subsequent collapse of the humeral head. A review of the literature has suggested that no form of treatment is universally accepted. Open reduction and internal fixation with plates and screws may restore the anatomy of the proximal humerus, but additional compromise of the vascularity of the head may result in avascular necrosis and a poor outcome. However, studies that have reported poor results with this approach have often been performed in patients with poor bone quality. The clinical and radiologic outcomes of open reduction and internal fixation for the treatment of complex fractures of the proximal humerus were reviewed.

Methods.—Thirty-four consecutive articular fractures of the proximal humerus were treated in 33 patients with good bone quality by open reduction and internal fixation. Follow-up examinations were conducted with the use of a structured interview, physical examination, and photographic documentation of shoulder functioning. Radiologic assessment included anteroposterior views in neutral and internal rotation and an axillary lateral and a Neer scapular lateral view.

Results.—Anatomical or nearly anatomical reduction was achieved in 30 fractures, at a mean follow-up of 63 months (range, 25-131 months). Complete or partial avascular necrosis occurred in 12 cases (35%). Arthroplasty was subsequently performed in 2 patients, and 6 additional patients required additional surgery. The 32 patients who did not require arthroplasty achieved a mean Constant score of 78 points or 89% of an age- and sex-matched normal score. Pain was absent in 22 of the 32 patients who did not require arthroplasty, 7 had mild pain, and 3 patients had moderate pain. The mean active anterior elevation was 156°.

Conclusions.—Internal fixation of complex fractures of the proximal humerus restored good shoulder functioning in patients who did not have avascular necrosis.

▶ The treatment of unstable, displaced fractures of the proximal humerus remains controversial. This is largely due to the generally disappointing results after hemiarthroplasty for a fracture. Contributing to the controversy is the relatively poor reliability of the current classifications of these fractures. Current trends are toward the surgical fixation of more complex fractures. The common complication of surgical fixation is the development of avascular necrosis (AVN) of the humeral head, which leads to pain and loss of function and necessitates another procedure.

The authors present a retrospective review of 34 consecutive unstable proximal humerus fractures treated with internal fixation. Follow-up averaged 63 months, and patients were evaluated by means of objective and subjective shoulder function scores. Radiographs evaluated the quality of the reduction, fracture healing, and the development of AVN, which was found in 35% of the patients. The authors did not correlate the development of AVN with the fracture type, although other studies document the development of AVN in the more complex fracture patterns.

Patients who maintained adequate reduction until healing occurred obtained the best results. Although the patients who developed AVN had significantly worse functional scores, their scores remained fair and similar to the published results after hemiarthroplasty.

Only patients with relatively good bone quality were included in this study. This selection bias influences the clinical applicability of this study because many of these fractures occur in the elderly population with osteoporosis.

This study is useful in guiding the surgeon in the treatment of proximal humerus fractures with good bone quality. Open reduction and internal fixation with maintenance of the reduction results in the best outcome. Patients who have AVN may obtain satisfactory results, similar to those after a hemiarthroplasty. Further studies are required to evaluate the differences between internal fixation and hemiarthroplasty directly, in patients with bone of good or poor quality.

J. Yao, MD

Midshaft Clavicular Fractures: The Role of Operative Treatment
Graves ML, Geissler WB, Freeland AE (Univ of Mississippi, Jackson)
Orthopedics 28:761-764, 2005   1–4

Background.—Usually, midclavicular fractures in children result from a direct blow to the shoulder or an indirect force transmitted to the shoulder girdle along an outstretched arm. Healing is generally uneventful with nonoperative management, rehabilitation is spontaneous, and no permanent loss of function results. In adults, the injury requires more severe and higher energy trauma, is more painful and debilitating, heals more slowly, and may require both surgery and more complex rehabilitation. The outcome can include complications and permanent compromise of function. The operative approaches to treatment and outcomes were reviewed.

Operative Approaches.—Surgery is generally undertaken to correct shoulder deformity, restore stability and function, and reduce pain. Patients who especially need a surgical approach are those with concurrent ipsilateral shoulder or extremity fractures, thoracic injuries, or pulmonary compromise. Stability can be restored with either intramedullary or plate fixation. Both approaches have high union and patient satisfaction rates, even for severely displaced midclavicular fractures and nonunions.

Results.—A review of the current literature found varied results after nonoperative approaches to midclavicular fractures. Permanent shortening often occurred, but it carried no clinical significance in a review of 100 nonsurgically treated patients followed up for 1 to 15 years. Another retrospective review of 225 patients with an average of 17 years of follow-up identified 18% who had some persistent complaints. A statistical relationship was noted between pain and clavicular shortening of 15 mm or greater. Operative approaches can run the risks of pneumothorax, air embolism, neurovascular injury, nonunion, symptomatic or unsightly incisional scar, infection, osteomyelitis, pin migration, and implant loosening. In a comparison of closed versus immediate open reduction, 0.1% of the patients undergoing a closed method and 4.6% of those having open reduction had nonunion.

Conclusions.—Midclavicular fractures in adults can be handled nonoperatively or reduced with closed or pin or wire-assisted operative approaches as well as with plate fixation. The results with nonoperative approaches vary, but are largely successful. With operative approaches, many successful outcomes are also reported, but the potential for complications is increased.

▶ This is essentially a review article looking at the results of operative treatment for clavicle fractures. It includes an anatomy and a biomechanics section, which provides a good review of scapulohumeral motion and clavicular anatomy. The actual operative rationale portion of this article is rather short, but the discussion section includes a good review of the existing literature. Overall, there is a trend toward operative fixation of midshaft clavicular fractures with 1½ to 2 cm of overlap and absence of any bony apposition. Several long-term follow-up studies indicate that this amount of shortening leads to some long-term sequelae in terms of range-of-motion symptoms and function.

L. M. Galatz, MD

Long-term Outcomes of Clavicular Pseudoarthrosis Therapy
Petrovic I, Davila S, Premuzic I, et al (Clinical Hosp Ctr "Rebro," Zagreb, Croatia; Clinical Hosp "Sestre milosrdnice," Zagreb, Croatia)
J Surg Res 121:222-227, 2004   1–5

Background.—From 5% to 10% of all fractures involve the clavicle, but nonunion of these fractures is rare. Non-union causes notable pain and disability. Repair with open surgery with internal fixation and bone grafting often yields good results. Complications, surgical approaches, and outcomes for clavicular pseudoarthrosis were assessed.

Methods.—Fifteen patients had hospital admissions for clavicular nonunion from 1993 to 2002. The 13 available for further study, seven female and six male patients, ranged from age 14 to 52 years (mean 33 years). One had hematogenic osteomyelitis, and 12 had traumatic fractures occurring from falling from a standing position to severe motor vehicle accident. Eight patients had conservative treatment initially (figure-eight splint), four intramedullary fixation with Kirschner wire, and one multiple osteotomies. The non-union occurred in the clavicle's middle third in 12 patients and the outer lateral third in one. For surgery, patients were positioned in a "beach-chair" position, folded towel under the affected shoulder. Pseudoarthrotic tissue was removed; then the sclerotic bone ends were prompted to bleed. Cancellous autogeneous or heterogeneous bone grafts or bone-graft substitutes were used as needed.

Results.—Seven patients needed one surgical procedure, four patients two, and one patient three. Eleven patients healed properly, but some still had mild to moderate symptoms after surgery. For one patient, a dynamic-compression plate with autogeneous bone-graft implantation was used. Four required double plating, with autogeneous iliac crest bone used initially in one. After unsuccessful semitubular double plating, one patient had a third operation using heterogeneous bone graft. Intramedullary osteosynthesis with Kirschner wire was ineffective for one patient; a dynamic-compression plate with an iliac crest bone graft was then placed. Nine patients had osteosynthetic material removed after 10 to 26 months (average 11 months). The postoperative Constant score was 78%, with a range of 29% to 100% (affected versus unaffected side). Clavicle length was shortened 0.8 mm (range 0.1 to 1.7 mm). Preoperative neurologic problems (mild pain and paresthesia to brachial plexus palsy) were successfully ameliorated in three cases.

Conclusions.—With conservative treatment, clavicular fracture non-union occurs in 0.1% to 0.8% of cases; with operative treatment the frequency is 3.7% to 4.6%. Thus the initial treatment should not be operative. Surgery is indicated for pain, instability, limited shoulder motion, and brachialgia (numbness or paresthesia of the arm with or without muscle weakness). Repair is better with more rigid options; the lightness and ease of modeling of the dynamic-compression plate make it a favorite. Wave plate osteosynthesis enhances bone healing in the mid-portion of the modified plate; wound healing is a problem. Two of three patients treated with Kirschner wire osteosynthesis had successful repairs. Wire migration led to replacement with a dynamic-compression plate in one. Patients with atrophic nonunion require autogeneous or heterogeneous bone grafting because greater subperiosteal dissection is needed to avoid injury to neurovascular structures. Severity of trauma and development of atrophic nonunion were not linked, with five of the six patients studied having had multiple trauma with atrophic nonunion. Patient satisfaction and objective improvement scores were high in the cases reported, but several needed multiple procedures.

▶ This paper attempts to look at the treatment of clavicular nonunion. The authors looked at 12 nonunions located in the middle third of the clavicle and one at the lateral third of the clavicle. Seven of these nonunions were atrophic, while six were hypertrophic. A variety of various fixation techniques were utilized. These included K-wires, reconstruction plates, semitubular plates, and dynamic compression plates. Their series showed that they were able to obtain union, but this may take two or three attempts at surgery. The other significant finding from this study was that patients may continue to have residual symptoms of pain, stiffness, and neurologic compromise, especially if there had been preoperative brachial plexus problems. They do recommend using bone graft material. Their conclusion that a reconstruction plate is superior to the dynamic compression plate, however, is not borne out by the data that they present in the article. Overall, this paper outlines the challenge of treating these fractures and provides evidence that the most rigid construct, as with almost any fracture, will most likely provide the optimal rates of union.

S. F. M. Duncan, MD, MPH

The Extended Anterolateral Acromial Approach Allows Minimally Invasive Access to the Proximal Humerus
Gardner MJ, Griffith MH, Dines JS, et al (Hosp for Special Surgery, New York)
Clin Orthop 434:123-129, 2005   1–6

Lateral approaches to the proximal humerus have been limited by the position of the axillary nerve. Extensive surgical dissection through a deltopectoral approach may further damage the remaining tenuous blood supply in comminuted fractures. The purpose of our study was to explore a direct anterolateral, less invasive approach to the proximal humerus. Twenty cadaver shoulders were dissected using the extended anterolateral acromial approach through the anterior deltoid raphe. Multiple parameters were measured regarding the axillary nerve. The nerve was easily palpable in all specimens as it exited the quadrilateral space, and predictably was found and protected deep to the raphe, approximately 35 mm from the prominence of the greater tuberosity. Examination of the entire anterior nerve revealed that no branches besides the main motor trunk crossed the deltoid raphe. Subsequently, this approach was used in 16 patients with proximal humerus fractures, none of whom has had complications related to the surgical approach. This minimally invasive surgical approach seems to be safe, and may be useful in treating proximal humerus fractures.

▶ Plate fixation of proximal humerus fractures is increasingly common with the advent of new, stronger implants. Yet the standard deltopectoral approach for open reduction and internal fixation for 3- and 4-part fractures has a relatively high rate of avascular necrosis of the humeral head.

In this article, the authors have detailed an anatomical study and a case series that provide an alternative approach to proximal humerus fractures. They recommend splitting the deltoid between the anterior and middle heads of the deltoid through the anterior deltoid raphe. The axillary nerve and posterior humeral circumflex artery are identified within this interval and a plate is placed deep to these neurovascular structures. Although there is no electrophysiology to detail preservation of deltoid function, postoperative physical examination confirms deltoid function in all patients who did not have neural injury at the time of injury.

The authors have detailed the anatomical location of the axillary nerve relative to both the acromion and greater tuberosity. Although this technique is not likely to replace the standard deltopectoral approach for many proximal humerus fractures, this surgical technique is a useful tool that all reconstructive surgeons should have in their armamentarium when tackling difficult proximal humerus fractures. This technique warrants further research with a larger number of patients to determine if there is a significant reduction in the rate of avascular necrosis after surgical management of proximal humerus fractures.

R. Gupta, MD

Failure of Reamed Nailing in Humeral Non-Union: An Analysis of 26 Patients

Verbruggen JPAM, Stapert JWJL (Univ Hosp Maastricht, The Netherlands)
Injury 36:430-438, 2005   1–7

Summary.—The use of an intramedullary nail in the treatment of humeral non-unions remains controversial. This study evaluated the treatment of humeral delayed and non-unions with reamed nailing and compression. In a retrospective analysis of prospectively gathered data from 26 cases all treated with the Telescopic Locking Nail® (TLN®), the healing rate after the first intervention for non-union was 58%.

After one or more re-interventions combined with an external cancellous bone graft at some time during follow-up, 90% of the 21 patients with complete follow-up eventually healed after a mean of 22 months. A total of 49 procedures with a mean of 1.9 per patient were needed. After a mean follow-up of 65 (range 24-88) months, we conducted a study to assess the functional results in the shoulder and elbow. Twelve patients were suitable for inclusion. We used the Neer and Morrey score for shoulder and elbow function, respectively. For the Neer score the median was 91 points and for the Morrey score 94 points.

The outcome suggests that simple reamed nailing of humeral non-union is insufficient. Reamed interlocked nailing is feasible, provided that the primary intervention for non-union is combined with an external cancellous bone graft.

▶ A device called the telescoping locking nail® (TLN®) was used in 26 patients to treat delayed union or nonunion of the humerus, and the results of treatment were retrospectively reviewed. The theory behind the TLN® was that it would allow for "closed" treatment of nonunions because intramedullary reaming used to insert it combined with the compression achieved with the device would be sufficient to promote healing.

Instead, the authors found this was not the case. Healing occurred only 58% of the time after the initial treatment. Additional procedures were required, most importantly debridement of fibrous tissue and the addition of cancellous bone graft directly at the nonunion site in order to achieve healing in 90% of cases. The authors correctly point out that plate fixation with bone grafting remains the gold standard for treating nonunions of the humerus (healing rates of 94%-100% reported).

Intramedullary nailing can be used as a treatment option but should be combined with supplemental bone grafting. The authors speculate on why this may be the case in the upper, and not the lower, extremities.

R. R. Slater, Jr, MD

2 Shoulder: Anatomy and Instability

Pathomechanics in Atraumatic Shoulder Instability: Scapular Positioning Correlates With Humeral Head Centering
von Eisenhart-Rothe R; Matsen FA III, Eckstein F, et al (Univ of Frankfurt, Germany; Univ of Washington, Seattle; Ludwig-Maximilians-Universität, Munich)
Clin Orthop 433:82-89, 2005   2–1

The objective was to analyze three-dimensional scapular positioning and glenohumeral centering of normal and atraumatic unstable shoulders. We hypothesized that changes of humeral head position correlate with alterations of scapular positioning. The shoulders of 28 healthy volunteers and 14 patients with atraumatic instability were examined in various arm positions using open magnetic resonance imaging. After segmentation and three-dimensional reconstruction, three-dimensional analyses of scapular positioning and humeral head position relative to the glenoid were done. The coefficient of correlation (r) between both parameters was determined using the correlation z test. The glenohumeral to scapulothoracic ratio in the scapular plane was increased in nine of 14 patients and decreased in three patients, whereas the scapular internal rotation in the transverse plane was increased in all unstable shoulders. The unstable shoulders also had malcentering (greater than two times the standard deviation in the healthy volunteers) of the humeral head in the direction of instability during various arm positions. In healthy and unstable shoulders, the correlation between scapular position and glenohumeral positioning was high during passive elevation ($r = 0.60–0.87$). The high correlation suggests that scapular positioning is relevant for humeral head decentering. Therefore, physiotherapeutic strategy should consider the malpositioning of the scapula and be adapted to the direction of instability.

▶ The authors hypothesized that patients with atraumatic shoulder instability show an increased scapulohumeral rhythm and internal rotation of the scapula and have malcentering of the humeral head. To prove their hypothesis they used their well-developed and described 3-dimensional MRI technique and examined healthy volunteers and patients with atraumatic shoulder instability without any previous surgery. They could show that indeed there is increased scapulohumeral rhythm in the scapular plane and increased internal rotation in the transverse plane. Patients with atraumatic instability also showed a malcentering of the humeral head in the direction of their main instability. These results occurred during muscle relaxation. Interestingly, during isometric muscle activity a sufficient repositioning of the scapula or recentering of the head did not occur, leading them to suggest that beside the scapular insuffiency, muscular insufficiency would also be a factor for this type of instability.

They conclude that in patients with atraumatic instability, scapular malpositioning is at least one important factor for this entity, leading to the suggestion that these kind of patients should first be treated by physiotherapy emphasizing not only strengthening of the rotator cuff muscles, but also of the scapular stabilizing muscles. One weak point of this work is that the authors did not take into account the different degree of capsular laxity between patients and the control volunteers. Further, they did not discuss the influence of laxity on the inability to recenter the head during isometric muscle activity. With their excellent study, the authors have proven what is obvious in clinical practice every day. Patients with atraumatic shoulder instability have a lack of scapular control in addition to a hyperlaxity of the glenohumeral ligaments. The first step of therapy should, therefore, be the regaining of muscular control and strength of scapular position and then of the humeral head centering muscles, the rotator cuff.

S. Lichtenberg, MD

A Modified Capsular Shift for Atraumatic Anterior-Inferior Shoulder Instability
Marquardt B, Pötzl W, Wit K-A, et al (Univ Hosp of Münster, Germany; Shoulder and Sportsmedicine Practice-Clinic, Münster, Germany)
Am J Sports Med 33:1011-1015, 2005   2–2

Purpose.—To evaluate the long-term outcome of a modified inferior capsular shift procedure in patients with atraumatic anterior-inferior shoulder instability by analyzing a consecutive series of patients who had undergone a modified inferior capsular shift for this specific type of shoulder instability.

Study Design.—Case series; level of evidence, 4.

Methods.—Between 1992 and 1997, 38 shoulders of 35 patients with atraumatic anterior-inferior shoulder instability that were unresponsive to nonoperative management were operated on using a modified capsular shift procedure with longitudinal incision of the capsule medially and a bony fixation of the inferior flap to the glenoid and labrum in the 1 o'clock to 3 o'clock position. The patient study group consisted of 9 men and 26 women with a mean age of 25.4 years (range, 15-55 years) at the time of surgery. The mean follow-up was 7.4 years (range, 4.0-11.4 years); 1 patient was lost to follow-up directly after surgery. The study group was evaluated according to the Rowe score.

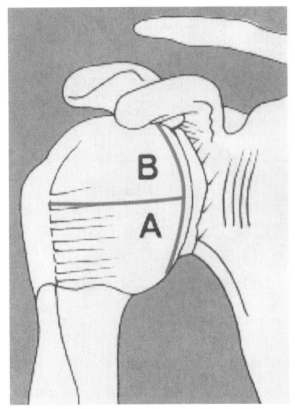

FIGURE 1.—Medially-based T-like incision for the capsular shift. **A** and **B**, suture anchor position. (Courtesy of Marquardt B, Pötzl W, Wit K-A, et al: A modified capsular shift for a traumatic anterior-inferior shoulder instability. *Am J Sports Med* 33:1011-1015, 2005.)

Results.—After 7.4 years, 2 patients experienced a single redislocation or resubluxation, 1 patient had recurrent dislocations, and 1 patient had a positive apprehension sign, which is an overall redislocation rate of 10.5%. The average Rowe score increased to 90.6 (SD = 19.7) points from 36.2 (SD = 13.5) points before surgery. Seventy-two percent of the patients participating in sports returned to their preoperative level of competition.

Conclusions.—Results in this series demonstrate the efficacy and durability of a modified capsular shift procedure for the treatment of atraumatic anterior-inferior shoulder instability (Figs 1 and 3).

▶ This article provides a follow-up to previous results published by the authors about a specific subset of patients who have atraumatic anterior-inferior shoulder instability. They found that even at a longer follow-up, an average of 7.4 years, good results were maintained, unlike many other reports in the literature where results deteriorated with time. Their procedure was done through an open capsular shift, which is a good option. It will be interesting to see how the more commonly used arthroscopic capsule plication and shift pro-

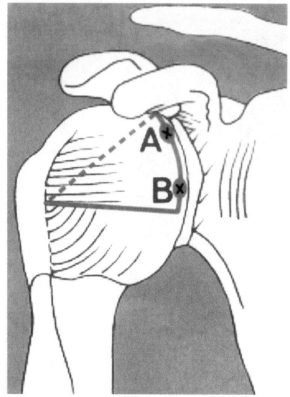

FIGURE 3.—Bony fixation of the inferior capsular flap. **A** and **B**, suture anchor position. (Courtesy of Marquardt B, Pötzl W, Wit K-A, et al: A modified capsular shift for atraumatic anterior-inferior shoulder instability. *Am J Sports Med* 33:1011-1015, 2005.)

cedures compare in the future. They do use suture anchors rather then pure plication even when the labrum is intact. It appears that the use of suture anchors provides some bleeding and improved scar formation to decrease recurrence even when the labrum is intact. As in many shoulder problems, correct diagnosis is especially important with this entity to differentiate atraumatic anterior-inferior instability from true multidirectional instability.

T. R. McAdams, MD

Effect of Simulated Shoulder Thermal Capsulorrhaphy Using Radiofrequency Energy on Glenohumeral Fluid Temperature
Lu Y, Bogdanske J, Lopez M, et al (Univ of Wisconsin-Madison; Rush Univ, Chicago)
Arthroscopy 21:592-596, 2005   2–3

Purpose.—To determine joint fluid temperatures at different time intervals during treatment with radiofrequency energy (RFE) applied in intermittent and continuous treatment manners under flow or no-flow conditions using a simulated shoulder joint model.

Type of Study.—In vitro measurement of simulated joint fluid temperature during RFE treatment.

Methods.—A custom-built jig with a chamber (volume size, 25 mL) was used to mimic the adult human shoulder. Three RFE systems: Vulcan EAS plus TAC-S probe (Smith & Nephew Endoscopy, Andover, MA); VAPR II plus End-Effect Electrode (Mitek, Westwood, MA); and ArthroCare 2000 plus TurboVac 90° probe (ArthroCare, Sunnyvale, CA) were tested in the chamber with saline solution initially set at 23°C. Each RFE probe was applied in a paintbrush pattern on the capsular tissue in the chamber and a fluoroptic thermometry probe was placed 1 cm above the RFE treatment probe to record the fluid temperature. Both intermittent and the continuous treatment manners were tested under flow and no-flow conditions. For each probe/manner/flow combination, 6 bovine capsular tissue specimens were tested (n = 6). All data were recorded using a HyperTerminal software program (Hilgraeve Inc, Monroe, MI) into a personal computer.

Results.—When using intermittent and continuous treatment manners with flow, all recorded chamber fluid temperatures for all tested RFE probes at each time interval were below 40°C. Under no-flow conditions, with intermittent treatment, the ArthroCare probe caused joint fluid temperatures to exceed 50°C after 70 seconds of RFE treatment. With the continuous treatment, the ArthroCare caused chamber fluid temperatures to exceed 65°C after 2 minutes of treatment. The highest mean recorded chamber fluid temperature was caused by ArthroCare probe, which reached 80°C at 3 minutes. For all probes, continuous treatment caused significantly higher chamber fluid temperatures than intermittent treatment.

Conclusions.—The results of this study indicate that using flow during thermal capsulorrhaphy could lower joint fluid temperature to prevent heated joint fluid from killing chondrocytes of articular cartilage, and the intermittent treatment manner caused lower fluid temperature compared with continuous treatment within the RFE-treated shoulder joint.

▶ Chondrocytes in articular cartilage begin to die at 45°C and completely die at 65°C. This study shows that RFE is safe so long as there is fluid flow and intermittent rather than continuous use. Therefore, during thermal capsulorrhaphy and, for that matter, any intra-articular application, care must be taken to avoid elevation of glenohumeral fluid temperatures so that the risk of chondrolysis is minimized. The results of this study probably indicate that similar caution is warranted when RFE is used during smaller joint arthroscopy (eg, for the wrist), during which flow rates are typically less and continuous use is more likely.

M. Tomaino, MD

Treatment of Glenohumeral Subluxation Using Electrothermal Capsulorrhaphy

Wong KL, Getz CL, Yeh GL, et al (Univ of Pennsylvania, Philadelphia; Cleveland Clinic Found, Ohio)
Arthroscopy 21:985-991, 2005   2–4

Purpose.—The purpose of this study was to review the results of a relatively homogenous group of patients with glenohumeral subluxation without labral pathology who were treated with an electrothermal capsulorrhaphy procedure.

Type of Study.—Case series without controls.

Methods.—From 1997 to 1998, 42 patients underwent electrothermal capsulorrhaphy using a monopolar radiofrequency probe (Oratec Interventions, Menlo Park, CA). Patients with prior capsular repairs, labral pathology that required repair, or capsular avulsion injuries were excluded from the study. Thirty-one patients met the inclusion criteria. Patients had a minimum of 2 years of follow-up (mean, 25 months), and a mean age of 25 years (range, 16 to 38 years). All of the patients had previously failed conservative treatment. There were 25 patients with unidirectional anterior instability, 2 patients with unidirectional inferior instability, 1 patient with unidirectional posterior instability, and 3 patients with multidirectional instability. The patients were assessed using a modified American Shoulder and Elbow Surgeons (ASES) score that examined pain (30 points), function (60 points), and patient satisfaction (10 points). In addition, subjective stability was assessed using a 10-point scale.

Results.—The average modified ASES score increased to 88 points from 56 preoperatively ($P < .01$). The average subjective stability scale increased to 8.5 from 4.4 preoperatively ($P < .01$). Nineteen patients (61%) had an excellent result, 4 (13%) had a good result, 5 (16%) had a fair result, and 3 (10%) had a poor result; 22 of 26 patients who participated in sports were able to return to their preinjury level of play. The subset of patients with isolated anterior instability had results similar to the overall group. There were no instances of axillary neuritis or other neurologic injury.

Conclusions.—In carefully selected patients with shoulder instability, including unidirectional anterior instability without associated labral pathology, electrothermal capsulorrhaphy was effective and had few complications.

▶ The article by Wong et al represents one of the few published series on the outcome of thermal shrinkage for glenohumeral instability. This study consists of 31 patients with a minimum 2-year follow-up who were treated with thermal shrinkage for glenohumeral instability. The authors demonstrate that in carefully selected patients thermal shrinkage may represent an effective treatment option.

J. W. Sperling, MD

Anterior Shoulder Instability: Accuracy of MR Arthrography in the Classification of Anteroinferior Labroligamentous Injuries

Waldt S, Burkart A, Imhoff AB, et al (Technische Universität München, Germany)

Radiology 237:578-583, 2005   2–5

Purpose.—To retrospectively evaluate the accuracy of magnetic resonance (MR) arthrography in the classification of anteroinferior labroligamentous injuries by using arthroscopy as the reference standard.

Materials and Methods.—Ethical committee approval and informed consent were obtained. MR arthrograms obtained in 205 patients, including a study group of 104 patients (74 male and 30 female; mean age, 28.2 years) with arthroscopically proved labroligamentous injuries and a control group of 101 patients (65 male and 36 female; mean age, 31.4 years) with intact labroligamentous complex, were reviewed in random order. MR arthrograms were analyzed for the presence and type (Bankart, anterior labral periosteal sleeve avulsion [ALPSA], Perthes, glenolabral articular disruption [GLAD], or nonclassifiable lesion) of labroligamentous injuries by two radiologists in consensus. Results were compared with arthroscopic findings. Sensitivity, specificity, accuracy, and corresponding 95% confidence intervals for the detection and classification of anteroinferior labroligamentous lesions with MR arthrography were calculated.

Results.—At arthroscopy, 104 anteroinferior labroligamentous lesions were diagnosed, including 44 Bankart lesions, 22 ALPSA lesions, 12 Perthes lesions, and three GLAD lesions. Twenty-three labral lesions were nonclassifiable at arthroscopy, all of which occurred after a history of chronic insta-

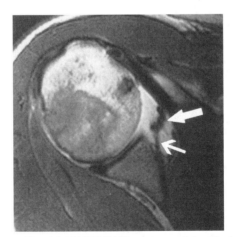

FIGURE 5.—Transverse T1-weighted (650/14) MR arthrogram of the right shoulder in a 37-year-old man demonstrates detachment and anterior displacement of the labroligamentous attachment (*thick arrow*). The medially stripped intact periosteum (*thin arrow*) is clearly delineated with contrast medium. The lesion was correctly categorized as a Perthes lesion. (Courtesy of Waldt S, Burkart A, Imhoff AB, et al: Anterior shoulder instability: Accuracy of MR arthrography in the classification of anteroinferior labroligamentous injuries. *Radiology* 237:578-583, 2005. Radiological Society of North America.)

bility. Nineteen (83%) of these 23 lesions were also nonclassifiable at MR arthrography. With arthroscopy used as the reference standard, labroligamentous lesions were detected and correctly classified at MR arthrography with sensitivities of 88% and 77%, specificities of 91% and 91%, and accuracies of 89% and 84%, respectively. Bankart, ALPSA, and Perthes lesions were correctly classified in 80%, 77%, and 50% of cases, respectively. The three GLAD lesions were all correctly assessed.

Conclusion.—MR arthrography is accurate in enabling classification of acute and chronic anteroinferior labroligamentous injuries, although correct interpretation of Perthes lesions remains difficult (Fig 5).

▶ This helpful article focuses on the accuracy of direct gadolinium arthrography of the shoulder for evaluating the anteroinferior labroligamentous complex in patients with shoulder instability. This includes specific entities such as Bankart, ALPSA, Perthes, and GLAD lesions, in addition to less well-defined processes such as degeneration and localized tears. The overall sensitivity of MR arthrography was 88%, the specificity was 91%, and the accuracy was 89% when compared with arthroscopy. The accuracy for correctly identifying Perthes lesions, that is, avulsion of the labrum with medial periosteal stripping, was the worst, at only 50%. The technique was 100% accurate for the 3 GLAD lesions included in this study. The authors conclude that MR arthrography of the shoulder is an effective tool for classifying anteroinferior labroligamentous problems in patients with unidirectional instability and suggest that it is a useful study for preoperative planning and the selection of open versus arthroscopic interventions.

K. K. Amrami, MD

Glenoid Dysplasia: Incidence and Association With Posterior Labral Tears as Evaluated on MRI

Harper KW, Helms CA, Haystead CM, et al (Duke Univ, Durham, NC)
AJR 184:984-988, 2005   2–6

Background.—Most shoulder joint abnormalities are currently assessed with MRI. Evaluation of the structural abnormalities of the shoulder has suggested a link between glenoid dysplasia or deficiency of the inferoposterior glenoid rim and posterior labral tears. Shoulders were assessed with MRI to determine the overall observed incidence of glenoid dysplasia and whether it is associated with posterior labral tears.

Methods.—The MRI scans of 98 patients (69 male, 29 female) were evaluated. Patients ranged in age from 15 to 81 years, with an average age of 43 years. The criteria for diagnosing glenoid dysplasia were posterior sloping or rounding of the posteroinferior glenoid rim, excluding the lowest axial image, along with abnormally thick or hypertrophied overlying posterior labral tissues. The radiologists who reviewed the scans determined whether the study was normal or indicated mild, moderate, or severe dysplasia. Statistically, the normal and mild groups were combined, as were the moderate and severe groups. The MRI studies were then examined for posterior labral tears, which were diagnosed by the presence of joint fluid or intra-articular gadolinium either between the bony glenoid and posterior labrum or in the substance of the posterior labrum, or by the presence of a posterior paralabral cyst.

Results.—Moderate to severe dysplasia was detected in 14 patients (14.3%), with 84 patients (85.7%) having normal or mild dysplasia. The normal group had 9 posterior labral tears (10.7%), as did the moderate to severe group (64.3%). The difference was statistically significant. Only 5 (8.5%) of the normal cases had labral tears, whereas 13 (33.3%) of the dysplasia cases had labral tears; the difference was statistically significant. Surgery proved the presence of posterior labral tears in 15 cases analyzed retrospectively. Eleven patients (73%) had moderate or severe posterior glenoid dysplasia.

Conclusions.—Of patients whose MRI results indicated moderate to severe posterior glenoid deficiency, 64.3% had posterior labral tears, which is a high incidence compared with other studies. Patients with no glenoid dysplasia or mild dysplasia had labral tears in only 10.7% of cases. Among the cases surgically proved to have labral tears, 73% had moderate to severe posterior glenoid dysplasia. These results indicate a correlation between the 2 findings, with patients who have glenoid dysplasia on MRI having a much higher incidence of posterior labral tears than patients whose MRI results are normal.

▶ This is an MRI study looking at the incidence and association of posterior labral tears with posterior instability. The authors evaluated 103 consecutive shoulder MR arthrograms. They had stringent criteria for diagnosing mild, moderate, and severe posterior glenoid insufficiency. They found the prevalence of glenoid hypoplasia is 14.3% in their patient population. There was a higher prevalence of posterior labral tears in the moderate and severe dysplasia group. As a separate portion of this study, 15 surgically proven cases of posterior labral tears were retrospectively analyzed for glenoid morphology. Of the 15 cases, 11 (73%) were graded as having moderate or severe posterior glenoid dysplasia. This study brings attention to an aspect of glenoid morphology that has recently received a lot of attention. Evidence supports an association between posterior glenoid rim insufficiency (or glenoid dysplasia) and posterior instability, posterior labral tears, and possibly even early arthritic changes. Strengths of this study include the strict criteria for radiographic evaluation. A possible weakness is bias in the patient population given that the MR arthrograms were presumably all obtained in patients with pathologic shoulders, so this may not represent a true cross-section of the normal population.

L. M. Galatz, MD

Posterior Humeral Avulsion of the Glenohumeral Ligament as a Cause of Posterior Shoulder Instability: A Case Report

Safran O, DeFranco MJ, Hatem S, et al (Cleveland Clin Found, Ohio)
J Bone Joint Surg Am 86:2732-2736, 2004   2–7

Background.—The shoulder suffers traumatic forces during sports activities and can develop glenohumeral instability. Few cases of posterior humeral avulsion of the glenohumeral capsule are reported.

Case Report.—Man, 19, had intermittent clicking and pain in the left shoulder for 2 years. He suffered a blow to the anterior aspect of the left shoulder trying to tackle another football player in a high school game. The left shoulder slipped out of place and returned spontaneously, but clicking, pain, and looseness of the shoulder occurred thereafter when playing sports and during normal activities. The pain was located in the posterior aspect and was worse with forward elevation of the arm to shoulder height and throwing motions. Five more episodes of shoulder slippage and spontaneous reduction also occurred, each producing pain and limited range of motion lasting several days. The worsening symptoms eventually precluded sports participation. The patient was prescribed a supervised exercise program to strengthen the deltoid and rotator cuff muscles, rest, and physical therapy, but symptoms remained.

The physical examination revealed equal passive and active range of glenohumeral motion with normal scapulothoracic rhythm bilaterally. Palpation produced tenderness along the posterior glenohumeral joint line and posterior humeral head translation. Although radiographs were normal, magnetic resonance arthrography revealed multiple abnormalities, including a posterior labral tear, deformity of the posterolateral part of the humeral head extending inferiorly to the neck, and subtle changes in the anterior labrum superiorly and the infraspinatus. A superior labral anterior-to-posterior (SLAP) lesion indicated posterior impingement. Arthroscopy was performed and revealed a minor cleavage crack in the anteroinferior aspect of the glenoid labrum and a similar lesion in the posterior inferior part of the labrum, but no labral detachment. Complete detachment of the posterior glenohumeral ligament and capsule at the site of humeral insertion was also noted. Arthroscopic repair was accomplished, then the shoulder was immobilized in a gunslinger brace with 25° of abduction and 0° of arm rotation for 5 weeks. Physical therapy was begun, with posterior capsular stretching exercises added later to strengthen the rotator cuff, deltoid, and scapulothoracic muscles. The patient's pain, clicking, and subjective symptoms resolved within 16 weeks of surgery. After 12 months, the patient could perform all activities of daily living and participated in recreational sports with no symptoms or limitations.

Conclusions.—Posterior instability is a seldom encountered shoulder disability in young patients. The patient described had posterior humeral avulsion of the posterior portion of the glenohumeral ligament after a sports injury. The diagnosis was based on magnetic resonance arthroscopy, and repair was achieved arthroscopically. Physical therapy helped in rehabilitation, after which the patient was able to return to sports participation without symptoms.

▶ This case report is an important contribution to our expanding knowledge of the pathology of the shoulder joint. The increasing use of shoulder arthroscopy to diagnose and treat shoulder problems has led to more refined pathological diagnoses. Fortunately this will allow us to better treat patients and address their specific problems more accurately. Whereas in the past this patient's problem may have been treated with an open posterior stabilization, today the specific pathology can be addressed arthroscopically.

In addition, the study correlates magnetic resonance imaging findings to arthroscopic anatomy. This, along with other studies, will certainly benefit our patients through more accurate magnetic resonance imaging and clinical diagnosis.

Finally, this report reminds us that a complete diagnostic arthroscopy is critical in all cases. Using multiple viewing portals and having a systematic approach will ensure that no pathology is left undiagnosed or untreated.

D. I. Ilan, MD

Manipulative Therapy in Addition to Usual Medical Care for Patients With Shoulder Dysfunction and Pain: A Randomized, Controlled Trial

Bergman GJD, Winters JC, Groenier KH, et al (Univ of Groningen, The Netherlands; Maastricht Univ, The Netherlands; Vrije Universiteit, Amsterdam; et al)
Ann Intern Med 141:432-439, 2004   2–8

Background.—Dysfunction of the cervicothoracic spine and the adjacent ribs (also called the shoulder girdle) is considered to predict occurrence and poor outcome of shoulder symptoms. It can be treated with manipulative therapy, but scientific evidence for the effectiveness of such therapy is lacking.

Objective.—To study the effectiveness of manipulative therapy for the shoulder girdle in addition to usual medical care for relief of shoulder pain and dysfunction.

Design.—Randomized, controlled trial.

Setting.—General practices in Groningen, the Netherlands.

Patients.—150 patients with shoulder symptoms and dysfunction of the shoulder girdle.

Interventions.—All patients received usual medical care from their general practitioners. Only the intervention group received additional manipulative therapy, up to 6 treatment sessions in a 12-week period.

Measurements.—Patient-perceived recovery, severity of the main complaint, shoulder pain, shoulder disability, and general health. Data were collected during and at the end of the treatment period (at 6 and 12 weeks) and during the follow-up period (at 26 and 52 weeks).

Results.—During treatment (6 weeks), no significant differences were found between study groups. After completion of treatment (12 weeks), 43% of the intervention group and 21% of the control group reported full recovery. After 52 weeks, approximately the same difference in recovery rate (17 percentage points) was seen between groups. During the intervention and follow-up periods, a consistent between-group difference in severity of the main complaint, shoulder pain and disability, and general health favored additional manipulative therapy.

Limitations.—The sample size was small, and assessment of end points was subjective.

Conclusion.—Manipulative therapy for the shoulder girdle in addition to usual medical care accelerates recovery of shoulder symptoms.

▶ This study shows, by subjective outcomes scores, that manipulative therapy for the shoulder girdle in addition to usual medical care can be beneficial to patients with shoulder pain. Since it was not possible to blind this study, bias upon the part of the patient, therapist, and general practitioner could have affected the subject's responses on the patient-perceived recovery scale. A more valid and standardized outcome measure, such as the DASH, might have provided more objective data for analysis for this study.

M. Outzen, MD, OTR/L

3 Shoulder: Rotator Cuff

Variation in Orthopaedic Surgeons' Perceptions About the Indications for Rotator Cuff Surgery
Dunn WR, Schackman BR, Walsh C, et al (Hosp for Special Surgery, New York)
J Bone Joint Surg Am 87-A:1978-1984, 2005   3–1

Background.—Epidemiologic studies have demonstrated substantial variations in per capita rates of many surgical procedures, including rotator cuff repair. The purpose of the current study was to characterize orthopaedic surgeons' attitudes concerning medical decision-making about rotator cuff surgery and to investigate the associations between these beliefs and reported surgical volumes.

Methods.—A survey was mailed to randomly selected orthopaedic surgeons listed in the American Academy of Orthopaedic Surgeons directory. Only individuals who had treated patients for a rotator cuff tear, or had referred patients for such treatment, within the previous year were asked to complete the two-page survey. The survey comprised fifteen questions regarding clinical opinion, including four regarding hypothetical cases. Clinical agreement was defined as >80% of the respondents answering similarly.

Results.—Of the 1100 surveys that were mailed, 539 were returned (a response rate of 49%). Of the 539 respondents, 316 (58.6%) had treated or referred patients with a rotator cuff tear in the previous year. There was a significant negative correlation between the surgeon's estimation of the failure rate of cuff repairs in the United States and that surgeon's procedure volume (r = −0.21, p = 0.0003), indicating that surgeons with a lower procedure volume are more pessimistic about the results of surgery than are those with a higher procedure volume. Arthroscopic, mini-open, and open cuff repairs were preferred by 14.5%, 46.2%, and 36.6% of the respondents, respectively. Surgeons who performed a higher volume of procedures were less likely to perform open surgery (p < 0.0001). There was clinical agreement regarding only four of the nine clinical questions and none of the four questions about the hypothetical vignettes.

Conclusions.—We found significant variation in surgical decision-making and a lack of clinical agreement among orthopaedic surgeons about rotator cuff surgery. There was a positive correlation between the volume of procedures performed by the surgeon and the surgeon's perception of outcome, with surgeons who had a higher procedure volume being more enthusiastic about rotator cuff surgery than those who had a lower procedure volume.

▶ We generally embrace the notion that higher surgical volume leads to increased experience with a given procedure and that this will lead to better outcomes. This study intimates this, but it should be acknowledged that the study measured "perception" not "reality." That higher volumes of rotator cuff surgery did, indeed, result in superior outcomes and that superior outcomes may have inspired those high-volume surgeons to rely on surgical interventions more commonly—rather than being secondary merely to overly optimistic, "surgery-happy" docs—would have required the reporting of objective outcomes in this study.

M. Tomaino, MD

Accuracy of CT Arthrography in the Assessment of Tears of the Rotator Cuff
Charousset C, Bellaïche L, Duranthon LD, et al (AFTS, Paris)
J Bone Joint Surg Br 87-B:824-828, 2005   3–2

CT arthrography and arthroscopy were used to assess tears of the rotator cuff in 259 shoulders. Tear size was determined in the frontal and sagittal planes according to the classification of the French Arthroscopy Society.

CT arthrography had a sensitivity of 99% and a specificity of 100% for the diagnosis of tears of supraspinatus. For infraspinatus these figures were 97.44% and 99.52%, respectively and, for subscapularis, 64.71% and 98.17%. For lesions of the long head of the biceps, the sensitivity was 45.76% and the specificity was 99.57%.

Our study showed an excellent correlation between CT arthrography and arthroscopy when assessing the extent of a rotator cuff tear. CT arthrography should, therefore, be an indispensable part of pre-operative assessment. It allows determination of whether a tear is reparable (retraction of the tendon and fatty degeneration of the corresponding muscle) and whether this is possible by arthroscopy (degree of tendon retraction and extension to subscapularis).

▶ When patients present with shoulder pain, a thorough history and physical examination are routinely performed and may lead to the presumed diagnosis of a rotator cuff tear. Usually, an MRI study is ordered to confirm this diagnosis. In certain patients such as those with metal implants, this noninvasive imaging modality cannot be performed. In this situation, the physician may consider alternative studies such as US or CT arthrography.

The authors have provided data that support the use of CT arthrography as an imaging modality to document rotator cuff pathology by correlating the data with findings from surgical arthroscopy. This study detailed the fact that CT arthrography is limited to identifying pathology of the supraspinatus and infraspinatus. In the latter group, CT arthrography overreads longitudinal intratendinous cleavages, as this pathology is not readily detectable by arthroscopy. Furthermore, it cannot reliably detect pathology of the subscapularis or long head of the biceps. As such, CT arthrography is unlikely to replace MRI as the primary imaging modality, but rather may serve an adjunct role for those patients who cannot have an MRI.

R. Gupta, MD

Sonography of Full-Thickness Supraspinatus Tears: Comparison of Patient Positioning Technique With Surgical Correlation
Ferri M, Finlay K, Popowich T, et al (McMaster Univ and Hamilton Health Sciences, Ont, Canada; St Joseph's Hosp, Hamilton, Ont, Canada; Guelph Gen Hosp, Ont, Canada; et al)
AJR 184:180-184, 2005   3–3

Objective.—Sonography has become a popular technique for the assessment of musculoskeletal disorders. Patient positioning is crucial to a thorough and accurate assessment of rotator cuff tendons. Two positions, the Crass and modified Crass, have been routinely used in the research and clinical settings to examine the supraspinatus tendon. Our study was a prospective trial to determine whether the Crass or the modified Crass position affords the most accurate measure of supraspinatus tears when compared with surgical findings.

Subjects and Methods.—Twenty-one patients with full-thickness supraspinatus tears underwent shoulder sonography in both the Crass and the modified Crass positions. Measurements of supraspinatus tears were performed in the sagittal and transverse dimensions. Patients subsequently underwent either arthroscopic or open supraspinatus repair. Intraoperative measurements were made in two dimensions and were compared with sonographic findings.

Results.—Sonography had 100% specificity in detecting full-thickness supraspinatus tears. No statistically significant difference was seen between the size of supraspinatus tears in the Crass and modified Crass positions and surgical findings in the transverse plane ($p = 0.55$ and 0.61, respectively). In the sagittal dimension, no statistically significant difference was seen between surgical findings and the Crass position ($p = 0.14$); however, a difference existed when the modified Crass position was used ($p = 0.03$).

Conclusion.—Sonography reliably detects and quantifies supraspinatus tears. Both the Crass and the modified Crass positions reflected the true size of supraspinatus tears in the transverse plane. In the sagittal plane, the Crass position is the more useful to quantify supraspinatus tears because the modified Crass position overestimates the size of such tears.

▶ This is a radiographic study examining the accuracy of measuring the size of rotator cuff tears using 2 different positions, the Crass and modified Crass positions. The authors' conclusion was that the Crass position is better, as the modified Crass position had a tendency to overestimate tear size. All full-thickness tears based on sonography were confirmed intraoperatively, resulting in 100% specificity of the detection of full-thickness supraspinatus tears. Overall, this is an excellent study that had surgical correlation to apply to the results and good data to support the conclusion. This information may be helpful to an orthopedic surgeon who plans to use sonography in the clinical office setting.

L. M. Galatz, MD

Cyclic Loading of Rotator Cuff Repairs: An In Vitro Biomechanical Comparison of Bioabsorbable Tacks With Transosseous Sutures
Bicknell RT, Harwood C, Ferreira L, et al (Univ of Western Ontario, London, Canada)
Arthroscopy 21:875-880, 2005   3–4

Purpose.—This study compares rotator cuff repair strength after cyclic loading of bioabsorbable tacks and traditional transosseous sutures, and correlates the results with bone density, age, and gender. The hypotheses were that tack repair strength would be inferior to transosseous sutures and that repair strength would be directly related to bone quality.

Type of Study.—In vitro randomized biomechanical study.

Methods.—Eight paired cadaveric shoulders with a standardized supraspinatus defect were randomized to tack or suture repair and subjected to step-wise cyclic loading. Repair migration was measured by quantifying the motion of markers affixed to tendon and bone using a digital camera. Failure mode, cycles, and load were measured for 50% and 100% loss of repair. Results were correlated with bone density, age, and gender.

Results.—Tack repairs failed at the tack-tendon interface, whereas suture rupture was the mode of failure for the suture repairs. Mean values for 50% loss of repair were 206 ± 88 cycles and 44 ± 15 N for the sutures, and 1,193 ± 252 cycles and 156 ± 20 N for the tacks ($P < .05$). The corresponding values for 100% loss of repair were 2,458 ± 379 cycles and 294 ± 27 N for the sutures, and 2,292 ± 333 cycles and 263 ± 28 N for the tacks ($P > .05$). These results did not correlate with bone density, age, or gender.

Conclusions.—This study has shown that bioabsorbable tacks provide improved repair strength in comparison with traditional suture techniques. Repair strength did not correlate with bone quality, and this may be attributed to failure primarily through the repair construct or at the tack-tendon interface and not through bone. This report describes a new high-resolution optical method of measuring tendon repair strength that should be a useful model for future studies.

▶ The study by Bicknell et al is an innovative study comparing the use of bioabsorbable tacks versus sutures to repair rotator cuff tears. The authors showed that bioabsorbable tacks actually provided improved repair strength in comparison to traditional suture techniques. The study demonstrates the potential advantages of a sutureless tack device for rotator cuff repair.

J. W. Sperling, MD

Arthroscopic Side-to-Side Rotator Cuff Repair
Wolf EM, Pennington WT, Agrawal V (California Pacific Med Ctr, San Francisco; St Luke's Med Ctr, Milwaukee, Wis; Central Indiana Orthopedics, Muncie)
Arthroscopy 21:881-887, 2005   3–5

Background.—Purely arthroscopic techniques are being used more frequently to repair full-thickness rotator cuff tears. In the surgical approach, the anatomy of the intact rotator cuff is recreated, reinserting and fixing the tendon to the greater tuberosity of the humerus. This generally involves securing the repair to the proximal humerus with suture through bone tunnels or with anchor-based fixation. A unique method of achieving repair using a side-to-side fixation without anchoring the repair to bone was performed in tears identified as amenable to this approach after thorough arthroscopic visualization and assessment.

Patients.—Forty-two patients had side-to-side repairs done between 1990 and 1996. The 24 men and 18 women ranged in age from 42 to 79 years at the time of surgery; all had injuries that had not responded to conservative approaches.

Technique.—Patients were placed in a lateral decubitus position for routine shoulder arthroscopy to inspect the area and remove all frayed, devitalized tissue from the rotator cuff tendon. After realignment to visualize the subacromial space, a decompression was performed to remove all bursal tissue over the rotator cuff so the extent of the tear was obvious. A full-radius shaver and burr were used to abrade the region of the greater humeral tuberosity so the cuff would heal more readily to the tuberosity. The mobility of the rotator cuff was determined. Repairs were performed by using a side-to-side technique and not fixing the repair to bone. Nerve hook evaluation was undertaken to assess the anatomic relationship between the margins of the torn cuff edges and to ensure optimal restoration of normal anatomy without tension on the repair. Sutures were used to approximate the tendon edges, closing the entire defect over the bleeding trough of bone on the proximal humerus. A suture placed in the anterior corner of the posterior leaf of the tear and passing under the transverse humeral ligament and through the coracohumeral ligament helped advance the posterior leaf anteriorly, promoting a more secure approximation. In general, 4 sutures per repair were needed.

Results.—Good and excellent results were reported for 98% of the patients. All but one of the patients deemed the repair satisfactory and successful. With the use of the UCLA shoulder scoring system, patients graded their strength as 4.6 (range, 2-5), their pain as 9.0 (range, 2-10), and their mean perceived function as 9.3 (range, 1-10). Forward flexion of the shoulder averaged a grade of 4.9 (range, 1-5). Three patients had previous repair procedures assisted arthroscopically. All rated the current surgery as more satisfactory and with a faster recovery and return to function than with the open repair.

Conclusions.—Patients whose full-thickness defect of the rotator cuff tendon was amenable to purely arthroscopic repair fared well with the side-to-side technique. During a follow-up period of 4 to 10 years, 98% of the patients reported good to excellent results.

▶ This study evaluated the outcome of 42 patients who underwent a repair of a full-thickness rotator cuff tear using a side-to-side repair technique. No anchors or tendon-to-bone fixation was used. The authors evaluated the patients by using UCLA scores and reported that 55% of the results were excellent, 43% were good, and 2% were poor. All but one of the patients were satisfied with their surgery and felt that it was a success. The authors do not have any preoperative UCLA shoulder ratings, so it is difficult to compare preoperative and postoperative results. The study does not include range-of-motion and strength data. In addition, there is no information regarding tear size and radiographic evaluation preoperatively. There is no postoperative radiographic evaluation, so we have no information as to whether any of these tears healed. Studies exist that report good results after simple debridement of massive tears. It is difficult to apply this particular study to clinical practice because we don't know how big these tears were, how much functional improvement they actually gained, and whether this method results in anatomic healing of a rotator cuff tear.

L. M. Galatz, MD

Rotator Cuff Repair in Patients With Rheumatoid Arthritis
Smith AM, Sperling JW, Cofield RH (Mayo Clinic, Rochester, Minn)
J Bone Joint Surg Am 87:1782-1787, 2005   3–6

Background.—The literature on rotator cuff tear repair in patients with rheumatoid arthritis is sparse. Personal clinical experience was reviewed retrospectively.

Methods.—A database search for persons with rheumatoid arthritis needing rotator cuff repair between 1988 and 2002 yielded only 31 shoulders and only 21 patients (23 shoulders) with a follow-up over 2 years. The median age of the 10 men and 11 women was 65 years (range 35 to 79 years). Follow-up extended at least 3 years; no patient had previous shoulder surgery or rotator cuff repair combined with shoulder arthroplasty. All took medication to control rheumatoid arthritis symptoms preoperatively. Patients completed a questionnaire on shoulder function and satisfaction to complement the data from medical records and imaging studies. The Simple Shoulder Test (SST) and patient section of the American Shoulder and Elbow Surgeons (ASES) instrument yielded additional data. Functional capacity status reflected the patients' ability to perform activities of daily living (ADL) preoperatively. Surgery was performed for rotator cuff tears plus unrelenting shoulder pain and dysfunction affecting ADL performance. Nine shoulders had partial-thickness tears (subdivided as >50% or <50% of the thickness of the intact cuff) confirmed by magnetic resonance imaging, arthrography, or arthroscopy. Full-thickness tears were also subdivided by size. In 18 shoulders, tendon-to-tendon and tendon-to-bone repairs were done. All had acromioplasty, 18 had bursectomy, seven distal clavicular excision, three synovectomy, two biceps tendon debridement, and one biceps tendon tenodesis. For rehabilitation, a shoulder immobilizer with the arm at the side (18) or slightly abducted (5) was used per surgeon preference. Patients noted satisfaction on a scale from 1 (poor) to 10 (excellent) before and after surgery and at the latest follow-up examination. Statistics were reported as median and range (minimum to maximum). For tear thickness and ordered Neer-rating results, an exact test for ordered categorical data was used; level of significance was $p < 0.05$.

Results.—Patients with partial-thickness repairs had better scores for pain, active elevation, and satisfaction when last followed up than preoperatively. Active elevation improved from 155° before to 165° after surgery and external rotation from 50° before to 60° after surgery, but these were not statistically significant. Manual strength did not improve. Over a median follow-up of 9.7 years, 20 patients needed no revision. Eight unsatisfactory results were attributed to revision surgery (3 shoulders), decreased motion only (3), pain only (1), and decreased motion and pain (1). Neither active elevation nor external rotation improved significantly in full-thickness tears. Two shoulders, one with partial-thickness and the other medium full-thickness tear, required revision to a total shoulder arthroplasty; these were done 9 and 6 years, respectively, after initial repair. Before revision, these patients and one needing debridement and drainage of an acromioclavicular cyst, humeral head bone contouring, and synovectomy 4 years after massive tear repair had functionally intact rotator cuffs.

Conclusions.—Pain, active elevation, and patient satisfaction improved after rotator cuff repair in two of nine shoulders with partial-thickness tears and six of 14 with full-thickness tears. Neer, ASES, and SST scores were less predictable in partial-thickness than full-thickness tears. The latter showed a nonsignificant trend toward less shoulder function after repair. Three patients needed revision, but had healed rotator cuff tendons at that point. Patients thus reported pain relief and satisfaction with results, but not functional gains with full-thickness rotator cuff tears. Surgeon bias was possible, since patient selection was not randomized but focused on less severe radiographic changes. This may reflect a less severe inflammatory phase of the rheumatoid arthritis, yielding a healthier rotator cuff and adjacent soft tissue that permitted effective repair. Many patients had additional procedures, especially acromioplasty, done routinely with the open rotator cuff repair. History has proved that sacrificing the coracoacromial ligament, compromising the coracoacromial arch, because of concern for rheumatoid progression, loss of humeral head containment, and rotator cuff insufficiency is inadvisable.

▶ The authors have performed a retrospective review looking at rotator cuff repairs in patients with underlying rheumatoid arthritis. They looked at patients over approximately a 15-year period, and this involved 23 shoulders and 21 patients. They had a minimum duration of follow-up of three years. They evaluated the patients utilizing a simple shoulder test as well as the American Shoulder and Elbow Surgeons Instrument. The operative indications included unrelenting shoulder pain and dysfunction that interfered with daily activities. Conservative measures were exhausted. The group included nine shoulders with a partial-thickness tear. Full-thickness tears were divided based on their size. Eighteen shoulders had open treatment only, whereas five had combined arthroscopic and open treatments. All patients had an acromioplasty, and seven had a distal clavicular excision. Two had biceps tendon debridement, and one had a biceps tendon tenodesis and three had a synovectomy. The most significant finding of this paper was that even though their pain was likely to improve with the use of the surgical intervention, their motion did not improve substantially, and their strength was essentially unchanged as well. This was especially true with the full-thickness tear patient group. Also of interest is that of the 23 shoulders that underwent rotator cuff repair, two did require revision to a total shoulder arthroplasty. Of note is that the rotator cuff was found to be functionally intact in all three patients at the time of repeat surgery. In summary, pain relief and patient satisfaction are achievable in this group. Functional gain should not be expected in patients with full-thickness rotator cuff tears.

S. F. M. Duncan, MD, MPH

Long-term MRI Findings in Operated Rotator Cuff Tear
Kyrölä K, Niemitukia L, Jaroma H, et al (Kuopio Univ Hosp, Finland)
Acta Radiol 45:526-533, 2004   3–7

Background.—MRI is able to demonstrate full-thickness rotator cuff (RC) tears readily. Differentiating partial-thickness tears from degenerative tendinosis can be more challenging. MRI without fat saturation was used to evaluate 28 operated shoulders, and the findings were correlated with long-term outcomes after tendon repair.

Methods.—The patients ranged in age at the time of surgery from 36 to 68.5 years (mean age, 55.8 years). Twenty-four right and 4 left shoulders were evaluated. The standard sequences in the oblique coronal, oblique sagittal, and axial planes were obtained. Two observers evaluated the RC, including repeat tears and tendon degeneration. Measurements of the thickness of the supraspinatus tendon and narrowing of the subacromial space were taken. Clinical outcome was determined by using the Constant score.

Results.—MRI was unable to detect any visible RC tendon lesions in 11 patients (39%). These patients had significantly less pain, better active abduction motion and abduction force, and better Constant scores than patients who had either tendinosis or RC tendon tears. The size of the tears in patients with a normal MRI result varied. However, their primary tears were significantly smaller than those of patients whose MRI revealed a full-thickness tear. Seven patients (25%) had full-thickness tears demonstrated on MRI; 6 patients (21%) had partial-thickness tears. Tendinosis was revealed in another RC tendon in 1 patient with a full-thickness and 2 with partial-thickness tears. Thirteen patients (46%) had narrowing of the subacromial space, which was correlated with a repeat tear of the RC.

Conclusions.—Standard MRI sequences without fat saturation proved capable of evaluating the status of the RC after repair procedures. Good clinical outcome was demonstrated as a normal appearance of the RC on MRI. Repeat tear and tendinosis were also demonstrated.

▶ In this study, the authors randomly selected 28 shoulders after RC repair to reexamine with MRI. Their purpose was to evaluate the postoperative findings and correlate this to clinical outcome. Of the 28 shoulders, 39% had normal RC tendons on MRI with good clinical outcomes. Fourteen patients had findings of tendinosis, and a full-thickness tear was found in 25%. Twenty-one percent had partial-thickness RC tears. The size of the tear was determined by the surgeon at the time of surgery. Overall, the authors found that the tears that healed were smaller tears to start with, and healing was associated with better outcomes.

This study has several weaknesses. One weakness is a possible inconsistency in measuring the size of RC tears. No preoperative MRI findings are reported. Thus, there is no assessment of muscle atrophy.

This article has several strong points. It reinforces the finding that smaller tears heal better than larger tears, and tears that heal have a better outcome than tears that are not healed.

L. M. Galatz, MD

Three-Dimensional Scapulothoracic Motion During Active and Passive Arm Elevation

Ebaugh DD, McClure PW, Karduna AR (Drexel Univ, Philadelphia; Arcadia Univ, Glenside, Pa; Univ of Oregon, Eugene)
Clin Biomech 20:700-709, 2005   3–8

Background.—Scapulothoracic muscle activity is believed to be important for normal scapulothoracic motion. In particular, the trapezius and serratus anterior muscles are believed to play an important role in the production and control of scapulothoracic motion. The aim of this study was to determine the effects of different levels of muscle activity (active versus passive arm elevation) on three-dimensional scapulothoracic motion.

Methods.—Twenty subjects without a history of shoulder pathology participated in this study. Three-dimensional scapulothoracic motion was determined from electromagnetic sensors attached to the scapula, thorax, and humerus during active and passive arm elevation. Muscle activity was recorded from surface electrodes over the upper and lower trapezius, serratus anterior, anterior and posterior deltoid, and infraspinatus muscles. Differences in scapulothoracic motion were calculated between active and passive arm elevation conditions.

Findings.—Scapular motion was observed during the trials of passive arm elevation; however, there was more upward rotation of the scapula, external rotation of the scapula, clavicular retraction, and clavicular elevation under the condition of active arm elevation. This was most pronounced for scapular upward rotation through the mid-range (90–120°) of arm elevation.

Interpretation.—The upper and lower trapezius and serratus anterior muscles have an important role in producing upward rotation of the scapula especially throughout the mid-range of arm elevation. Additionally, it appears that capsuloligamentous and passive muscle tension contribute to scapulothoracic motion during arm elevation. Assessment of the upper and lower trapezius and serratus anterior muscles and upward rotation of the scapula should be part of any shoulder examination.

▶ This article provides additional information in evaluation of the role of scapular thoracic mechanics in shoulder activity. Much confusion exists in the literature in regard to "normal" scapular thoracic motion as this often varies in throwing athletes with different types of shoulder pathology. Regardless, this article emphasizes the importance of improved understanding of scapular thoracic motion. The authors show the difference between active and passive elevation, specifically, in regard to scapular upward rotation, which, if too great, can increase the risk for impingement. One should also consider the scapular retraction test described by Kibler in patient evaluation in which increased rotator cuff strength may be seen when the scapula is held in a retracted position during supraspinatus testing. As additional information is gleaned from studies such as this, we will continue to improve our understanding of the importance of scapular stabilization in rehabilitation and management of shoulder injuries.

T. R. McAdams, MD

4 Shoulder: Arthroplasty

The Association Between Hospital Volume and Total Shoulder Arthroplasty Outcomes
Lyman S, Jones EC, Bach PB, et al (Hosp for Special Surgery, New York)
Clin Orthop 432:132-137, 2005   4–1

Background.—The outcomes of total hip and total knee arthroplasties have been better when performed by high-volume surgeons and hospitals than by surgeons and hospitals where few of these procedures are done. Better results include decreased risk of in-hospital complications and mortality, decreased length of stay, fewer posthospital complications, less need for revision surgery, and fewer posthospital deaths. A similar evaluation was carried out for total shoulder arthroplasties done in New York.

Methods.—Length of stay, hospital costs, readmission within 60 days, revision surgery within 24 months, and death within 60 days were the variables measured for patients undergoing total shoulder arthroplasty at various institutions and under the care of various surgeons in New York. Data were obtained from the Statewide Planning and Research Cooperative System database of the New York State Department of Health. The data covered the period 1996-1999, when 1307 total shoulder arthroplasties were performed in that state.

Results.—Fifty-seven percent of the patients were women, and 10% were ethnic or racial minorities. Most patients (63.3%) were hospitalized for fewer than 4 days and had adjusted hospital costs under $10,000. The 5 high-volume hospitals accounted for 46.8% of the patients, averaging 41.6 patients per study year. The middle-volume hospitals averaged 6.6 patients per study year, and the low-volume hospitals averaged 2.0 patients per study year. Readmission to the hospital within 60 days was required for 87 patients; 3 patients died during the same period. Revision total shoulder arthroplasties were performed for 30 patients within 2 years of the initial surgery, with 21 done in the first year postoperatively. Younger patients were more likely to have surgery at the high-volume hospitals. Patients at the low-volume hospitals had more comorbid conditions than those at high-volume hospitals and had a longer length of stay than at middle-volume hospitals. High-volume hospitals had the highest charges. These charges were significantly higher than those at middle-volume hospitals, which had the lowest charges. Readmission within 60 days was associated with hospital volume, with patients from the low-volume hospitals having the highest readmission rates and patients from the high-volume hospitals the lowest. High-volume hospitals had the lowest rates for revision surgery and death within 60 days. No deaths occurred in the high-volume hospitals, although nearly half of the surgeries were performed there. Statistical analysis revealed a reduction in readmission risk within 60 days for all hospitals with volumes of at least 16 cases, with significance reached when the high-volume category of 48+ cases was attained.

Conclusions.—The most significant variable for comparing hospital volume and improved outcome of total shoulder arthroplasty was readmission to the hospital within 60 days. This outcome reflects inconvenience to the patient and can be related to a significant adverse health event. In this category, high-volume hospitals had a significant advantage, with lower readmission rates than either low-volume or middle-volume hospitals even with adjustments for age and comorbidity. The other variables measured occur infrequently and did not differ widely between the institutions. Surgeon volume was not addressed.

▶ This article looked at the relationship between hospital volumes and total shoulder arthroplasty outcomes. Over 1300 total shoulder arthroplasties were performed in New York State during a 4-year period. Almost one half were done at 5 hospitals in the New York City region. Patients at hospitals with greater volumes of total shoulder arthroplasties were at a lower risk of patient readmission within 60 days. There were no data on individual surgeon volume or clinical data on pain and function of the patients. Of interest is that over 100 hospitals performed less than 5 total shoulder arthroplasties per year and provided more than half of the study patients. If each of these hospitals had 2 to 3 surgeons performing total shoulder arthroplasty, then the majority of total shoulder arthroplasties in New York State were performed by surgeons who do perhaps 2 a year.

S. P. Steinmann, MD

Shoulder Arthroplasty for the Treatment of Inflammatory Arthritis
Collins DN, Harryman DT II, Wirth MA (Arkansas Specialty Orthopaedics, Little Rock; Univ of Washington, Seattle; Univ of Texas, San Antonio)
J Bone Joint Surg Am 86-A:2489-2496, 2004   4–2

Background.—Prosthetic replacement of the glenohumeral joint can relieve pain and improve shoulder function for patients with end-stage inflammatory arthritis. The purpose of this study was to prospectively analyze the clinical, functional, and radiographic outcomes of shoulder reconstruction with hemiarthroplasty or total shoulder arthroplasty.

Methods.—In this multicenter prospective study, clinical history, physical examination, and self-assessment tools including a visual analogue scale, the Simple Shoulder Test, and an activities questionnaire were used to measure comfort, quality of life, and function. Radiographic outcome was determined by assessing the severity of the disease, the adaptation of the prosthesis to the anatomy, the implant position and relationships, and the restoration of glenohumeral alignment.

Results.—At the time of follow-up, at a minimum of twenty-four months (mean, thirty-nine months), the thirty-six shoulders treated with a hemiarthroplasty and the twenty-five treated with a total shoulder arthroplasty showed significant improvement (p < 0.0001) as demonstrated by the visual analogue scale and the Simple Shoulder Test as well as improvements in the components of the activities questionnaire. Active forward elevation was significantly better (p < 0.004) after the total shoulder arthroplasties than after the hemiarthroplasties. The presence of extremely severe disease did not affect the clinical outcome. Prosthetic adaptation to the anatomy and restoration of glenohumeral alignment resulted in significant improvement in certain motion parameters and were associated with one another (p < 0.001). Restoration of glenohumeral alignment resulted in significant improvements in overall quality of life (p = 0.038), use of the arm for work and play (p = 0.014), and range of motion (p = 0.0004) compared with those parameters when alignment had not been restored. Glenoid erosion occurred in four of the shoulders treated with hemiarthroplasty. Two of the glenoid components used in the total shoulder arthroplasties loosened.

Conclusions.—Patients with inflammatory arthritis treated with hemiarthroplasty or total shoulder arthroplasty can be expected to have improved comfort, range of motion, and function. Restoration of glenohumeral alignment appears to lead to even greater improvement in these clinical parameters.

▶ This excellent study examines the role of total shoulder arthroplasty and hemiarthroplasty in the care of the patient with inflammatory arthritis. In 71 patients with 2-year follow-up the authors compared the results and found little difference between the 2 groups with respect to their radiographic and clinical outcomes. Multiple surgeons were used to accumulate the numbers. Patients with intact rotator-cuff function and those with good glenoid bone stock had optimal results with a total shoulder replacement. Restoration of glenohumeral alignment should be the goal of the surgeon, as the patients in whom this was achieved had the best clinical outcomes from their surgery. Although a significant number of patients were excluded due to short-term follow-up, the authors present a good study that should be a reference for future surgeons. The authors should be encouraged to provide longer-term analysis of the reported group and analyze the patients that were excluded.

C. Carroll IV, MD

Shoulder Hemiarthroplasty in Patients With Juvenile Idiopathic Arthritis
Thomas S, Price AJ, Sankey RA, et al (Heatherwood and Wexham Park Hosps, England)
J Bone Joint Surg Br 87-B:672-676, 2005   4–3

Replacement of the shoulder in juvenile idiopathic arthritis is not often performed and there have been no published series to date.

We present nine glenohumeral hemiarthroplasties in eight patients with systemic or polyarticular juvenile idiopathic arthritis. The mean follow-up was six years (59 to 89 months). The mean age at the time of surgery was 32 years. Surgery took place at a mean of 27 years after diagnosis. The results indicated excellent relief from pain. There was restoration of useful function, which deteriorated with time, in part because of progression of the systemic disease in this severely affected group. No patient has required revision to date and there has been no radiological evidence of loosening or osteolysis around the implants.

We discuss the pathoanatomical challenges unique to this group. There was very little space for a prosthetic joint and, in some cases, bony deformity and the small size necessitated the use of custom-made implants.

▶ The study by Thomas et al represents one of the few published series on the results of hemiarthroplasty in patients with juvenile idiopathic arthritis. This series of 8 patients with a mean follow-up of 6 years demonstrates significant improvement in pain and improvement in function. The authors report that no patient has required revision to date.

J. W. Sperling, MD

A Comparison of Pain, Strength, Range of Motion, and Functional Outcomes After Hemiarthroplasty and Total Shoulder Arthroplasty in Patients With Osteoarthritis of the Shoulder: A Systematic Review and Meta-Analysis
Bryant D, Litchfield R, Sandow M, et al (McMaster Univ, Hamilton, Ont, Canada)
J Bone Joint Surg Am 87-A:1947-1955, 2005   4–4

Background.—A systematic review of the literature was performed to estimate the impact of hemiarthroplasty compared with total shoulder arthroplasty on function and range of motion in patients suffering from osteoarthritis of the shoulder.

Methods.—We conducted an electronic search for relevant studies published in any language from 1966 to 2004, a manual search of the proceedings from five major orthopaedic meetings from 1995 to 2003, and a review of the reference lists from potentially relevant studies. Four randomized clinical trials, with similar eligibility criteria and surgical techniques, that compared hemiarthroplasty and total shoulder arthroplasty for the treatment of primary osteoarthritis of the shoulder were found to be eligible. Authors from three of the four studies provided original patient data. Analysis of co-variance focused on the two-year outcome and included a comparison of the aggregate University of California at Los Angeles shoulder score, four University of California at Los Angeles domain scores, and range of motion.

Results.—A total of 112 patients (fifty managed with hemiarthroplasty and sixty-two managed with total shoulder arthroplasty), who had a mean age of sixty-eight years, were included in this analysis. A significant moderate effect was detected in the function domain of the University of California at Los Angeles shoulder score ($p < 0.001$) in favor of total shoulder arthroplasty (mean [and standard deviation], 8.1 ± 0.3) compared with hemiarthroplasty (mean, 6.6 ± 0.3). A significant difference in the pain score was found in favor of the total shoulder arthroplasty group ($p < 0.0001$). However, the large degree of heterogeneity ($p = 0.006$, $I^2 = 80.2\%$) among the studies decreased our confidence that total shoulder arthroplasty provides a true, consistent benefit with regard to pain. There was a significant difference in the overall change in forward elevation of 13° (95% confidence interval, 0.5° to 26°) in favor of the total shoulder arthroplasty group ($p = 0.008$).

Conclusions.—At a minimum of two years of follow-up, total shoulder arthroplasty provided better functional outcome than hemiarthroplasty for patients with osteoarthritis of the shoulder. Since continuous degeneration of the glenoid after hemiarthroplasty or glenoid loosening after total shoulder arthroplasty may affect the eventual outcome, longer-term (five to ten-year) results are necessary to determine whether these findings remain consistent over time.

▶ Using the Cochrane strategy for randomized clinical trials, these authors performed a meta-analysis comparing pain, strength, range of motion, and functional outcomes between hemiarthroplasty (HA) and total shoulder arthroplasty (TSA) for primary osteoarthritis of the shoulder in patients with an intact rotator cuff and concentric glenoid. Using strict criteria, they were only able to identify one published study out of 311 abstracts that was eligible for inclusion. TSA patients had significantly less pain, less restriction of activity, and improved internal rotation and were able to work above shoulder level better than HA patients. Average forward elevation improved 43° for TSA and 31° for HA patients. Unsatisfactory results were 5 times greater in the HA group. The key points were that 20% of the HA group crossed over to TSA, the majority after 24 months. Long-term results (>10 years) are necessary to determine how rates of symptomatic glenoid erosion with HA or symptomatic glenoid loosening with TSA affect the difference in outcome between the 2 groups.

K. J. Renfree, MD

The Effect of Humeral Component Anteversion on Shoulder Stability With Glenoid Component Retroversion

Spencer EE Jr, Valdevit A, Kambic H, et al (Cleveland Clinic Found, Ohio)
J Bone Joint Surg Am 87-A:808-814, 2005   4–5

Background.—Posterior glenoid bone loss is often seen in association with glenohumeral osteoarthritis. This posterior asymmetric wear can lead to retroversion of the glenoid component and posterior instability after total shoulder arthroplasty. Options for the treatment of this asymmetric wear include eccentric reaming of the so-called high side, bone-grafting, and/or anteverting the humeral component. Although anteverting the humeral component has been advocated by many, it has not been substantiated on the basis of biomechanical data. The purpose of the present study was to determine whether anteverting the humeral component increases the stability of a total shoulder replacement with a retroverted glenoid component.

Methods.—A total shoulder arthroplasty was performed in eight human cadaveric shoulders. The glenoid component was placed in 15° of retroversion. Two humeral versions were tested for each specimen: anatomic version and 15° of anteversion relative to anatomic version. The specimens were mounted supine in a custom fixture on a servohydraulic testing system. The humerus was translated posteriorly by one-half of the width of the glenoid. Three positions of humeral rotation were tested for each position of humeral version. Both the energy and the peak load were analyzed as measures of joint stability.

Results.—There was no significant difference in either energy or peak load between the tests performed with the humeral component in 15° of anteversion and those performed with the component in anatomic version in any of the three rotational positions (p > 0.05).

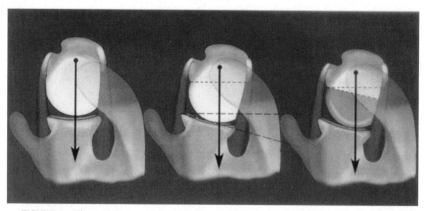

FIGURE 6.—Three axial views depicting the normal joint-reaction force and how this force translates posteriorly with glenoid retroversion. The third view (right) demonstrates how this translation is not affected by compensatory humeral component anteversion. (Courtesy of Spencer EE Jr, Valdevit A, Kambic H, et al: The effect of humeral component anteversion of shoulder stability with glenoid component retroversion. *J Bone Joint Surg [Am]* 87-A:808-814, 2005. Reprinted by permission of the publisher via Copyright Clearance Center, Inc.)

Conclusions.—Although anteverting the humeral component during total shoulder arthroplasty to compensate for glenoid retroversion has been advocated, these data suggest that compensatory anteversion of the humeral component does not increase the stability of a shoulder replacement with a retroverted glenoid component (Fig 6).

▶ A laboratory study was performed to study the relationship between simulated posterior glenoid erosion and shoulder stability following total shoulder arthroplasty. Specimen preparation placed the glenoid component in 15° retroversion to simulate posterior erosion, and then a humeral component was implanted either in anatomical version or 15° anteversion. While a 40-N centering force was applied, the maximum force required to translate the humeral head posteriorly by one-half the width of the glenoid component was measured.

The energy required to create that translation was calculated. Measurements were made in simulated internal and external rotation as well as neutral. Significantly more force was required to translate the humeral head when the specimens were internally rotated 30° versus other positions, but it made no difference if the humeral component was set at 15° anteversion or anatomical alignment.

The study was technically well-done but is limited by all the problems inherent in any ex vivo study and, by design, ignores the complex array of muscle and soft tissue forces acting on the shoulder in vivo and how those may change over time. Spencer et al chose to model the scenario in which there is 15° glenoid retroversion because they assumed most surgeons would prefer to address that amount of bone loss by anteverting the humeral stem rather than adding a bone graft. That may or may not be true.

The authors conclude by writing that "restoring a neutral glenoid surface might be preferred in cases of posterior glenoid bone loss." While that may seem reasonable, that statement remains an unproven hypothesis not addressed directly or supported by the data presented. How much stability is "enough" and at precisely what point one should treat posterior glenoid erosion and with what technique are questions awaiting future research.

R. R. Slater, Jr, MD

Two-Year Results After Exchange Shoulder Arthroplasty Using Inverse Implants
Katzer A, Sickelmann F, Seemann K, et al (Endo-Klinik, Hamburg, Germany)
Orthopedics 27:1165-1167, 2004   4–6

Background.—Inverse implants are used in exchange shoulder arthroplasty to treat impingement, limited range of motion, joint instability, and infection. Indications for revision are impingement, prosthesis head dislocation, and periprosthetic infection. A prospective pilot study determined the outcomes of exchange shoulder arthroplasty for revision indications using a Delta Prosthesis (DePuy Orthopaedics Inc., Warsaw, Ind.).

Methods.—The first 21 of 84 patients followed up for at least 2 years were included in the current analysis. At the time of surgery, patient age ranged from 49 to 77 years. Three total and 17 hemi prostheses were exchanged. A total humerus replacement was needed in 1 patient. Indications for the procedure were impingement with pain and limited motion in 12 cases, cranioventral dislocation or subluxation in 5, periprosthetic infections in 3, and ankylosis from periarticular ossifications in 1.

Outcomes.—Eighty-one percent of the patients rated their surgical outcomes as very good. Fourteen percent judged the result to be good, and 5% satisfactory. Preoperatively, all patients needed analgesics regularly or sporadically; postoperatively, only 3 patients needed these medications sporadically. Shoulder range of motion improved markedly after surgery in all patients. At 3 months after operation, patients had achieved a degree of function nearly equal to the final maximum outcome. Radiographs showed no signs of loosening in any of the patients. In 1 patient, painless acromion pseudarthrosis developed, and in another 2, inferior glenoid notching of no pathologic importance was noted.

Conclusions.—Exchange shoulder arthroplasty using a Delta Prosthesis for revision indications can produce functional outcomes corresponding to those of primary implantation. The high cost of the implant is a disadvantage of this procedure.

▶ This study reveals what has garnered increasing interest in Europe over the last 6 to 8 years, treating failed arthroplasties with an inverse implant. The indication for an inverse prosthesis is the loss of rotator cuff function (tear arthropathy, secondary cuff insufficiency, infections) and severe bone loss, including the insertion sites of the rotator cuff (posttraumatic cases with loss of the tuberosities, nonunions of the tuberosities). It is not correct to call the upward migration of the prosthetic head impingement, because the term is definitely used for another entity. We should use the same language when talking about rotator cuff insufficiency. The study shows that the inverse prothesis developed by Paul Grammont is a viable option for such difficult cases where the rotator cuff gets insufficient secondarily or loss of its insertion occurs. The patients are usually pain free and very satisfied with their shoulder function. As a shoulder surgeon you have to keep the advantages of this technique in mind to counsel the patients, but you should also be aware of the possible complications of this prosthesis that usually cause deterioration of the results after 4 to 5 years, which could not be covered by this short-term study.

S. Lichtenberg, MD

The Reverse Shoulder Prosthesis for Glenohumeral Arthritis Associated With Severe Rotator Cuff Deficiency: A Minimum Two-Year Follow-up Study of Sixty Patients

Frankle M, Siegal S, Pupello D, et al (Florida Orthopaedic Inst, Tampa)
J Bone Joint Surg Am 87-A:1697-1705, 2005   4–7

Background.—Patients who have pain and dysfunction from gleno-humeral arthritis associated with severe rotator cuff deficiency have few treatment options. The goal of this study was to retrospectively evaluate the short-term results of arthroplasty with use of the Reverse Shoulder Prosthesis in the management of this problem.

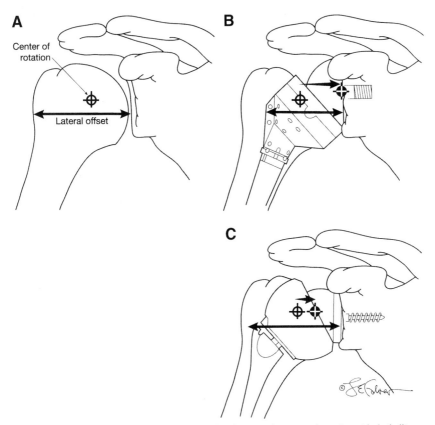

FIGURE 4.—**A**, Anatomical drawing of a shoulder, depicting the center of rotation with the bull's-eye and the lateral offset with the *bold arrow*. **B**, A drawing of a Delta-III device implanted in a shoulder, demonstrating how it causes the center of rotation and lateral offset to shift medially with respect to the anatomical shoulder. **C**, A drawing of the Reverse Shoulder Prosthesis implanted in a shoulder, demonstrating how the device causes the center of rotation and lateral offset to shift medially with respect to the anatomical shoulder but to a smaller degree than with the Delta-III prosthesis. (From Frankle M, Siegal S, Pupello D, et al: The reverse shoulder prosthesis for glenohumeral arthritis associated with severe rotator cuff deficiency: A minimum two-year follow-up study of sixty patients. *J Bone Joint Surg Am* 87-A:1697-1705, 2005. Courtesy of Lewis E. Calver. Reproduced by permission of the publisher via Copyright Clearance Center, Inc.)

Methods.—We report the results for sixty patients (sixty shoulders) with a rotator cuff deficiency and glenohumeral arthritis who were followed for a minimum of two years. Thirty-five patients had no previous shoulder surgery, whereas twenty-three had had either an open or arthroscopic rotator cuff repair, one had had a subacromial decompression, and one had had a biceps tendon repair. All patients were assessed preoperatively and postoperatively with the American Shoulder and Elbow Surgeons scoring system for pain and function and with visual analog scales for pain and function. They were also asked to rate their satisfaction with the outcome. The shoulder range of motion was measured preoperatively and postoperatively.

Results.—The average age of the patients was seventy-one years. The average duration of follow-up was thirty-three months. All measures improved significantly (p < 0.0001). The mean total score on the American Shoulder and Elbow Surgeons system improved from 34.3 to 68.2; the mean function score, from 16.1 to 29.4; and the mean pain score, from 18.2 to 38.7. The score for function on the visual analog scale improved from 2.7 to 6.0, and the score for pain on the visual analog scale improved from 6.3 to 2.2. Forward flexion increased from 55.0° to 105.1°, and abduction increased from 41.4° to 101.8°. Forty-one of the sixty patients rated the outcome as good or excellent; sixteen were satisfied, and three were dissatisfied. There were a total of thirteen complications in ten patients (17%). Seven patients (12%) had eight failures, requiring revision surgery to another Reverse Shoulder Prosthesis in five patients (one shoulder had two revisions) and revision to a hemiarthroplasty in two patients because of deep infection.

Conclusions.—The data from this study suggest that arthroplasty with the Reverse Shoulder Prosthesis may be a viable treatment for patients with glenohumeral arthritis and a massive rotator cuff tear. However, future studies will be necessary to determine the longevity of the implant and whether it will provide continued improvement in function (Fig 4 and Table 1).

TABLE 1.—Clinical Results for Pain, Function, and Range of Motion*

	Preoperative	Follow-up	Improvement
American Shoulder and Elbow Surgeons system scores *(points)*			
Total	34.3 (0 to 65)	68.2 (15 to 100)†	33.9
Pain	18.2 (0 to 45)	38.7 (10 to 50)†	20.5
Function	16.1 (0 to 40)	29.4 (0 to 50)†	13.3
Visual analog scale scores *(points)*			
Pain	6.3 (1 to 10)	2.2 (0 to 8)†	4.1
Function	2.7 (0 to 9)	6.0 (1 to 10)†	3.3
Range-of-motion measurements *(deg)*			
Forward flexion	55.0 (0 to 120)	105.1 (30 to 180)†	50.1
Abduction	41.4 (0 to 110)	101.8 (30 to 180)†	60.4
External rotation	12.0 (−15 to 45)	41.1 (10 to 65)†	29.1

*The values are given as the mean, and the range is in parentheses.
†The difference was significant ($P < .0001$).

(Courtesy of Frankle M, Siegal S, Pupello D, et al: The reverse shoulder prosthesis for glenohumeral arthritis associated with severe rotator cuff deficiency: A minimum two-year follow-up study of sixty patients. *J Bone Joint Surg Am* 87-A:1697-1705, 2005. Reproduced by permission of the publisher via Copyright Clearance Center, Inc.)

▶ The article by Frankle et al represents one of the first large reported series on the outcome of a reverse prosthesis for glenohumeral arthritis associated with severe rotator cuff deficiency. The study consisted of 60 shoulders with a minimum 2-year follow-up. The authors noted significant improvement in patients' American Shoulder and Elbow Surgeons scores and visual analog pain scale scores, as well as improvements in elevation. The overall rate of complications was 17%. This study demonstrates that the reverse prosthesis may be a viable treatment option for patients with massive rotator cuff tears and glenohumeral arthritis.

J. W. Sperling, MD

Analysis of a Retrieved Delta III Total Shoulder Prosthesis
Nyffeler RW, Werner CML, Simmen BR, et al (Univ of Zurich, Switzerland)
J Bone Joint Surg Br 86-B:1187-1191, 2004   4–8

Background.—The Delta III total shoulder is a reversed semi-constrained prosthesis used in the treatment of painful glenohumeral arthritis associated with irreparable rotator cuff tear. The shapes of the scapular and humeral joint surfaces are transposed by this prosthesis to medialize the center of rotation of the joint. Good short-term and mid-term results for pain relief, active elevation, and patient satisfaction have been reported. The post-mortem and histologic findings regarding notching, fixation, and stability of a reversed Delta III total shoulder prosthesis retrieved 8 months after implantation were reported.

Methods.—A fresh frozen left shoulder specimen from a 91-year-old man, who died after a severe brain injury resulting from a fall, was examined post-mortem. The patient's left glenohumeral joint had been replaced with a Delta III shoulder prosthesis 8 months before his death. The joint replacement had been performed because of a painful, pseudoparalytic shoulder with an irreparable rotator cuff tear. Radiographs 6 weeks post-operatively showed a small notch at the lateral border of the scapula and a radiolucent line on the posterior aspect of the glenoid component.

Results.—Gross inspection revealed an intact deltoid muscle. Histologic examination showed a chronic foreign body reaction in the joint capsule. True anteroposterior radiographs were taken under fluoroscopic control with the proximal humerus in adduction and neutral rotation and revealed a small radiolucent line of less than 1 mm between cement and bone of the humeral shaft. The synovium was of a normal color and the capsule was thick and hard. The inferior pole of the glenoid and the scapular neck were eroded, corresponding to the radiographic notch on the lateral border of the scapula (Fig 3). However, there were no histologic signs of loosening of the glenoid base plate. The stability of the prosthetic articulation was only slightly reduced by the eroded rim of the cup. Testing of the range of motion showed that maximum abduction in the scapular plane was 70° with respect to the plane of the glenoid component.

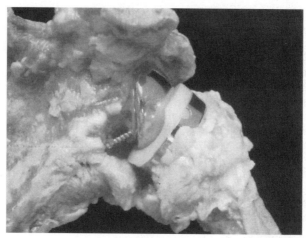

FIGURE 3.—Photograph showing the erosion around the inferior pole of the glenoid and the scapular neck. The inferior screw and the inferior part of the glenoid base plate are denuded of bone. The polyethylene liner is worn. (Courtesy of Nyffeler RW, Werner CML, Simmen BR, et al: Analysis of a retrieved Delta III total shoulder prosthesis. *J Bone Joint Surg Br* 86-B:1187-1191, 2004).

Conclusions.—The Delta III reversed shoulder prosthesis is recommended for use in older patients with irreparable rotator cuff tears and osteoarthritis. An inferior notch often develops within the first months after the operation but may not progress thereafter. In the present case, mechanical impingement between epiphyseal polyethylene and the inferior screw was present but had not led to loosening of the glenoid component. Positioning of the glenoid component more inferiorly on the glenoid could reduce the risk of inferior glenoid impingement.

▶ The study by Nyffeler is a case report that is an analysis of a retrieved Delta III reverse prosthesis. This study examines the histologic response of the native shoulder to the prosthesis. In addition, this study provides potential insight into positioning the glenoid component in a more inferior position to potentially decrease the risk of inferior glenoid impingement and notching.

J. W. Sperling, MD

Incidence of Early Radiolucent Glenoid Lines in Patients Having Total Shoulder Replacements

Klepps S, Chiang AS, Miller S, et al (Montana Orthopedics and Sports Medicine, Billings; Hosp for Joint Diseases, New York; Pro Sports Orthopedics, Inc, Brookline, Mass; et al)
Clin Orthop 435:118-125, 2005

4–9

Glenoid loosening is the most common long-term complication occurring after total shoulder replacement. Imprecise cement technique and glenoid preparation may result in early radiolucent glenoid line formation. Early radiolucent lines may indicate inadequate initial fixation, which may contribute to early loosening. Improved cement techniques, refined instrumentation, and glenoid component design all may reduce early radiolucent lines. In our study, postoperative anteroposterior and axillary radiographs were obtained after 68 total shoulder replacements done by one surgeon using either an old free-hand, manual packing technique before November 1998 (n = 28) or a new instrument preparation and pressurization technique since November 1998 (n = 40). Three orthopaedic surgeons blindly reviewed the radiographs for the presence and thickness (mm) of radiolucent lines. The newer instrumented pressurization group had a lower incidence of radiolucent lines than the old manually packed group. In the new subgroup, pegged components had a lower incidence of radiolucent lines than keeled components. The incidence of radiolucent lines seems to be reduced using specially designed instruments, new glenoid designs, and modern cement techniques, which may lead to reduced long-term glenoid loosening.

▶ The long-term success of total shoulder arthroplasty (TSA) relies primarily on the longevity of its individual components. A common cause of revision of TSA is glenoid loosening. The factors that influence glenoid loosening include the morphology and the positioning of the glenoid and the humeral components, as well as glenoid preparation and cementation. Although radiolucent lines surrounding other joint arthroplasties are useful in diagnosing significant loosening of the implant, the presence of radiolucent lines around glenoid components has not, to date, correlated with symptomatic loosening.

The authors present a retrospective cohort study of 68 patients to delineate any difference between 2 generations of cement technique as well as 2 types of glenoid components in the development of significant radiolucency seen on postoperative radiographs. Patients treated prior to November 1998 were treated with hand-packing of cement and a keeled component. Thereafter, patients were treated with either keeled or pegged glenoids with pressurization of the cement. Any radiolucency greater than 1 mm around the glenoid seen on postoperative radiographs was considered significant.

The authors found a decreasing trend toward significant radiolucency around the glenoid component following the use of the newer-generation cement technique. Similarly, they found that the pegged components had fewer radiolucent lines. However, radiolucency has not correlated with symptomatic loosening and the current results for keeled components remain excellent.

Certainly, as cement technique improves, the longevity of these implants is expected to improve. The clinical difference between keeled and pegged implants remains to be seen. It is my preference to use pegged implants as they appear more stable and resistant to edge loading, with uniform dispersion of stress among the 3 fixation points. With adequate glenoid exposure, pegged components are equally simple to implant. However, longer-term studies are necessary to differentiate the clinical outcome between the 2 components.

J. Yao, MD

Stability of Cemented All-Polyethylene Keeled Glenoid Components: A Radiostereometric Study With a Two-Year Follow-up

Rahme H, Mattsson P, Larsson S (Uppsala Univ, Sweden)

J Bone Joint Surg Br 86-B:856-860, 2004   4–10

We studied the stability of cemented all-polyethylene keeled glenoid components by radiostereometric analysis (RSA) in 16 shoulders which had received a total shoulder replacement. There were 14 women (one bilateral) and one man with a mean age of 64 years. The diagnosis was osteoarthritis in eight and rheumatoid arthritis in seven. Two of the shoulders were excluded from the RSA study because of loosening of the tantalum markers.

Three tantalum markers were inserted in the glenoid socket, two in the coracoid process and two in the acromion. The polyethylene keeled glenoid component was marked with three to five tantalum markers. Conventional radiological and RSA examinations were carried out at five to seven days, at four months and at one and two years after operation. Radiolucent lines were found in all except three shoulders. Migration was most pronounced in the distal direction and exceeded 1 mm in four shoulders. In ten shoulders rotation exceeded 2 degrees in one or more axes with retroversion/anteversion being most common. No correlation was found between migration and the presence of radiolucencies on conventional radiographs (Fig 1).

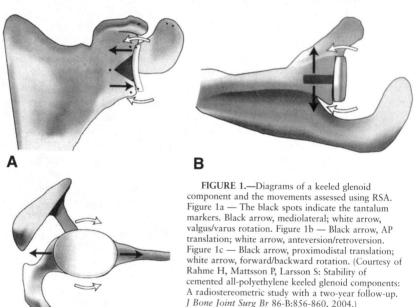

A   **B**

C

FIGURE 1.—Diagrams of a keeled glenoid component and the movements assessed using RSA. Figure 1a — The black spots indicate the tantalum markers. Black arrow, mediolateral; white arrow, valgus/varus rotation. Figure 1b — Black arrow, AP translation; white arrow, anteversion/retroversion. Figure 1c — Black arrow, proximodistal translation; white arrow, forward/backward rotation. (Courtesy of Rahme H, Mattsson P, Larsson S: Stability of cemented all-polyethylene keeled glenoid components: A radiostereometric study with a two-year follow-up. *J Bone Joint Surg Br* 86-B:856-860, 2004.)

▶ The study by Rahme et al represents one of the first series published on the use of radio stereometric analysis in total shoulder replacement. This is a study of 16 shoulders that underwent a total shoulder arthroplasty with placement of these markers. The study demonstrated no relation between the appearance of radiolucencies and migration of the markers. Further long-term studies will be necessary to further evaluate this technique to determine loosening of glenoid components.

J. W. Sperling, MD

5 Shoulder: Arthroscopy

Determining the Relationship of the Axillary Nerve to the Shoulder Joint Capsule From an Arthroscopic Perspective

Price MR, Tillett ED, Acland RD, et al (Univ of Louisville, Ky)

J Bone Joint Surg Am 86-A:2135-2142, 2004

5–1

Background.—The axillary nerve is out of the field of view during shoulder arthroscopy, but certain procedures require manipulation of capsular tissue that can threaten the function or integrity of the nerve. We studied fresh cadavers to identify the course of the axillary nerve in relation to the glenoid rim from an intra-articular perspective and to determine how close the nerve travels in relation to the glenoid rim and the inferior glenohumeral ligament.

Methods.—We dissected nine whole-body fresh-tissue shoulder joints and exposed the axillary nerve through a window in the inferior glenohumeral ligament. Then we cut coronal sections through the glenoid fossa of ten unembalmed, frozen shoulder specimens after the axillary nerve had been stained with Evans blue dye. All specimens were studied with the joint secured in the lateral decubitus position used for shoulder arthroscopy.

Results.—Microsurgical dissection through the inferior glenohumeral ligament from within the joint capsule revealed the axillary nerve as it traversed the quadrangular space. In each dissection, the teres minor branch was the closest to the glenoid rim. The coronal sectioning of the unembalmed shoulder specimens demonstrated that the closest point between the axillary nerve and the glenoid rim was at the 6 o'clock position on the inferior glenoid rim. At this position, the average distance between the axillary nerve and the glenoid rim was 12.4 mm. The axillary nerve lay, throughout its course, at an average of 2.5 mm from the inferior glenohumeral ligament.

Conclusions.—We used two novel approaches to map the axillary nerve from an intra-articular perspective. Our analysis of the position of the nerve with use of these methods provides the shoulder arthroscopist with essential information regarding the location, route, and morphology of the nerve as it passes inferior to the glenoid rim and shoulder capsule (Fig 11).

▶ This article presents improved techniques to evaluate the axillary nerve in reference to shoulder arthroscopy. The authors use both an infraglenoid window open dissection and a staining of the axillary nerve with coronal frozen

49

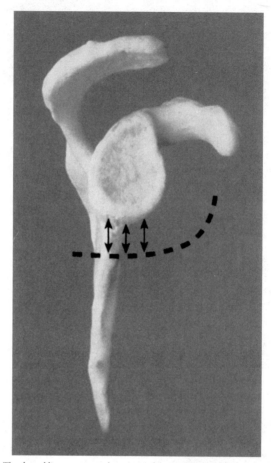

FIGURE 11.—The *dotted line* represents the course of the axillary nerve running inferior to the glenoid rim. The *arrows* depict the approximate distances measured from the axillary nerve to the glenoid rim at the 6 o'clock position and in the 5-mm cuts made anterior and posterior to the 6 o'clock position. The nerve lies closest to the glenoid rim at the 6 o'clock position. (Courtesy of Price MR, Tillett ED, Acland RD, et al: Determining the relationship of the axillary nerve to the shoulder joint capsule from an arthroscopic perspective. *J Bone Joint Surg Am* 86-A:2135-2142, 2004. Reproduced by permission of the publisher via Copyright Clearance Center.)

sections to evaluate the course of the nerve as it relates to the inferior labrum. The excellent figures show the course of the nerve including its branching into sensory and separate motor branches. The take-home message from all studies that evaluate the course of the nerve in reference to arthroscopy is to stay within 1 cm of the rim of the inferior glenoid when working in this area to avoid problems. The 1 limitation of this particular study is that the shoulder is not distended, a fact that would likely move the nerve even farther away than the authors' findings.

T. R. McAdams, MD

Arthroscopic Removal of the Glenoid Component for Failed Total Shoulder Arthroplasty: A Report of Five Cases

O'Driscoll SW, Petrie RS, Torchia ME (Mayo Clinic, Rochester, Minn)
J Bone Joint Surg Am 87-A:858-863, 2005   5–2

Background.—Total shoulder arthroplasty has been shown to be effective in pain relief and improvement of function, but significant concerns exist regarding the prevalence of glenoid lucent lines and, thus, the possibility of loosening of the glenoid component over the long term. Among the options for treatment of symptomatic glenoid loosening is revision of the component or conversion to a hemiarthroplasty by removal of the loose glenoid component with or without bone-grafting of the glenoid. Removal of the glenoid component is based on reports of humeral hemiarthroplasty that have indicated that it is possible to obtain pain relief without a glenoid component. In the current study, an arthroscopic method is described for removal of a symptomatic loose glenoid component and the underlying cement mantle.

Methods.—Arthroscopic removal of the glenoid component was performed in 5 patients from June 1995 through May 2000. All patients had a painful failed total shoulder prosthesis with isolated loosening of the glenoid component. In the first cut, the glenoid prosthesis was transected diagonally from anteroposterior to posteroinferior (Fig 2). The remaining intact polyethylene between the cut portion of the faceplate and the underlying keel was then divided. The superior third of the glenoid faceplate was then withdrawn through the anterior portal (Fig 3). The osteotome was then passed beneath the remaining middle third of the faceplate, which separated it from the keel (Fig 4). The keel was removed with strong graspers. After removal of the cement in pieces, a curet was used to clean the glenoid cavity. A total syn-

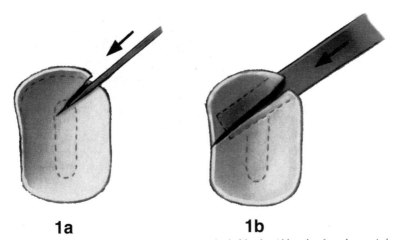

1a   **1b**

FIGURE 2.—Cut 1a separates the superior–posterior third of the glenoid faceplate from the remainder of the faceplate, leaving a small attachment to the underlying keel. Cut 1b separates the component fragment from the keel to permit removal. (Courtesy of O'Driscoll SW, Petrie RS, Torchia ME: Arthroscopic removal of the glenoid component for failed total shoulder arthroplasty: A report of five cases. *J Bone Joint Surg Am* 87-A:858-863, 2005. Reproduced by permission of the publisher via Copyright Clearance Center, Inc.)

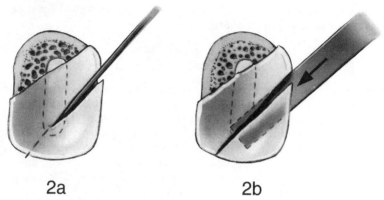

2a   2b

FIGURE 3.—Cuts 2a and 2b are similar to cuts 1a and 1b. They separate the anterior–inferior third of the faceplate from the middle portion and from the keel. (Courtesy of O'Driscoll SW, Petrie RS, Torchia ME: Arthroscopic removal of the glenoid component for failed total shoulder arthroplasty: A report of five cases. *J Bone Joint Surg Am* 87-A:858-863, 2005. Reproduced by permission of the publisher via Copyright Clearance Center, Inc.)

ovectomy may be necessary if extensive synovitis is present. A capsulotomy may also be performed if improved motion is required. After surgery, the patients were given a sling for comfort for the first few days but were encouraged to move the limb on the day after surgery and to pursue activities as tolerated.

Results.—The operations were successful in all 5 patients. The average duration of follow-up was 49 months. The procedures were all determined to be clinically beneficial. No additional surgical procedures were performed in any of the 5 shoulders. Subjective pain relief was partial in 2 patients and complete in 3 patients. No operative or perioperative complications oc-

FIGURE 4.

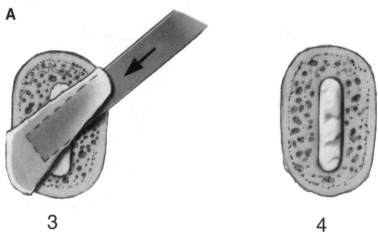

A

3   4

(Continued)

FIGURE 4 (cont.)

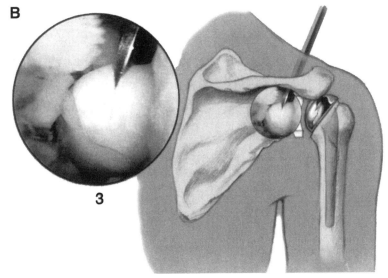

FIGURE 4.—The third and fourth segments of the glenoid component (the middle portion of the face-plate and the keel, respectively) are separated by cut 3 with the osteotome. (Courtesy of O'Driscoll SW, Petrie RS, Torchia ME: Arthroscopic removal of the glenoid component for failed total shoulder arthroplasty: A report of five cases. *J Bone Joint Surg Am* 87-A:858-863, 2005. Reproduced by permission of the publisher via Copyright Clearance Center, Inc.)

curred, except for temporary exacerbation of pre-existing lymphedema in 1 patient.

Conclusions.—The current indications for arthroscopic removal of a loose glenoid component and its cement are painful loosening of a polyethylene glenoid component in the presence of a large rotator cuff defect or a relative contraindication to a revision arthroplasty. This approach might also be considered in a patient in whom reimplantation of a glenoid component is expected to be exceptionally difficult, such as in an obese individual with a nonmodular humeral component.

▶ Revision of a failed total shoulder arthroplasty is a difficult problem that plagues surgeons who work on the upper extremities. O'Driscoll and colleagues provide a unique treatment option for this challenging condition. They provide a case series and a surgical technique that details how to arthroscopically remove a loose glenoid component. This technique should be considered when the patient has either significant comorbidities that prohibit a revision shoulder arthroplasty or a massive rotator cuff tear along with the failed total shoulder arthroplasty. As the authors caution, this treatment option should only be performed by a surgeon proficient in shoulder arthroscopy because this procedure is technically demanding. The polished humeral head often creates mirror reflections that make orientation within the glenohumeral joint difficult during the procedure. Furthermore, this procedure should not be performed if the glenoid component is backed with metal. In the appropriately selected patient, this procedure is a valuable surgical option that provides significant pain relief after a failed total shoulder arthroplasty.

R. Gupta, MD

Arthroscopic Bicipital Sheath Repair: Two-Year Follow-up With Pulley Lesions
Bennett WF (Sarasota, Fla)
Arthroscopy 20:964-973, 2004   5–3

Purpose.—The purpose of this study was to evaluate arthroscopic repair in patients who had lesions of both the subscapularis insertion/medial head of the coracohumeral ligament and the lateral head of the coracohumeral ligament and supraspinatus tendon (a type 5 biceps subluxation/instability classification), and to determine if primary repair of the torn structures used to reconstruct the bicipital sheath was associated with a high biceps rupture rate. The null hypothesis, that there is no difference between preoperative and postoperative outcomes, was tested.

Type of Study.—Prospective cohort.

Methods.—Since 1995, the author has had 18 patients who had lesions that affected both the medial and lateral wall of the bicipital sheath. An adjunct was added if tendonitis was present with fraying, and the biceps tendon was debrided if the fraying consisted of 50% or less the width of the tendon. This was chosen arbitrarily. Greater than 50% fraying of the biceps tendon was treated with repair of the supraspinatus and subscapularis. The biceps tendon was treated with tenotomy or tenodesis in these cases and these patients were not included in this study. This article reports on the repair technique and results having a minimum of 2-year follow-up.

Results.—There were 12 male patients (age range, 45 to 80 years; average, 62 years) and 6 female patients (age range, 50 to 85 years; average, 66 years). The dominant extremity was involved in 12 of the 16 extremities. Preoperative, ASES Index, Total Constant scores, Subjective Constant scores, Objective Constant scores, visual analog pain scales, and percent function were 31 ± 19, 53 ± 13, 12 ± 8, 41 ± 8, 7 ± 3, and 42 ± 17, respectively. Postoperative scores were 80 ± 14, 77 ± 10, 30 ± 4, 47 ± 7, 2 ± 2, and 84 ± 14, respectively. The null hypothesis was rejected at a level of $P = .001, .001, .001, .05, .001,$ and $.001$, respectively.

Conclusions.—There was 1 biceps disruption in this cohort following repair, for an incidence rate of 6%. There were 2 patients, active tennis players, who had recurrence of biceps inflammation in the follow-up period with no evidence of biceps subluxation. The arthroscopic technique reported is a primary repair used to reconstruct the normal structures of the groove. This may explain why previous recommendations not to reconstruct the groove because of the high biceps disruption rate have been noted previously. This study did not deepen the groove, tubulize the biceps tendon, or close the rotator interval in nonanatomic fashion. This arthroscopic technique is tech-

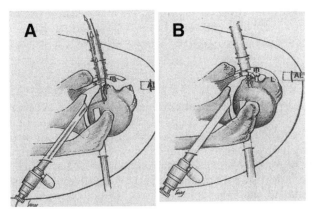

FIGURE 9.—The retrieval (A) and the final repair (B) of the medial side of the bicipital sheath. *Abbreviations: s*, Subscapularis; *m*, medial head coracohumeral ligament; *L*, lateral head coracohumeral ligament; *AL*, anterolateral portal. (Courtesy of Bennett WF: Arthroscopic bicipital sheath repair: Two-year follow-up with pulley lesions. *Arthroscopy* 20:964-973. Copyright 2004, with permission from The Arthroscopy Association of North America.)

nically feasible and can alleviate the symptoms of biceps tendon inflammation and/or subluxation in the majority of cases in this cohort (Fig 9).

▶ The soft tissue structures of the shoulder are interrelated, and an injury to one structure may be associated with an injury to another. For example, a tear of the subscapularis tendon from its insertion on the lesser tuberosity is often associated with rupture of the coracohumeral ligament, which leads to the subluxation of the long head of the biceps brachii tendon out of the bicipital groove. Subluxation of this tendon may lead to biceps irritation, attrition, and tendinosis.

While repair of the subscapularis tendon is important to restore internal rotation strength of the shoulder, the treatment of the unstable or torn biceps tendon remains controversial. The role of the long head of the biceps remains under debate, and treatment of an injured tendon ranges from debridement to tenolysis to tenodesis, with limited outcomes data available.

The author expands on his previous work on biceps subluxation and stability by presenting his 2-year follow-up of arthroscopic repair of the bicipital sheath with a concomitant rotator cuff repair. The author reports a significant improvement in the objective and subjective functional scores following the surgery. Biceps tendon rupture, a previously reported complication of open bicipital stabilization procedures (up to 33%), was reported as 6% in this series.

Limitations of this study include its retrospective nature and the lack of blinding and randomization. The rotator cuff repair is also a confounding variable as the study does not control for the improvement of symptoms following the rotator cuff repair alone. The author's work is useful for reintroducing the concept of long head biceps tendon stabilization, but its clinical significance awaits further studies. Further study will justify the routine use of this technically demanding technique.

J. Yao, MD

Assessment of Clavicular Translation After Arthroscopic Mumford Procedure: Direct Versus Indirect Resection—A Cadaveric Study

Miller CA, Ong BC, Jazrawi LM, et al (New York Univ—Hosp for Joint Diseases)
Arthroscopy 21:64-68, 2005   5–4

Background.—Arthroscopic distal clavicle revision (DCR) has the advantage of decreased morbidity compared to open resection. A superior (direct) or bursal (indirect) approach can be employed arthroscopically. If pain persists after DCR, the diagnosis may have been in error, resection inadequate or too extensive, or stability lacking because of disruption of the acromioclavicular or coracoclavicular ligament. The horizontal stability of the distal clavicle after arthroscopic resection of its lateral end was compared between the direct and indirect approaches.

Methods.—Twelve fresh-frozen human cadaveric shoulders underwent arthroscopic DCR, with the direct approach used in half and the indirect in the other half. In each, an arthroscopic burr was used to resect 5 mm of distal clavicle; then specimens were mounted on a materials testing (MTS) device permitting translation of the clavicle along the anteroposterior axis (Fig 3). Posterior translation was determined from the maximum anterior displacement of the clavicle.

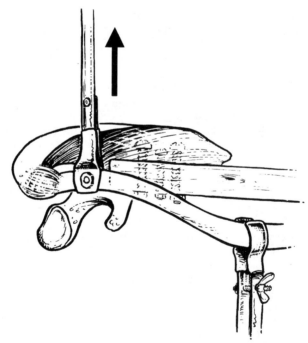

FIGURE 3.—Specimen mounted in the MTS device with posteriorly directed force being applied (*arrow*). (Courtesy of Miller CA, Ong BC, Jazrawi LM, et al: Assessment of clavicular translation after arthroscopic Mumford procedure: Direct versus indirect resection—a cadaveric study. *Arthroscopy* 21:64-68. Copyright 2005, with permission from The Arthroscopy Association of North America.)

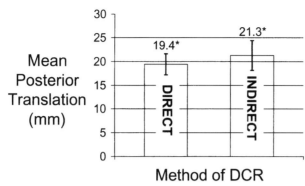

FIGURE 4.—Mean posterior translation in specimens. *$P = 0.27$. (Courtesy of Miller CA, Ong BC, Jazrawi LM, et al: Assessment of clavicular translation after arthroscopic Mumford procedure: Direct versus indirect resection—a cadaveric study. *Arthroscopy* 21:64-68. Copyright 2005, with permission from The Arthroscopy Association of North America.)

Results.—The direct group had a range of posterior translation between 18.2 and 23.1 mm, whereas the indirect group's range was 18.2 to 24.9 mm. Neither group suffered a catastrophic failure. The mean posterior translation was 19.4 mm for the direct group and 21.3 mm for the indirect group (Fig 4). The difference between groups was not statistically significant.

Conclusions.—The degree of posterior translation did not differ significantly between arthroscopic DCR performed by the direct or indirect approach. Thus the anteroposterior stability of the clavicle would be equivalent regardless of approach. Biomechanically, no concern should arise over the possibility of increased instability using one or the other technique.

▶ The authors of this paper performed a biomechanical study to compare the horizontal stability of two different arthroscopic techniques for distal clavicle resection. They specifically tried to examine whether there was any difference between the direct technique and the indirect technique. They used six cadavers in each group, and 5 mm of distal clavicle was resected with an arthroscopic burr. The soft tissues were stripped away and the specimens mounted on a materials testing device. A posterior directed force was then placed to try and measure the posterior translation. Specimens were cycled three times, and the displacement was measured and averaged. The difference they found was not statistically significant. It measured an average of 19.4 mm for the direct group and 21.3 mm for the indirect group. Excessive posterior translation of the clavicle following resection of the lateral end has been associated with a poor postoperative outcome. The authors did note that on gross examination, they found that specimens that had undergone direct resection had more disruption of the posterior capsule than those done using the indirect method. There were several limitations to this study, and these were discussed by the authors. There is the fact that unpaired specimens were used; also, the power of the study was diminished by its small sample size. The other criticism is that the specimens were stripped, leaving only the osseous and soft tissue structures about the acromioclavicular joint. This study showed that there was no significant difference in the degree of posterior translation of the distal clavicle after resection of a standard amount of bone by utilizing either the direct or indirect arthroscopic methods of resection.

S. F. M. Duncan, MD, MPH

6 Brachial Plexus

Glenohumeral Arthrodesis in Upper and Total Brachial Plexus Palsy: A Comparison of Functional Results

Chammas M, Goubier JN, Coulet B, et al (Lapeyronie Univ, Montpellier, France)

J Bone Joint Surg Br 86-B:692-695, 2004   6–1

We have compared the functional outcome after glenohumeral fusion for the sequelae of trauma to the brachial plexus between two groups of adult patients reviewed after a mean interval of 70 months. Group A (11 patients) had upper palsy with a functional hand and group B (16 patients) total palsy with a flail hand.

All 27 patients had recovered active elbow flexion against resistance before shoulder fusion. Both groups showed increased functional capabilities after glenohumeral arthrodesis and a flail hand did not influence the postoperative active range of movement. The strength of pectoralis major is a significant prognostic factor in terms of ultimate excursion of the hand and of shoulder strength. Glenohumeral arthrodesis improves function in patients who have recovered active elbow flexion after brachial plexus palsy even when the hand remains paralysed.

▶ The authors have presented their outcomes of glenohumeral fusions in 2 adult populations of patients with brachial plexus injuries: those with upper lesions and those with global palsies. They reach a number of interesting and informative conclusions, as follows:

1. Shoulder fusion does not help the pain of deafferentiation but will eliminate pain associated with subluxation. Thus, if the patient still complains of pain, even when the affected arm is well supported by a good-fitting sling, this surgery is unlikely to affect his or her pain.
2. If the patient has regained elbow flexion by whatever means, the patient senses postoperatively that elbow flexion strength is improved when the shoulder is stabilized. Many authors have reported this, but this study provides the best evidence to date to support this contention.
3. The gains, even in those with no hand function, outweigh the risks.
4. This procedure should not be recommended if good scapular control cannot be confirmed.

V. R. Hentz, MD

Transfer of Fascicles From the Ulnar Nerve to the Nerve to the Biceps in the Treatment of Upper Brachial Plexus Palsy
Teboul F, Kakkar R, Ameur N, et al (Bichat Hosp, Paris)
J Bone Joint Surg Am 86-A:1485-1490, 2004   6–2

Background.—The transfer of one or more ulnar nerve fascicles to the nerve to the biceps can restore elbow flexion in patients with upper brachial plexus palsy. The purposes of the present retrospective study were to evaluate the results of this procedure, to measure the delay in reinnervation of the biceps muscle, and to define the indications for a secondary Steindler flexorplasty.

Methods.—Thirty-two patients with an upper nerve-root brachial plexus injury were reviewed at an average of thirty-one months after the nerve fascicle transfer. The average age of the patients was twenty-eight years. The average time between the injury and the operation was nine months. Patients were evaluated with regard to reinnervation of the biceps, ulnar nerve function, elbow flexion strength, and grip strength.

Results.—The average time required for reinnervation of the biceps after nerve fascicle transfer was five months. No motor or sensory deficits related to the ulnar nerve were noted clinically. The average grip strength at the time of the last follow-up was 25 kg (an improvement of 9 kg compared with the preoperative value). After the nerve transfer, twenty-four patients achieved grade-3 elbow flexion strength or better according to the grading system of the Medical Research Council. A Steindler flexorplasty was performed as a secondary procedure in ten patients with persistent grade-3 flexor strength or worse. In eight of these cases, elbow flexion strength improved after nerve transfer and flexorplasty. Overall, thirty of the thirty-two patients achieved a good result (grade-4 strength) or a fair result (grade-3 strength).

Conclusions.—We recommend this procedure for brachial plexus injuries involving the C5-C6 or C5-C6-C7 nerve roots. This procedure spares the C5 nerve root and other nerves for grafting or transfer elsewhere. A secondary Steindler flexorplasty is indicated for patients who have persistent grade-3 elbow flexion strength or worse for at least twelve months after nerve fascicle transfer.

▶ There are now many reports extolling the virtues of this transfer in properly selected patients. It is now a key element in the brachial plexus surgeon's armamentarium. More recent studies have opined that innervating the brachialis muscle using expendable motor fascicles of the median nerve results in even greater recovery of elbow flexor force and may decrease the need to perform subsequent adjunctive procedures such as the Steindler flexorplasty.

Nerve transfers have now become the surgical paradigm for severe (avulsion and high rupture) plexus injuries, replacing the 30-year-old or greater paradigm of multiple plexo-plexal nerve grafts. Reinnervation distances are short, key muscles are precisely targeted, co-contractures minimized, and operative times considerably shortened. For example, my protocol for the patient with preoperative C5-C6 or C5–7 avulsions is exploration of the plexus and confirmation of the pathology, followed by spinal accessory to suprascapular nerve, ulnar (and for the next patient) median transfers to biceps and brachialis, and branch to triceps into the axillary nerve.

V. R. Hentz, MD

Selection of Grip Function in Double Free Gracilis Transfer Procedures After Complete Paralysis of the Brachial Plexus
Takka S, Doi K, Hattori Y, et al (Ogori Daiichi Gen Hosp, Yamaguchi, Japan)
Ann Plast Surg 54:610-614, 2005   6–3

Abstract.—Double free gracilis transfer (DFGT) procedures introduced by Doi et al have resulted in significant improvement in maintaining functional prehensile hand after total brachial plexus injury (TBPI). However, not all patients with satisfactory recovery of finger motion could improve their prehensile function. The use of reconstructed hand in daily activities was examined retrospectively to plan individual grip function, depending on the patient's own demand.

Thirty patients who had had reconstruction with DFGT procedures were evaluated retrospectively according to total active motion (TAM), power grip, hook grip, and pinch function. Power grip was evaluated by holding a bottle and hook grip by lifting a weight. Only 11 patients (36%) had very light pulp-to-pulp pinch, 11 (36%) had power grip, and 25 (83%) had hook grip. The mean weight that could be carried by hook grip was 1.3 kg. The mean TAM was 43 degrees. Pain sensation was the only encouraging sensation recovery, radiating to the chest.

Fine movements of the hand like pinching require well-developed exquisite control of movements. TBPI patients have the contralateral normal limb, which they always prefer, only using their reconstructed hand when the activity requires both hands, such as when holding a bottle to open its cap or lifting bags when the contralateral normal hand is already engaged. For performance of these actions, hook grip and power grip are the useful prehensile hand functions that can be obtained after DFGT. Selection of grip functions should be done according to patient needs, and the late-stage reconstructive hand operations should be decided according to preferred grip function.

▶ DFGT, as introduced by Doi et al, is a unique procedure and offers the opportunity for hand surgeons to reconstruct complete paralysis of the brachial plexus. Results were variable. Hook grip was the most useful and available function after DFGT procedures. Power grip was less functional, and powerful pinch was useless. The authors recommend that the selection of grip functions, hook grip or power grip, should be done according to the patient's needs. The authors reported that DFGT has resulted in significant improvement in maintaining functional prehensile hand after TBPI. However, they defined that more than 40° of TAM was satisfactory. The average hook grip strength was 1.3 kg. I wonder whether this TAM is useful. A little is a lot for a patient with nothing, but I wonder which kinds of activities in daily life patients could perform after these procedures. TBPI patients can still perform most activities with the contralateral normal limb without difficulty.

T. Ogino, MD, PhD

Protein Abnormality in Denervated Skeletal Muscles From Patients With Brachial Injury
Jia L, Xu L, Jiang M, et al (Fudan Univ, Shanghai, People's Republic of China)
Microsurgery 25:316-321, 2005   6–4

Background.—Rapid atrophy of skeletal muscle fibers is the process by which skeletal muscle responds to a variety of stimuli. Each atrophy-inducing stimulus has a unique initiation signal, but it is generally believed that a common mechanism of protein loss occurs independent of the inducing stimulus. Brachial plexus root avulsion is one of the main causes of serious skeletal muscle atrophy of the upper limb. It has been reported that, in patients suffering from brachial plexus root avulsion, irreversible atrophy has occurred in some target muscles, such as the intrinsic muscle of the hand, before regaining nerve stimulation.

The current treatment for brachial plexus root avulsion has improved with the development of microsurgical techniques for nerve transfer and nerve graft, but the outcomes have not been completely satisfactory because of a poor understanding of the molecular mechanism involved in muscle atrophy. Protein expression was compared between normal sternocleidomastoid muscle and denervated muscle using proteomic analysis.

Methods.—Muscle biopsy samples were obtained from 9 patients (mean age, 31.1 ± 1.6 years) who had suffered from brachial plexus injuries and C5 to T1 root avulsion for 3 to 5 months. Atrophic hypothenar and biceps muscle samples were obtained when the patients were admitted to hospital for surgical procedure on the contralateral C7 nerve root for neurotization, bridged by the ipsilateral vascularized ulnar nerve, for treatment of root avulsions of the brachial plexus. In the incision of healthy C7 dissections, normal sternocleidomastoid muscle was taken as control samples before neurorrhaphy between the healthy C7 and ipsilateral ulnar nerve.

Results.—Two-dimensional electrophoresis of muscle proteins showed that 26 proteins among about 800 spots in 2-dimensional electrophoresis gel displayed a decrease and 6 proteins an increase in expression of muscles with denervation atrophy compared with normal controls. The identified proteins that were abnormally expressed could be grouped as metabolic proteins, chaperone proteins, and contractile-apparatus proteins.

Conclusion.—The decrease in human tumor protein 54 may reduce the activity of transmembrane signaling in atrophied muscle, whereas the disregulation of the molecular chaperone protein DnaJC1 may indicate a role for molecular chaperone proteins in the functional recovery of atrophied muscles.

▶ This study characterized dynamic changes in denervated skeletal muscle proteins in human tissues. The authors compared protein expression between normal skeletal muscle and denervated muscle taken by biopsy from patients with brachial plexus injury. They found 30 proteins with differential expression between normal muscle and denervated muscle. Furthermore, they also found 7 proteins whose expression patterns in the denervated and atrophied biceps versus hypothenar muscles were different. It is well known that the recovery response of different muscles after nerve repair is different. The differential expression of protein in each muscle may reflect the prognosis of functional recovery of atrophied muscles after nerve repair.

T. Ogino, MD, PhD

Trapezius Transfer in Brachial Plexus Palsy: Correlation of the Outcome With Muscle Power and Operative Technique
Rühmann O, Schmolke S, Bohnsack M, et al (Hannover Med School, Germany)
J Bone Joint Surg Br 87-B:184-190, 2005   6–5

Background.—Shoulders with paralyzed deltoid and supraspinatus muscles may benefit from trapezius transfer. Functional results can vary, with improvements from 75° of abduction and forward flexion to only 40° or less. Experience has shown that reducing joint instability with brachial plexus palsy is an important consideration, leading to better control of the paralyzed arm and less pain. Between 1994 and 2003, the trapezius transfer technique developed by Saha was used in 58 patients; a modification was used for another 22 patients. All patients had brachial plexus palsy. The results with these 2 methods were compared.

Patients.—The 11 women and 69 men had a mean age of 31 years (range, 18-69 years). For all patients, a full evaluation of muscle function in the affected arm was conducted preoperatively. Forty-six percent of the patients had a completely flail arm; 54% had some peripheral function of the elbow and hand. None had full active motion of the elbow plus adequate hand function. Follow-up lasted 0.8 to 8 years (mean, 2.4 years).

Results.—All patients had an increase in function, with 74 patients (92.5%) having less multidirectional shoulder instability. Mean active abduction increased from 6° preoperatively to 34° postoperatively. Mean forward flexion increased from 12° preoperatively to 30° postoperatively. The mean deficit of external rotation was not significantly affected by surgery. Nineteen patients had a slight increase, 11 a decrease, and 50 no change in external rotation. All patients who had reasonable function of the biceps, coracobrachialis, and triceps improved their multidirectional shoulder instability. Flail shoulders with a power of MRC 0 to 2 demonstrated improved multidirectional instability that was considerably less. In the first 58 cases, complications included 14 patients who had persistent inferior subluxation of the humeral head and 4 patients who had no improvement in multidirectional instability. The modified technique produced no further cases of these complications and yielded slightly better abduction and forward flexion results and more improved stability.

Conclusions.—Both function and stability were improved in patients having trapezius transfer for flail shoulder. Better results occurred when patients retained some degree of function of the biceps, coracobrachialis, pectoralis major, and triceps. Modifying Saha's technique to use the atrophied deltoid to carry over the force of the trapezius provided improved joint stability and increased functional results.

▶ This is a study of 80 patients with brachial plexus palsy who underwent previous nerve surgery for reconstruction of the brachial plexus palsy, and then with failure of shoulder function underwent a trapezius transfer for the following indications: (1) multidirectional shoulder instability; (2) insufficient or weak abduction and forward flexion; and (3) poor function of the hand and elbow secondary to shoulder function. Before considering a trapezius transfer, the deltoid must demonstrate complete denervation, the trapezius must show full strength against resistance, and preoperative passive shoulder abduction must be to at least 80°.

This prospective study, carried out between 1994 and 2003, included 80 patients with brachial plexus injuries who met the indications for trapezius transfer. Sixty-two of these patients had undergone previous neurosurgical procedures before their trapezius transfer. The first 58 operations were performed in the manner according to Saha's original description. This included the detachment of the trapezius with a piece of distal acromion, and the insertion of the distal acromion onto the proximal humerus by a deltoid splitting approach. The shoulder was abducted 80° to 90°. The acromion was fixed to the humerus with two 6.5-mm cancellous screws, and the deltoid was sutured on top of the trapezius. In the last 22 cases, the authors modified Saha's technique and sutured the deltoid muscle under maximum tension on top of the trapezius and as far medially as possible. Overall, they performed this procedure in 37 patients who had a completely flail arm and in 18 patients who had some function in the flexors and extensors of the hand and wrist. Elbow flexion was noted in 15 patients.

The overall results demonstrated that 92.5% of the patients who underwent a trapezius transfer had a decrease of multidirectional instability of the shoulder. Patients had a mean increase of active abduction from 6° to 34°, a mean increase in forward flexion of 18°, and no improvement of external rotation. Complications included 2 intraoperative fractures of the head of the humerus, 2 cases of pressure-induced skin necrosis from the abduction splint, 4 infections, 2 cases of paralysis of the musculocutaneous nerve, and 2 cases of persistent shoulder instability that required arthrodesis. With respect to muscle power, 90% of patients had an MRC grade 0 to 2 deltoid power, and the surgery resulted in stabilization of their shoulder subluxation. The remaining trapezius muscle strength after surgery ranged from grade 4 to 5 in 96% of patients. The authors noted that if patients had reasonable function of the biceps, coracobrachialis, and triceps, the multidirectional instability of the shoulder was improved. However, in flail shoulders, in which these muscles and the pectoralis major had an MCR of 0 to 2, the gain in motion was much less. The authors then compared the 58 patients who had undergone a standard Saha technique with the 22 patients who had undergone a modified Saha technique. The modified Saha technique provided greater improvement in abduction and forward flexion compared with the standard Saha technique. The modified technique resulted in an overall increase of 5° of abduction and 2° of forward flexion. No statistical results were reported. In fact, no statistical reports were reported for the entire article. The authors conclude that trapezius transfer for the flail shoulder produces a satisfactory outcome.

Of note, it is important to understand the previous neurosurgical procedures performed on these patients before trapezius transfer. A standard nerve transfer for restoration of shoulder function in patients with brachial plexus injuries includes the use of the terminal branch of the spinal accessory nerve, preserving the proximal first rami of the trapezius. Typically, the distal portion of the spinal accessory nerve is used to neurotize the suprascapular nerve or other target. It would be interesting to know how many of the authors' 80 patients had the distal portion of the spinal accessory nerve transferred and whether this affected the outcome. Secondarily, it is difficult to ascertain whether the gain in motion was statistically significant, especially since the authors subdivided the 80 patients and compared 19 of the 58 patients who had undergone the standard Saha with 15 of the 22 patients who had undergone the modified procedure. The statistical analysis lacks a power analysis as well, and therefore, any changes that the authors describe are difficult to compare.

Overall, trapezius transfer is effective in reducing shoulder instability. However, the gain in motion that is described in this report was not statistically proven.

A. Y. Shin, MD

Reconstruction of the Spinal Accessory Nerve With Autograft or Neurotube? Two Case Reports

Ducic I, Maloney CT Jr, Dellon AL (Georgetown Univ, Washington, DC; Univ of Arizona, Tucson; Johns Hopkins Univ, Baltimore, Md)
J Reconstr Microsurg 21:29-33, 2005   6–6

Background.—The timing for intervention and the results of reconstruction of an injured accessory spinal nerve have not been widely addressed. Two patients had iatrogenic injury to cranial nerve XI and underwent reconstruction 3 months after shoulder function was lost. The techniques and outcomes were reported.

Case 1.—Woman, 40, was unable to lift her arm normally immediately after surgery that was performed to biopsy a lymph node of the right posterior cervical triangle. Electrodiagnostic evaluation demonstrated acute denervation of the upper and lower trapezius with injury to the spinal accessory nerve. The patient required an interposition autograft from the greater auricular nerve to reconstruct a length of fibrotic cranial nerve XI. Four months after reconstruction, some reinnervation of the upper trapezius was detected; after 6 months her ability to shrug the shoulder was nearly normal. Her arm abduction remained abnormal as a result of glenohumeral adhesions. The upper trapezius had good function, but the lower trapezius showed only partial recovery after 9 months.

Case 2.—Woman, 63, underwent posterior cervical lymph node biopsy and could not lift her shoulder normally immediately afterward. Electrodiagnostic evaluation revealed injury to the spinal accessory nerve. Function had not returned 14 weeks after the lymph node biopsy, and she had developed shoulder pain and limited function (only 40° of shoulder abduction). Reconstruction of cranial nerve XI was accomplished by using a 2.5-cm Neurotube. Full shoulder abduction returned 4 months after surgery.

Conclusions.—The 2 techniques shared several aspects, including early recognition of the nerve injury, surgical exploration when neural regeneration techniques were unsuccessful, and the use of microneurosurgery for reconstruction. These shared aspects indicate that appropriate postoperative treatment of cranial nerve XI injury begins with the use of supportive measures within 3 months, obtaining electrodiagnostic studies 3 to 6 weeks after injury, and educating the patient concerning the possibility that nerve function may recover spontaneously but reconstruction may be needed. A second electrodiagnostic evaluation is needed 12 weeks after injury, when the decision to operate can be made. Microsurgical neurolysis is sufficient if intraoperative electrical stimulation evokes trapezius function. No further surgery is needed if there is strong function of the mid and lower trapezius. With poor distal trapezius function or function limited to upper trapezius contraction, resection of the in-continuity neuroma and reconstruction of the spinal accessory nerve are appropriate. Either a bioabsorbable neural conduit or an autograft can be used.

▶ This is a retrospective review of 2 patients with spinal accessory nerve injuries, one treated with a nerve graft and the second treated with a bioabsorbable nerve conduit called a Neurotube. Based on this, the result of surgery, both patients regained strength of their spinal accessory nerve. The patient who had a Neurotube reconstruction gained M5 strength by 3 months and had no donor site morbidity, whereas the patient who received an autograft reached M4 strength by 6 months and had persistent numbness of the ear lobe—both likely attributable to the harvesting of cervical plexus nerves. The surgeons basically state that this is a first case of a cranial motor nerve being reconstructed with a bioabsorbable conduit. It is an interesting article but has very little science behind it, and essentially it is a case report of 2 different techniques.

A. Y. Shin, MD

Brachial Plexus Palsy Secondary to Birth Injuries: Long-term Results of Anterior Release and Tendon Transfers Around the Shoulder

Kirkos JM, Kyrkos MJ, Kapetanos GA, et al (Kilkis Gen Hosp, Greece)
J Bone Joint Surg Br 87-B:231-235, 2005   6–7

Background.—Obstetric brachial plexus palsy is a complication in 0.4 to 2.5 per 1000 live births, and 75% to 95% of patients recover completely in the first year of life. Unfortunately the remaining patients have some permanent damage, most often in the shoulder. All children with obstetric brachial plexus palsy have damage to the fifth and sixth cervical nerves, and in almost half of patients the lesion is confined to these two nerves. The most common deformity of the arm is internal rotation and adduction because of the loss of muscle balance around the glenohumeral joint. The long-term results of anterior shoulder release combined with tendon transfer of the teres major and latissimus dorsi in a series of patients with obstetric brachial plexus palsy were described.

Methods.—From 1959 to 1975, 10 patients with limited active external rotation of the arm resulting from obstetric brachial plexus palsy underwent anterior shoulder release with tendon transfer of latissimus dorsi and teres major. The mean age of the patients at the time of surgery was 6 years (range 5-9 years). The tendons were transferred posteriorly and laterally to allow them to serve as external rotators. Before surgery, the patients were unable to actively rotate the arm externally beyond neutral, although this movement was passively normal. All of the patients showed decreased strength of the external rotator but had normal strength of the internal rotator muscles. Radiologic examination showed no severe bony changes in the glenohumeral joint.

Results.—There was no clinically detectable improvement of active abduction in any patient after surgery. The mean active external rotation after operation was 36.5°, which was maintained for a mean of 10 years, and then deteriorated in 8 patients. At latest follow up the mean active external rotation was 10.5°.

Conclusions.—The early satisfactory results of anterior release and tendon transfer in patients with obstetric brachial plexus palsy were not maintained in the long term. There was loss of active external rotation over time, possibly because of gradual degeneration of the transferred muscles, contracture of the surrounding soft tissues, and degenerative changes in the glenohumeral joint.

▶ Ten patients with a 30-year follow-up of tendon transfers done at an average age of 4 years showed that 80% deteriorated with time. The procedures also included a subscapularis release at the insertion and contracture releases, although the authors stress the need for passive range of motion to be present prior to tendon transfer.

M. Ezaki, MD

Long-term Results on Abduction and External Rotation of the Shoulder After Latissimus Dorsi Transfer for Sequelae of Obstetric Palsy

Pagnotta A, Haerle M, Gilbert A (Institut de la Main, Paris)
Clin Orthop 426:199-205, 2004
6–8

Transfer of the latissimus dorsi to the rotator cuff is widely used for restoring shoulder abduction and external rotation in sequelae of brachial plexus palsy; however, its long-term results are not well known. Because persistence of clinical benefits is crucial for children with brachial plexus palsy, the aim of our study was to evaluate retrospectively the long-term results of this transfer in 203 children. Patients were classified according to type of paralysis (C5-C6, C5-C6-C7, and complete), degree of preoperative shoulder function according to Gilbert, and age at surgery. Active abduction and external rotation were measured at 1, 3, 6, 10, and 15 years and the results were analyzed statistically. Children with sequelae of C5-C6 palsy gained in abduction and external rotation more than children with C5-C6-C7 or complete palsy. Patients with mild preoperative shoulder dysfunction achieved the best results. The data showed the clinical results were related to the type of paralysis and to preoperative shoulder function, but not to age at surgery. They also showed progressive deterioration of abduction began at 6 years despite preserved active external rotation.

▶ The authors report on 203 latissimus transfers in a large group of patients with brachial plexus palsies. They give details of functional recovery using Gilbert's scale and sort the patients by level of injury, age, and preoperative scores. The long-term results for function appear to deteriorate with time, even in the group that did well initially. The results also correlate with the original level of injury and not with other factors that were investigated.

M. Ezaki, MD

Restoration of Prehension Using Double Free Muscle Technique After Complete Avulsion of Brachial Plexus in Children: A Report of Three Cases

Hattori Y, Doi K, Ikeda K, et al (Yamaguchi Univ, Japan; Ogori Daiichi Gen Hosp, Yamaguchi, Japan)
J Hand Surg [Am] 30A:812-819, 2005
6–9

Purpose.—Brachial plexus injury in children, excluding birth palsy, is relatively rare and seldom reported. We report our technique, the results of this procedure, and problems we encountered in treating children with brachial plexus injury.

Methods.—From 1999 through 2002, we treated 3 children with complete avulsion of the brachial plexus due to trauma by using double free muscle technique (DFMT) with a nerve transfer procedure using the contralateral seventh cervical nerve root transfer to reconstruct prehensile function.

There were 2 boys aged 5 and 11 years and a girl aged 4 years. All patients were followed up for at least 3 years after the surgery.

Results.—All the transferred muscles survived without any vascular complications and were reinnervated successfully. The average active range of elbow flexion was 125° (range, 90°–145°). The average total active range of motion of the fingers was 69° (range, 40°–102°). All patients obtained voluntary prehensile function and could use the reconstructed hand for activities of daily living. They were able to lift and carry light objects with the reconstructed hand and heavy objects with both hands.

Conclusions.—The results of DFMT for reconstruction of BPI in children were encouraging. Appropriate postoperative rehabilitation under close supervision is important to obtain useful prehensile function.

▶ This small case series from Japan highlights the possibilities of free functional muscle transfer in children with traumatic BPIs. The literature on pediatric traumatic BPIs, as opposed to obstetric ones, is scarce. However, it is believed that children should have a greater potential for recovery. The authors present a systematic approach to these patients with panplexal injuries, combining the liberal use of contralateral C-7 transfers with vascularized ulnar nerve transfers. Free functional muscle transfers are done in 2 separate stages: the first stage is done for elbow flexion, and the second stage is for finger flexion. Sensory reinnervation is also a very important component of this reconstructive process. The authors stress the importance of biofeedback and a specialized rehabilitation program. The overall results were very encouraging: protective sensation returned in all patients between 1.5 and 2 years after the nerve transfers.

S. L. Moran, MD

Traumatic Major Muscle Loss in the Upper Extremity: Reconstruction Using Functioning Free Muscle Transplantation
Lin S-H, Chuang DC-C, Hattori Y, et al (Chang Gung Univ, Taipei, Taiwan)
J Reconstr Microsurg 20:227-235, 2004   6–10

Background.—Cases of destroyed or chronically denervated functional muscles or muscle groups may be addressed by using functioning free muscle transplantation (FFMT). Twenty FFMTs were performed in 14 patients between 1986 and 1996, and the indications, reconstructive strategies, and long-term results were reported.

Methods.—All the major muscle loss was primarily caused by muscle avulsion, avascularity, and necrosis. None involved nerve or ischemic injury. All patients were men aged 16 to 37 years (mean, 24.5 years). In 8 cases, the dominant hand was affected. Six patients had injuries involving the elbow flexors; 8, the forearm extensors; and 6, the forearm flexors. Five patients had multiple muscle compartments in the arm and forearm that were affected. Before FFMT, 8 patients required 9 free tissue transfers to cover extensive soft tissue defects. The length and morphology of the muscle were considered in choosing which should be transferred. Transferred muscles included 11 gracilis, 5 latissimus dorsi, 3 rectus femoris, and 1 soleus (lateral half). For innervation of biceps replacement, the musculocutaneous nerve was used; for the flexor digitorum profundus, the anterior interosseous nerve was used; and for the extensor digitorum communis, the posterior interosseous nerve was used.

Results.—Muscle transfers were all successful with no loss of skin flaps. Postoperatively, patients had no complications. Electrical stimulation and passive motion under the direction of physical therapists began 3 weeks postoperatively. Three weeks later, patients discarded their splints and began more vigorous therapy. With the use of the Medical Research Council scale, results were classified as M4 (excellent), M3 (good), or M2 (poor). Excellent results were achieved in 90.0% of the cases; poor results were noted in 2 patients. Neither of these patients achieved functional strength, but voluntary muscle twitching was present at final follow-up evaluation. Only these 2 failed cases required tenolysis, which was not successful.

Conclusions.—All but 2 patients had excellent results with FFMT. The muscle of first choice for these procedures is the gracilis because of its size, good excursion, long and single innervated motor nerve, single dominant vascular pedicle, reliable overlying skin flap, easy access, and hidden medial thigh scar. The rectus femoris has greater force-generating capacity, easy access, and preservation of a reliable, sizeable overlying skin flap and is the second choice. Access difficulty and large fan shape make the latissimus dorsi the third choice, although it is the second for biceps or forearm flexor digitorum profundus replacement. The rectus abdominis is an alternative not used in this series.

▶ This is a retrospective evaluation of patients who underwent FFMTs in the upper extremity for severe traumatic loss. The authors searched their database at Chang Gung Memorial Hospital in Taipei, Taiwan, a large trauma referral center. Between 1986 and 1999, they identified more than 200 patients who had FFMTs performed for severe injuries of the upper extremity. From this group, between 1986 and 1996, 14 patients were identified as having severe injury of the upper extremity with major muscle loss who underwent 20 FFMTs for reconstruction. Excluded from this analysis were patients with nerve injuries, such as brachial plexus, high-level median, ulnar, or radial nerve injuries, and patients with muscle loss secondary to vascular injuries or amputation. The average age of the 14 patients studied was 24.5 years, and the average follow-up was 8.3 years. All patients sustained major muscle losses. Patients underwent FFMTs that included 11 gracilis, 5 latissimus dorsi, 3 rectus femoris, and 1 lateral portion of the soleus. They were used as elbow flexors in 6 patients, forearm flexors in 6 patients, and forearm extensors in 8 patients. The donor nerve to neurotize the flap included the musculocutaneous nerve for elbow flexors, the anterior interosseous nerve for the wrist and finger flexors, and the posterior interosseous nerve for the wrist and finger extensors. Eighteen of the 20 free-functioning muscles obtained an M4 strength, an excellent outcome. Two had a poor outcome and it was deemed that they were done too early, 1 week after injury, as a primary reconstruction for wound coverage and simultaneous reconstruction of finger flexion.

The authors present a nice discussion on the use of muscle selection for the variety of functions they try to restore, and demonstrate excellent decision-making options for elbow flexors, forearm flexors, and forearm extensors. This is an important article for any hand surgeon dealing with cases of traumatic major loss in the upper extremity in terms of regaining function.

A. Y. Shin, MD

A Modified Coracoid Approach to Infraclavicular Brachial Plexus Blocks Using a Double-Stimulation Technique in 300 Patients
Minville V, N'Guyen L, Chassery C, et al (Toulouse Univ, France; Bicêtre Univ, Le Kremlin-Bicêtre, France)
Anesth Analg 100:263-265, 2005   6–11

Infraclavicular brachial plexus block is used less than other techniques of regional anesthesia for upper-limb surgery. We describe a modified coracoid approach to the infraclavicular brachial plexus using a double-stimulation technique and assess its efficacy. Patients undergoing orthopedic surgery of the upper limb were included in this prospective study. The landmarks used were the coracoid process and the clavicle. The needle was inserted in the direction of the top of the axillary fossa (in relation to the axillary artery), with an angle of 45 degrees. Using nerve stimulation, the musculocutaneous nerve was identified first and blocked with 10 mL of 1.5% lidocaine with 1:400,000 epinephrine. The needle was then withdrawn and redirected posteriorly and medially. The radial, ulnar, or median nerve was then blocked. The block was tested every 5 min for 30 min. The overall success rate, i.e., adequate sensory block in the 4 major nerve distributions at 30 min, was 92%, and 6% of the patients required supplementation. Five patients required general anesthesia. No major complications were observed. This modified infraclavicular brachial plexus block using a double-stimulation technique was easy to perform, had frequent success, and was safe in this cohort.

▶ The authors describe their approach to infraclavicular blockade of the brachial plexus. They use a neurostimulator to assess proper positioning of the needle to first locate and block the musculocutaneous nerve. The needle is repositioned so that stimulation results in activity either of the median, ulnar, or radial nerve. A quantity of local anesthetic (30 ml of 1.5% xylocaine and epinephrine) is placed here. The authors achieved a successful block in 92% of patients after 30 minutes.

Infraclavicular blockade has become the norm in my hospital. Few now perform axillary blocks. The key to success is still the same, however. Put a large enough volume of the anesthetic in the right spot and wait long enough before operating on the patient. More blocks are "unsuccessful" because of failure to wait sufficient time between injection and incision than fail because of improper location.

V. R. Hentz, MD

Neurologic Sequelae After Interscalene Brachial Plexus Block for Shoulder/Upper Arm Surgery: The Association of Patient, Anesthetic, and Surgical Factors to the Incidence and Clinical Course
Candido KD, Sukhani R, Doty R Jr, et al (Northwestern Univ, Chicago)
Anesth Analg 100:1489-1495, 2005   6–12

We determined the incidence, distribution, and resolution of neurologic sequelae and the association with anesthetic, surgical, and patient factors after single-injection interscalene block (ISB) using levobupivacaine 0.625% with epinephrine 1:200,000 in subjects undergoing shoulder or upper arm surgery, or both, in 693 consecutive adult patients. After a standardized ISB, assessments were made at 24 and 48 h and at 2 and 4 wk for anesthesia, hypesthesia, paresthesias, pain/dysesthesias, and motor weakness. Symptomatic patients were monitored until resolution. Subjects reporting pain or discomfort >3 of 10 and those with motor or extending sensory symptoms received diagnostic assessment. Six-hundred-sixty subjects completed 4 wk of follow-up. Fifty-eight neurologic sequelae were reported by 56 subjects. Symptoms were sensory except for two cases of motor weakness (lesions identified distant from the ISB site). Thirty-one sequelae with likely ISB association were reported by 29 subjects, including 14 at the ISB site, 9 at the distal phalanx of thumb/index finger, 7 involving the posterior auricular nerve, and 1 clinical brachial plexopathy. Sequelae not likely associated with the ISB were reported by 27 subjects with symptoms reported in the median ($n = 9$) and ulnar ($n = 4$) nerves, surgical neuropraxias ($n = 12$), and motor weakness ($n = 2$). Symptoms resolved spontaneously (median 4 wk; range, 2–16 wk) except in the two patients with motor weaknesses and the patient with clinical brachial plexopathy, who received therapeutic interventions. Variables identified as independent predictors of neurologic sequelae likely related to ISB were paresthesia at needle insertion and ISB site pain or bruising at 24 h. In contrast, surgery performed in the sitting position, as well as ISB site bruising, was identified as a predictor of neurologic sequelae not likely related to ISB. In conclusion, neurologic sequelae after single-injection ISB using epinephrine mainly involve transient minor sensory symptoms.

▶ This study shows how safe ISB anesthesia is in the majority of cases. Because paresthesias at needle insertion, greater than 3 attempts, and bruising appear to be correlated with neurologic sequelae, the use of newer imaging techniques to guide execution of the block seems warranted as a means to increase success, minimize multiple attempts, decrease local trauma, and avoid intentional provocation of paresthesias.

M. Tomaino, MD

7   Elbow: Trauma

Interference Kirschner Wires Augment Distal Humeral Fracture Fixation in the Elderly

Molloy S, Jasper LE, Burkhart BG, et al (Johns Hopkins Univ, Baltimore, Md; Union Mem Hosp, Baltimore, Md)

J Orthop Trauma 19:377-379, 2005   7–1

Objectives.—This study was designed to compare the biomechanical stability of a two-plate distal humerus fixation with and without Kirschner-wire (K-wire) augmentation of supracondylar osteotomies.

Design.—Ex vivo paired cadaveric study.

Setting.—Biomechanical laboratory.

Materials.—Five pairs of fresh, elderly cadaveric humeri.

Intervention.—Two 3.5-mm reconstruction plates were used to stabilize each humerus. This fixation model was selected solely to evaluate the effect of K-wire augmentation. Augmentation consisted of 2 K-wires placed in both the medial and lateral columns of the humerus to interdigitate with the plate screws. A posteriorly directed load was cyclically applied to the distal fragment for 5000 cycles or until failure, and osteotomy site motion was tracked optically.

Main Outcome Measurements.—Fixation survival was defined as 5000 cycles or the number of cycles until osteotomy site motion reached >2 mm.

Results.—K-wire augmented fixations survived significantly more cycles than did controls (4410 ± 875 vs. 1114 ± 2182, respectively; paired t test, $P < 0.05$).

Conclusions.—Augmentation with K-wires may decrease the incidence of loss of fixation in distal humeral fractures.

▶ This small biomechanical study seeks to evaluate the augmentation of adjunctive percutaneous stabilization to 2 distal humeral plates. Biomechanical integrity is optimized with the use of 3 plates, but the associated periosteal stripping and devitalization of tissue in the osteoporotic setting, the authors note, is potentially hazardous. They comment on similar lines of reasoning adopted in treatment of the osteoporotic distal radius.

Intrafocal pinning, known as Kapandji pinning, is one of the more common techniques for improving biomechanical stability, and I, at first, thought this was what the authors used for their study. Instead, "interference" refers to small intramedullary pins/wires, rather than the use of them as biomechanical wedges in the fracture, at least in this model. It is not surprising that the additional wires add stability. Their clinical utility, as the authors point out, has yet to be shown.

A. L. Ladd, MD

Treatment of Distal Humerus Fractures in the Elderly
Hausman M, Panozzo A (Mount Sinai Med Ctr, New York)
Clin Orthop 425:55-63, 2004   7–2

Geriatric patients with osteopenic bone present unique challenges in the treatment of fractures of the distal humerus, and require different strategies from the traditional treatment philosophies. Fracture union, rather than motion, is the first priority, because motion can be restored reliably by subsequent contracture release, if necessary, as long as the fracture heals. Modifications in the surgical technique, combined with newer implants incorporating distal, transcondylar screws into the plate to improve distal fixation, may improve outcomes. The use of massive, tricortical autogenous bone grafts to replace very comminuted segments of the medial and lateral columns also is helpful. Finally, modification of olecranon osteotomy fixation will minimize healing and hardware problems at this site. For fractures that are judged intraoperatively not to be stable enough to commence early motion, the implementation of a short period of immobilization followed by early soft tissue release will avoid exposing the patient to the risk of nonunion, and result in a more predictable functional outcome.

▶ These authors have confirmed that open reduction and internal fixation of distal humerus fractures in the elderly is, in many cases, preferred to a primary total elbow replacement. Because of the significant medical advances seen in civilized countries, patients are living longer and are remaining very active, making it increasingly difficult to define "elderly." Furthermore, although the patients may be "low demand," dependence upon walking aids may not make them ideal candidates for a total elbow arthroplasty. Nonetheless, with the current locking plate/screw constructs available and parallel plating, good fixation can be often be achieved adequately for early mobilization, even in osteoporotic bone. In cases in which fixation is tenuous, postoperative immobilization, followed by secondary lysis of adhesions and joint contracture release will often produce acceptable motion. As the authors point out, the key is achieving healing of the distal fragments to the shaft. In very distal noncomminuted fractures, minimal fixation with columnar screws is also a reasonable option. Under no circumstance should cement be utilized to fill voids, but rather bone graft is preferred. Should the patient have a pre-existing inflammatory arthritis or severe osteoporosis with a high level of comminution, primary total elbow arthroplasty can achieve good results as well. It is not necessary to retain the condyles, however; an extended flange will provide improved rotational stability. It is often possible to place the prosthesis on either side of the triceps without detaching this structure from the olecranon or splitting it. Nonoperative treatment will typically result in poor motion, although pain may be minimal.

K. J. Renfree, MD

Distal Humeral Fractures Treated With Noncustom Total Elbow Replacement
Kamineni S, Morrey BF (Mayo Clinic, Rochester, Minn)
J Bone Joint Surg Am 86-A:940-947, 2004   7–3

Background.—The purpose of this study was to review the cases of patients with a distal humeral fracture that was treated with a noncustom total elbow arthroplasty. We hypothesized that, on the basis of the functional and clinical outcome, total elbow replacement is a reliable option for the treatment of elderly patients with a severe, comminuted fracture of the distal part of the humerus.

Methods.—We retrospectively reviewed forty-nine acute distal humeral fractures in forty-eight patients who were treated with total elbow arthroplasty as the primary option. The average age of the patients was sixty-seven years. Forty-three fractures were followed for at least two years. According to the AO classification, five fractures were type A, five were type B, and thirty-three were type C. The average age of the forty-three patients was sixty-nine years and the average duration of follow-up was seven years. Fourteen patients died during the review period. Postoperative clinical function was assessed with use of the Mayo elbow performance score, and anteroposterior and lateral radiographs made at follow-up examinations were reviewed.

Results.—At the latest follow-up examination, the average flexion arc was 24° (range, 0° to 75°) to 131° (range, 100° to 150°) and the Mayo elbow performance score averaged 93 of a possible 100 points. Heterotopic ossification was present to some extent in seven elbows, with radiographic abutment noted in two. Thirty-two (65%) of the forty-nine elbows had neither a complication nor any further surgery from the time of the index arthroplasty to the most recent follow-up evaluation. Fourteen elbows (29%) had a single complication, and most of them did not require further surgery. Ten additional procedures, including five revision arthroplasties, were required in nine elbows; five were related to soft tissue and five were related to the implant or bone.

Conclusions.—Complex distal humeral fractures should be assessed primarily for the reliability with which they can be reconstructed with osteosynthesis. When osteosynthesis is not considered to be feasible, especially in patients who are physiologically older and place lower demands on the joint, total elbow arthroplasty can be considered. This retrospective review supports a recommendation for total elbow arthroplasty for the treatment of an acute distal humeral fracture when strict inclusion criteria are observed.

▶ Distal humeral fractures in the elderly are often more distal and are associated with significant articular comminution. These fracture characteristics are associated with more osteopenic bone and can make fixation quite difficult, leading to extended immobilization and elbow stiffness. The use of a total elbow replacement results in immediate stability and initiation of motion when soft tissue healing allows. This retrospective study substantiates the use of a total elbow replacement for severe distal humeral fractures in elderly patients.

R. Goitz, MD

Revision Surgery for Nonunion After Early Failure of Fixation of Fractures of the Distal Humerus

Ali A, Douglas H, Stanley D (Northern Gen Hosp, Sheffield, England)
J Bone Joint Surg Br 87-B:1107-1110, 2005   7–4

Sixteen patients who underwent a revision operation for nonunion of fractures of the distal humerus following previous internal fixation were reviewed at a mean follow-up of 39 months (8 to 69).

The Mayo elbow performance score was excellent in 11, good in two, fair in two and poor in one. In 15 patients union was achieved and in one with an infected nonunion a subsequent bone graft was necessary in order to obtain union.

Age, gender, a history of smoking, mechanism of the injury and the AO classification of the initial fracture did not correlate with the development of nonunion. In 12 patients (75%), the initial fixation was assessed as being suboptimal. The primary surgery was regarded as adequate in only three patients. Our findings suggest that the most important determinant of nonunion of a distal humeral fracture after surgery is the adequacy of fixation.

▶ This study demonstrated that revision surgery for failed internal fixation of fractures of the distal humerus can produce excellent or good results in the majority of patients with respect to the union, stability, pain, and ultimate range of motion. Although the authors did not identify age, history of smoking, or the AO classification of the initial fracture (degree of comminution, etc.), the number of patients in the study group was probably too small (16) to realize these. Seventy-five percent of the patients who developed the nonunion were believed to have had inadequate treatment primarily. This underscores the importance of rigid internal fixation, typically using dual plating and bone grafting, when necessary, to achieve a good result in patients with this injury.

K. J. Renfree, MD

Supracondylar Fractures of the Humerus in Children

de las Heras J, Durán D, de la Cerda J, et al (Hosp Universitario La Paz, Madrid; Hosp Universitario Príncipe de Asturias, Madrid)
Clin Orthop 432:57-64, 2005   7–5

Supracondylar fractures of the humerus need a precise treatment in order to obtain a satisfactory result because of the low bone remodeling associated with these injuries. It is important to use a systematic procedure for closed reduction and percutaneous fixation. A retrospective review of fractures treated using two K-wires from the lateral side was done in 77 patients with a mean age of 6.7 years (range, 1-13 years). Displacement of the fracture was classified as Gartland Type II in 39 patients (50.6%) and Gartland Type III in 38 patients (49.4%). The results according to Flynn criteria were excellent in 70 patients (90.9%), fair in three patients (3.9%) and poor in four patients (5.2%), with overall satisfactory results in 96.1% of the cases. In four patients there was secondary displacement of the fragments in internal rotation and three of these patients were operated on again, increasing fixation with a third K-wire either from the lateral or medial side. There were two nerve lesions (2.6%), and four patients (5.2%) had a pulseless pink hand that recovered when the fracture was reduced. In three patients (3.9%) infection developed. To obtain satisfactory results using this procedure, enough stability should be achieved, avoiding iatrogenic damage of the ulnar nerve.

▶ The authors present a retrospective review of 77 surgically treated supracondylar fractures, all classified as Gartland II or III. The authors present a nice review of technical tips that may be helpful to some readers. The major limitation of the article is using only Flynn's criteria, which assess only cosmesis and range of motion to judge results, but the authors admit that not much else is available. The authors also stress the importance of carefully analyzing the so-called Type I fractures, because these frequently are the ones that malunite.

J. A. Katarincic, MD

Late Presentation of Supracondylar Fracture of the Humerus in Children

Devnani AS (Univ Sains Malaysia, Kubang Kerian, Kelantan)
Clin Orthop 431:36-41, 2005   7–6

In children with delayed presentation of displaced supracondylar fractures, closed or open reduction with K-wire fixation risks complications. Gradually reducing the fracture with traction potentially reduces these risks. An unacceptable deformity can be corrected later by an osteotomy. This concept was used for 28 children, with an average age of 7 years 6 months, who presented after an average delay of 5.6 days. Their stay in the hospital was 14 days on average. At followup (average, 24 months), five children (18%) who had cubitus varus greater than 10° had corrective osteotomy. There were no additional neurovascular injuries after treatment. The results are comparable with other methods of treatment.

▶ The author has carefully reviewed 28 children with displaced supracondylar humerus fractures that were reduced with gradual traction to reduce the risk of hardware-related complications. The children presented with an average delay of 5.6 days and had an average hospital stay of 14 days. Results were comparable to historic norms for this difficult fracture. Five (18%) of the children required a corrective osteotomy due to a cubitus varus of greater than 10°. The technique warrants consideration but may be difficult to apply in the United States due to the prolonged hospital stay. The orthopedists who care for these fractures should consider this technique when a difficult pediatric supracondylar fracture presents at any time, though it may be more appropriate if the facture presents a number of days after the event that caused the fracture.

C. Carroll IV, MD

Open Reduction, Ulnar Osteotomy and External Fixation for Chronic Anterior Dislocation of the Head of the Radius
Hasler CC, Von Laer L, Hell AK (Univ Children's Hosp, Basel, Switzerland)
J Bone Joint Surg Br 87-B:88-94, 2005   7–7

We reviewed 15 patients, nine girls and six boys, with chronic anterior dislocation of the radial head which was treated by ulnar osteotomy, external fixation and open reconstruction of the elbow joint but without repair of the annular ligament. Their mean age was 9.5 years (5 to 15) and the mean interval between the injury and reconstruction was 22 months (2 months to 7 years).

All radial heads remained reduced at a mean follow-up of 20 months (6 months to 5 years). Normal ranges of movement for flexion, extension, pronation and supination were unchanged in 96.1% (49/51) and worse in 3.9% (2/51). Limited ranges of movement were improved in 77.8% (7/9), unchanged in 11% (1/9) and further decreased in 11% (1/9). There were two superficial pin-track infections and two cases of delayed union but with no serious complications. Reconstruction of the radiocapitellar joint is easier using external fixation since accurate correction of the ulna can be determined empirically and active functional exercises started immediately. Only patients with a radial head of normal shape were selected for treatment by this method.

▶ This retrospective review shows outstanding functional outcomes after ulnar osteotomy with either closed or open radial head reduction, performed as late as 7 years after the injury. The authors emphasize that normal radial head and capitellar morphological features are critical success factors, that traumatic dislocation needs to be differentiated from congenital cases—which are less amenable to reconstruction—and that annular ligament reconstruction is not necessary if reorientation of the ulna is performed in all planes.

M. Tomaino, MD

Neglected Dislocation of the Elbow

Mahaisavariya B, Laupattarakasem W (Madihol Univ, Bangkok, Thailand; Khon Kaen Univ, Thailand)
Clin Orthop 431:21-25, 2005   7–8

We retrospectively review the intermediate-term to long-term results of 24 patients treated after late open reduction of neglected posterior elbow dislocation in terms of the elbow, particularly noting joint mobility. The mean interval from injury to operation was 7.9 months (range, 1–60 months). The posterior approach with V-Y muscleplasty was used in most patients with 2 to 3 weeks postoperative immobilization. The average preoperative arc of elbow flexion was from 17° with an average maximum flexion of 27° (range, 5–60°) and an average flexion contracture of 10° (range, 0–30°). The mean followup was 48.3 months (range, 12–132 months). At the time of final followup, the average arc of elbow flexion was 82° with an average of maximum flexion of 122° (range, 90–150°) and an average flexion contracture of 40° (range, 0–75°). There was no correlation between the postoperative arc of elbow motion and preoperative parameters including patient age, preoperative arc of elbow motion, or duration of untreated dislocation.

▶ This study comprises a very heterogenic group of patients with a wide range of age and a high standard deviation. With the exception of 2 patients who had a neglected elbow dislocation for 60 weeks, all patients were treated with open reduction and a V-Y-plasty of the triceps within 6 weeks. The authors did not perform any reconstructive surgery, as for example, palmaris longus or triceps transplants for ligament reconstruction. They simply sutured the remnants of the collateral ligaments. The results in terms of extension and flexion are acceptable but show some bad results, with a total range of motion of only 30° or 45°. Taking into account that the patients come from rural areas in a developing country, it is interesting to see how a surgeon can achieve decent results with a simple surgical technique. One has to consider that the demand of the patients may be lower than in a highly developed country, in which the patients not only need their elbow for work, but also for the leisure time activities such as sports, leaving the study not quite transferable to Western countries. Still, it is a study that deserves attention due to the difficult problem of neglected elbow dislocation, which in this described extent would not happen in Europe or the United States, but rather would lead to a malpractice suit.

S. Lichtenberg, MD

Effective Treatment of Fracture-Dislocations of the Olecranon Requires a Stable Trochlear Notch

Doornberg J, Ring D, Jupiter JB (Massachusetts Gen Hosp, Boston)
Clin Orthop 429:292-300, 2004   7–9

Abstract.—Our goal with this study was to better define and characterize fracture-dislocations of the olecranon and to provide additional data regarding complications and elbow function after operative treatment. Twenty-six patients with fracture-dislocations of the elbow were reviewed retrospectively. Ten had anterior and 16 had posterior fracture-dislocations. Five of 10 patients with anterior injuries and all of the patients with posterior injuries had an associated fracture of the coronoid process of the ulna. One of 10 patients with anterior and 13 of 16 patients with posterior injuries had fracture of the radial head. Only one patient had a true dislocation of the ulnohumeral joint. In the other 25 patients the articular surfaces remained apposed. All 26 patients were treated operatively and followed up for at least 3 years (average, 6 years). The results were good or excellent in 21 of 26 patients according to the system of Broberg and Morrey. The five unsatisfactory results were related to inadequate fixation of the coronoid with subsequent arthrosis (three patients), proximal radioulnar synostosis (three patients), and a subsequent fracture of the distal humerus (one patient). Fracture-dislocations of the olecranon occur in anterior and posterior patterns with specific injury characteristics and pitfalls. The key to effective treatment is stable restoration of the trochlear notch.

▶ This is a retrospective review of the treatment of fracture-dislocations of the olecranon by a center that has great experience with treating these difficult fractures. The authors' vast experience in this area provides certain recommendations that clinicians can use to treat these difficult injuries.

The authors emphasize the importance of differentiating between anterior versus posterior dislocation. The posterior dislocations can be "bad actors." In addition, they stress the importance of the coronoid fixation. Although they describe several different methods of coronoid fixation, I prefer the custom coronoid plates that are available because these provide a spring loaded-type buttress to provide the important medial support for large type III coronoid fractures.

The authors did not specifically identify and evaluate the lateral ligament complex in most of their patients. I would stress that this should be an important part of the treatment plan for all elbow fracture dislocations, because this can be quite troublesome if addressed late.

T. R. McAdams, MD

Impaired Forearm Rotation After Tension-Band-Wiring Fixation of Olecranon Fractures: Evaluation of the Transcortical K-wire Technique

Candal-Couto JJ, Williams JR, Sanderson PL (Freeman Hosp, Newcastle-upon Tyne, England)
J Orthop Trauma 19:480-482, 2005   7–10

Summary.—The tension-band-wiring technique is a well-accepted method of internal fixation of olecranon fractures. In addition, it is suggested that transcortical placement of the k-wires results in lower rates of wire migration. We encountered two clinical cases in which transcortical placement of the k-wires led to impairment of forearm rotation. An anatomic study was conducted to study the effect of transcortical wire placement to avoid similar future complications. Using specimens from 10 embalmed cadavers, we found that transcortical wires inserted in <30° of ulnar angulation in the coronal plane to the medial ridge of the olecranon, impinged on the radial neck, supinator muscle, or biceps tendon. This was avoided in all 10 specimens when the wires were inserted, with the forearm in supination, at 30° of ulnar angulation. We recommend this technique to be adopted to avoid forearm rotation impairment.

▶ In an attempt to decrease wire migration and hardware complications after tension band wiring of olecranon fractures, some have advocated transcortical K-wire technique. The authors designed a cadaver model to assess the effect of the transcortical K-wire technique on forearm rotation. They concluded that limitations of forearm rotation were more likely to occur if the forearm was pronated during K-wire insertion. When the K-wire is inserted at a 30° angle to the posteromedial ridge of olecranon (flexor carpi ulnaris origin) with the forearm in supination, no restriction to motion was noted. If the wire was inserted at 0° to the posteromedial ridge of olecranon, with the forearm in pronation, the wire consistently encountered the radius or anterior soft tissue structures. The authors did not standardize the length of penetration through the cortex, nor did they study how far the wires can safely protrude through the anterior cortex, although they recommend the absolute minimal degree of penetration. This study is useful in describing a methodology to avoid impingement of hardware when using tension band wiring of olecranon fractures. The complication of limited forearm rotation when treating these fractures with tension band wire fixation utilizing a transcortical technique is unreported, but may occur with injudicious wire placement.

S. H. Berner, MD

Bilateral Radial Head Fractures With Elbow Dislocation

Raman R, Srinivasan K, Matthews SJE, et al (St James's Univ, Leeds, England)
Orthopedics 28:503-505, 2005   7–11

Background.—Isolated radial head fracture is the most common type of elbow fracture and accounts for one third of all elbow fractures in adults.

The fracture occurs most often after a fall on the outstretched hand. From 5% to 10% of patients with elbow dislocations have associated radial head fractures. The outcome of these fractures is usually dependent on the type of fracture, the involvement of the articular surface, the degree of comminution, and treatment method. However, management is further complicated by the presence of bilateral injury. A case of bilateral elbow dislocations associated with Mason type 4 radial head fractures was presented.

> *Case Report.*—A 34-year-old right-hand dominant police officer presented with a closed injury to both elbows after a fall on his outstretched hands while chasing a suspect. He had clinical deformity of both elbows, with no neurovascular compromise. Conventional radiographs showed bilateral elbow dislocations with radial head fractures—Mason type 4 fractures. The elbows were reduced in the operating room. No intra-articular fragments were present. Kocher's approach was used to stabilize both radial head fractures using AO mini T plates. Intraoperative screening showed no ligamentous instability. The elbows were splinted for a few days, followed by gradual mobilization. The patient underwent physiotherapy treatment 3 weeks after injury. At 5 months, both fractures were clinically and radiologically united. At final review 18 months later, the patient had excellent range of motion in both elbows, despite the presence of minor heterotopic ossification in the left elbow and a fatigue failure of the T plate in the right elbow. The patient had 15° to 130° of flexion and full rotation in the right elbow and 10° to 135° of flexion and full rotation in the left elbow.

Conclusions.—Bilateral radial head fracture associated with elbow dislocation is an extremely rare injury. Prompt reduction of the dislocated elbow is mandatory to relieve pain and prevent the development of neurovascular compromise, including compartment syndrome. In the present case elbow reduction was followed by reconstruction of the radial head fractures using AO T plates. There are many relative indications either for reconstruction of radial head fractures or replacement of the radial head. The bilateral nature of radial head fractures associated with elbow dislocations should be considered a relative indication for surgical intervention.

▶ Radial head fractures have been classified by Mason types I-IV; type III (intra-articular) and type IV (intra-articular with elbow instability or dislocation) indicate open reduction and internal fixation or prosthetic replacement. Much effort should be made to retain the radial head.

In this article, an unusual case of bilateral Mason Type IV radial head fractures is presented. While we agree with internal fixation, the mini "T" plates chosen are too small to resist the forces across the radiocapitellar joint. We recommend a larger plate with 2.7-mm small fragment screws. An appropriate surgical approach with avoidance of the posterior interosseous nerve is well described by Hotchkiss and Smith.[1]

W. P. Cooney, MD

Reference

1. Smith GR, Hotchkiss RN: Radial head and neck fractures: Anatomic guidelines for proper placement of internal fixation. *J Shoulder Elbow Surg* 5:113-117, 1996.

Failure of Fresh-Frozen Radial Head Allografts in the Treatment of Essex-Lopresti Injury: A Report of Four Cases
Karlstad R, Morrey BF, Cooney WP (Mayo Clinic, Rochester, Minn)
J Bone Joint Surg Am 87-A:1828-1833, 2005   7–12

Background.—Reconstructive management of Essex-Lopresti injury has been difficult, yielding variable, mostly unfavorable results. Described were outcomes in 4 patients with established symptomatic proximal radial translation secondary to prior trauma and radial head excision treated with a total of 5 frozen radial head allografts.

Case 1.—A 33-year-old man suffered a fracture of the right radial head in an automobile accident in January 1998, and a radial head excision was performed. The patient subsequently experienced elbow and wrist pain and loss of elbow motion and forearm rotation. Six months after the injury the range of elbow motion was 35° to 138°, and the patient had 0° of forearm supination and 80° of pronation. Radiographs showed 13 mm of positive ulnar variance. The patient underwent an allograft radial head replacement with miniplate fixation and an ulnar shortening osteotomy. At 3 months postoperatively, the patient had no pain or instability. Several years after surgery, the range of elbow motion was from 15° to 135°, and pronation and supination were 75° and 70°, respectively.

Case 2.—A 27-year-old man sustained a right radial head fracture in 1987. He was treated with radial head excision and insertion of a silicone radial head implant. By 1991 the silicone implant had failed, and it was excised. An ulnar shortening osteotomy was also performed at that time. The patient was found to have a range of elbow motion of 5° to 140°, with 80° of pronation and 80° of supination. He underwent an allograft radial head replacement with double-mini-plate fixation in 1995. At 17 months there was frank nonunion of the allograft. The range of elbow motion was now limited to 50° to 105°, with 70° of pronation and no supination. The patient underwent another allograft radial head replacement in October 1998. Radiographs 18 months later showed nonunion of this allograft, and autogenous bone grafting was performed. Nonunion persisted, and the second radial head allograft was resected 19 months later. The arc of elbow flexion was 30° to 145° after removal, with 80° of pronation and 20° of supination.

Case 3.—A 26-year-old construction worker fell from a height of 4.6 m and suffered a fracture-dislocation of the right elbow and a fracture of the right radial head and neck. He was treated immediately with radial head excision and silicone radial head replacement. The patient experienced discomfort in the wrist and forearm 6 months after injury. Radiographs demonstrated proximal radial migration and bone loss attributable to silicone synovitis. The silicone replacement was removed at 18 months after the injury, and a radial head allograft was inserted and fixed with a 2.7-mm plate. Moderate pain continued, and revision fixation and autologous and allograft bone-grafting were performed in November 2001. Examination 8 months later showed a range of elbow flexion of 0° to 145°, with pronation and supination limited to 70° and 55°, respectively.

Case 4.—A 37-year-old male carpenter sustained a fracture of the left radial head in a fall. With nonoperative treatment he attained an arc of elbow motion of 30° to 100° and was unable to rotate the forearm. An allograft radial head replacement with fixation with a 2.7-mm plate and screws was performed 1 year later. The patient did not experience relief of pain, and at 7 months the range of motion was 15° to 130°, with 35° of pronation and 10° of supination. Radiographs showed resorption of the radial head allograft.

Conclusions.—The results in these patients were not optimal. The literature has documented an 80% failure rate for reconstruction in patients in whom an acute Essex-Lopresti lesion was initially missed. Allograft radial head replacement proved unreliable for the treatment of this injury.

▶ This is a retrospective report of 4 cases treated with allograft radial head insertion for Essex-Lopresti lesions with only one satisfactory outcome and 3 failures. The topic of treatment of Essex-Lopresti is interesting for the orthopaedic surgeon. The report of these 4 cases is very well presented and clear. The conclusions and the discussion are correct and instructive. The weakness of this case series could be the low number of patients. However, the conclusions seem to be appropriate, and a larger number of patients might neither be necessary nor justified considering the poor outcome using this method. Overall, this is an interesting and instructive study worthy of being published.

A. G. Schneeberger, MD

Fractures of the Radial Head and Neck Treated With Radial Head Excision
Herbertsson P, Josefsson PO, Hasserius R, et al (Malmö Univ, Sweden)
J Bone Joint Surg Am 86-A:1925-1930, 2004   7–13

Background.—The reported long-term outcomes of the treatment of radial head and neck fractures with excision of the radial head have been mixed. The purpose of the present study was to evaluate the long-term outcomes of primary or delayed radial head excision for the treatment of these fractures.

Methods.—Sixty-one individuals (mean age, forty-four years) with thirty-nine Mason type-II, ten Mason type-III, and twelve Mason type-IV fractures were evaluated subjectively, objectively, and radiographically at a mean of eighteen years (range, eleven to thirty-three years) after treatment. Forty-three fractures were treated with primary radial head excision, and the remaining eighteen were treated with delayed radial head excision at a median of five months (range, one to 238 months) after the injury.

Results.—At the time of follow-up, twenty-eight individuals had no symptoms, twenty-seven had occasional elbow pain, and six had daily pain. Four individuals with daily pain had had a Mason type-IV fracture. The range of motion of the formerly injured upper extremities was slightly less than that of the uninjured upper extremities in terms of flexion ($139° \pm 11°$ compared with $142° \pm 8°$), extension ($-7° \pm 12°$ compared with $-1° \pm 6°$), and supination ($77° \pm 20°$ compared with $85° \pm 10°$) (all $p < 0.01$). A higher percentage of formerly injured elbows than uninjured elbows had cysts, sclerosis, and osteophytes (73% compared with 7%; $p < 0.001$), but none had a reduced joint space. No differences were found between the outcomes for individuals treated with a primary radial head excision and those for individuals treated with a delayed excision.

Conclusions.—Following a displaced radial head or neck fracture, excision of the radial head often leads to a good or fair result. We found no differences in outcome between primary and delayed radial head excisions following a Mason type-II, III, or IV fracture. The outcomes are associated with the type of fracture, with Mason type-IV fractures having the worst results, rather than with the timing of the radial head excision (primary or delayed).

▶ This retrospective study shows the long-term results of surgically treated Mason type II, III, and IV radial head and neck fractures, with an average follow-up of 18 years. Due to the long follow-up period, many patients from the original number of 131 patients could not be included, leaving 61 cases for follow-up. They could not demonstrate significant differences in outcome (range of motion, strength, carrying angle) between patients that had primary or delayed excision of their radial head after fracture, and found that rather the type of fracture is responsible for the differences in outcome, with Mason type IV fractures showing the worst results. Furthermore, they saw no reduction in joint space. They conclude that it is feasible to attempt to save the radial head primarily, and in the case of persistent problems, to resect it later. On the other hand, their study could be interpreted to recommend primarily resecting the radial head, because degenerative changes in terms of joint space narrowing could not be detected, and therefore, no late complications would be expected. Unfortunately, the authors did not discuss why the Mason type IV fractures showed the worst results. The question is whether residual instability is responsible or not. Overall, this long-term follow-up study gives the elbow surgeon a reliable background on how to counsel patients when they present with an isolated Mason type II, III, or IV fracture of the radial head or neck.

S. Lichtenberg, MD

Comminuted Fractures of the Radial Head: Comparison of Resection and Internal Fixation

Ikeda M, Sugiyama K, Kang C, et al (Tokai Univ, Kanagawa, Japan)
J Bone Joint Surg Am 87-A:76-84, 2005   7–14

Background.—Satisfactory internal fixation of comminuted radial head fractures is often difficult to achieve, and radial head resection has been the accepted treatment. In this study, we compared the results of radial head resection with those of open reduction and internal fixation in patients with a comminuted radial head fracture.

Methods.—Twenty-eight patients with a Mason type-III radial head fracture (some with associated injuries) were enrolled in the study (Fig 1). Fifteen patients underwent radial head resection as the initial treatment (Group I), and thirteen patients underwent open reduction and internal fixation (Group II). The age at the operation averaged 41.1 and 38.2 years, respectively, and the duration of follow-up averaged ten and three years, respectively. The outcomes were assessed on the basis of pain, motion, radiographic findings, and strength measured with Cybex testing. The overall outcome was rated with the functional rating score described by Broberg and Morrey and with the American Shoulder and Elbow Surgeons Elbow Assessment Form.

Results.—Elbow motion averaged 15.5° (extension loss) to 131.4° (flexion) in Group I and 7.1° to 133.8° in Group II. The carrying angle and ulnar variance averaged 8.2° and 1.9 mm in Group I and 1.5° and 0.5 mm in Group II. Compared with Group II, Group I had a loss of strength in exten-

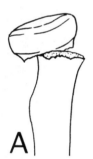 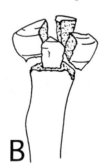 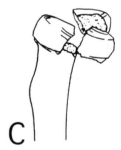

A   B   C

FIGURE 1.—Mason type-III radial head fracture patterns. **A,** A fracture of the entire radial neck, with the head completely displaced from the shaft. **B,** An articular fracture involving the entire head, which consists of more than two large fragments. Each fragment is completely displaced from the shaft. **C,** A fracture with a tilted and impacted articular segment, which must be reduced, and some articular fragments displaced from the shaft. (Courtesy of Ikeda M, Sugiyama K, Kang C, et al: Comminuted fractures of the radial head: Comparison of resection and internal fixation. *J Bone Joint Surg Am* 87-A:76-84, 2005. Reproduced by permission of the publisher via Copyright Clearance Center, Inc.)

sion, pronation, and supination (p < 0.01). The Broberg and Morrey functional rating score averaged 81.4 points in Group I and 90.7 points in Group II (p = 0.0034). The score on the American Shoulder and Elbow Surgeons Elbow Assessment Form averaged 87.3 points in Group I and 94.6 points in Group II (p = 0.0031).

Conclusions.—The patients in whom the comminuted radial head fracture was treated with open reduction and internal fixation had satisfactory joint motion, with greater strength and better function than the patients who had undergone radial head resection. These results support a recommendation for open reduction and internal fixation in the treatment of this fracture.

▶ Radial head fractures represent one of the most common fractures of the upper extremity, and their treatment has ranged from early motion to open reduction and internal fixation (ORIF), radial head resection, and implant arthroplasty. The radial head is important in forearm rotation and elbow motion, but also in elbow stability because of its role as a stabilizer against valgus stresses, and in wrist stability because of its role in preventing proximal migration of the radius.

The authors present their experience in treating displaced radial head and neck fractures (Mason III) in a retrospective study of 35 patients treated with resection of the radial head versus ORIF using small headless screws and low-profile plates. Consistent with other current literature, the authors found that patients treated with radial head resection alone had a higher carrying angle at the elbow, and less elbow extension, forearm rotation strength, and overall functional outcome than those treated with ORIF. They therefore concluded that preservation of the radial head should be pursued in the treatment of these comminuted radial head fractures.

Smaller low-profile plates and headless screws make ORIF of the radial head easier, but in the case of the severely comminuted fracture of the radial head, the advent of metal radial head replacements has changed the algorithm for the treatment of these difficult fractures. Ring et al[1] suggest that severely comminuted fractures of the radial head (with 3 or more fragments) are better treated with radial head replacement rather than ORIF.

Radial head ORIF remains the mainstay of treatment, with radial head replacements a viable option in the severely comminuted case. Radial head resection still serves a role in treating the infirm patient who may benefit from a shorter surgical procedure or who may have difficulty participating in the postoperative protocol.

J. Yao, MD

Reference

1. Ring D, Quintero J, Jupiter JB: Open reduction and internal fixation of fractures of the radial head. *J Bone Joint Surg Am* 84-A:1811-1815, 2002.

Standard Surgical Protocol to Treat Elbow Dislocations With Radial Head and Coronoid Fractures

Pugh DMW, Wild LM, Schemitsch EH, et al (St Michael's Hosp, London, Ont, Canada; Univ of Western Ontario, London, Canada)
J Bone Joint Surg Am 86-A:1122-1130, 2004   7–15

Background.—The results of elbow dislocations with associated radial head and coronoid fractures are often poor because of recurrent instability and stiffness from prolonged immobilization. We managed these injuries with a standard surgical protocol, postulating that early intervention, stable fixation, and repair would provide sufficient stability to allow motion at seven to ten days postoperatively and enhance functional outcome.

Methods.—We retrospectively reviewed the results of this treatment performed, at two university-affiliated teaching hospitals, in thirty-six consecutive patients (thirty-six elbows) with an elbow dislocation and an associated fracture of both the radial head and the coronoid process. Our surgical protocol included fixation or replacement of the radial head, fixation of the coronoid fracture if possible, repair of associated capsular and lateral ligamentous injuries, and in selected cases repair of the medial collateral ligament and/or adjuvant hinged external fixation. Patients were evaluated both radiographically and with a clinical examination at the time of the latest follow-up.

Results.—At a mean of thirty-four months postoperatively, the flexion-extension arc of the elbow averaged 112° ± 11° and forearm rotation averaged 136° ± 16°. The mean Mayo Elbow Performance Score was 88 points (range, 45 to 100 points), which corresponded to fifteen excellent results, thirteen good results, seven fair results, and one poor result. Concentric stability was restored to thirty-four elbows. Eight patients had complications requiring a reoperation: two had a synostosis; one, recurrent instability; four, hardware removal and elbow release; and one, a wound infection.

Conclusions.—Use of our surgical protocol for elbow dislocations with associated radial head and coronoid fractures restored sufficient elbow stability to allow early motion postoperatively, enhancing the functional outcome. We recommend early operative repair with a standard protocol for these injuries.

▶ Elbow dislocations with associated fractures of the radial head and coronoid are inherently difficult injuries to treat. Historically, the dilemma has been whether to allow early elbow motion (which may result in recurrent instability due to tenuous surgical stabilization) or to immobilize the elbow to allow healing of injured structures, which then may lead to unacceptable stiffness.

In an effort to address this dilemma, the authors of this report present their approach to treating the "terrible triad of the elbow." This is a retrospective review with all the biases found in such study designs. The authors point this out themselves, as well indicating where data are missing. The authors present an honest assessment of treatment results and complications, which were not insignificant. Given the concern for heterotopic ossification after such injuries, many surgeons would opt for prophylaxis against it. Only 1 of the 2 surgeons involved in this study did so, but the numbers were too small to prove that this had a significant effect on synostosis or stiffness.

Despite these shortcomings, Pugh et al have demonstrated that it is possible to achieve good results in treating such challenging injuries if the principles they outlined are followed. The essential point is that stability must be restored surgically, using whatever methods are necessary so that elbow range of motion can be initiated early.

R. R. Slater, Jr, MD

Surgical Treatment of Post-traumatic Stiffness of the Elbow
Park MJ, Kim HG, Lee JY (Sungkyunkwan Univ, Seoul, Korea)
J Bone Joint Surg Br 86-B:1158-1162, 2004   7–16

Surgical release of the elbow was performed in 27 patients with post-traumatic stiffness at a mean of 14.5 months after the initial injury. The outcome was related to whether there had been heterotopic ossification, which had occurred in 18 elbows and to whether, if there had been a fracture, it had involved the articular surface, which had occurred in 13 elbows. The final range of movement and the ratio of desired gain in each group were compared at a mean follow-up period of 22.5 months (12 to 43).

The arc of movement of the elbow improved in all patients after the operation. The mean final arc was 110° in those with heterotopic ossification and 86° in those without ($p = 0.001$). The ratios of desired gain were significantly higher in patients with heterotopic ossification (88.2% vs 54.9%; $p < 0.001$). There was no significant difference in relation to involvement of the articular surface. Careful assessment of the cause of stiffness is important in order to achieve a satisfactory result from surgery for post-traumatic stiffness of the elbow.

▶ This retrospective nonrandomized study reviews 27 patients after open elbow release through different approaches. Follow-up ranges from 1 to 3.5 years (average, 23 months). Stiffness caused by heterotopic ossification was found in 18 cases, and no heterotopic ossification was found in 9 cases.

The study reported a decrease of extension loss from 40° to 19° and an improvement of flexion from 86° to 121°, on average, along with a significant improvement in range of motion for patients treated with removal of heterotopic bone compared with those without removal of heterotopic bone. It shows that the results of open elbow release are better for those patients with heterotopic bone removal than for those without it.

The topic of elbow release is certainly of interest to the orthopedic surgeon. The authors included an analysis of the pathologic conditions of the elbow when analyzing the results.

However, the study did use a rather small number of cases. For example, the authors found no significant differences for gain of range of motion in patients that had an intra-articular injury compared with those who did not ($P = 0.051$). With a larger number of cases, this difference might have been significant.

Overall, the conclusions are somehow scarce, and the study might only be of average interest.

A. G. Schneeberger, MD

Anterior Release of the Elbow for Extension Loss
Aldridge JM III, Atkins TA, Gunneson EE, et al (Duke Univ, Durham, NC)
J Bone Joint Surg Am 86-A:1955-1960, 2004   7–17

Background.—There are many causes of elbow contracture. When non-operative techniques fail to increase the arc of motion of the elbow, surgical intervention may be indicated. The purpose of this study was to report the outcomes of surgical correction, predominantly with an anterior release, of elbow flexion contractures. In addition, we evaluated the efficacy of continuous passive motion in the immediate postoperative period.

Methods.—We retrospectively reviewed the outcomes of 106 consecutive patients who had undergone anterior elbow release for the treatment of a flexion contracture between July 1975 and June 2001. Twenty-nine patients were excluded because they had been followed for less than twelve months, leaving a study group of seventy-seven patients. Postoperatively, fifty-four of the seventy-seven patients were treated with continuous passive motion and the other twenty-three patients were treated with extension splinting. The average duration of follow-up was thirty-three months. The average patient age was thirty-four years. The results were evaluated on the basis of both preoperative and postoperative radiographs as well as clinical measurements of elbow motion, all performed by the same examiner using the same large (47-cm-long) goniometer.

Results.—The mean preoperative extension in the seventy-seven patients was 52°, which decreased to 20° postoperatively. The mean flexion increased from 111° preoperatively to 117° postoperatively, and the mean total arc of motion increased from 59° to 97°. The total arc of motion in the patients treated with continuous passive motion increased 45°, compared with an increase of 26° in those treated with extension splinting. There were eleven complications in ten patients. The majority were traction neuropathies. There were two infections (one superficial and one deep), both of which resolved following treatment.

Conclusions.—Release of a pathologically thickened anterior elbow capsule through a predominantly anterior approach to correct diminished elbow extension is a safe and effective technique. Furthermore, compared with splinting in extension alone, the utilization of continuous passive motion during the postoperative period increases the total arc of motion.

▶ This is a retrospective nonrandomized study reviewing 77 of 106 patients after open anterior elbow release through an anterior skin incision. Follow-up ranged from 1 to 10 years (average, 33 months). Patients were treated with physiotherapy rehabilitation for all elbows; in addition, 54 patients were allowed continuous passive motion (CPM), and 23 patients had extension splinting.

The study showed a decrease of extension loss from 52° to 20° and an improvement of flexion from 111° to 117°, on average, along with a significantly better improvement of range of motion for patients with CPM compared with those with extension splinting.

This study was well presented and clearly shows the results of open anterior elbow release. The patients were all treated by the same surgeon in the same institution, and the technique and the results are clearly described.

The weakness of this study is that it is retrospective and nonrandomized. Only 77 of 106 patients were reviewed. The conclusion that CPM yields superior results as compared with splinting in extension might be questioned because of the design of the study (ie, retrospective, nonrandomized).

One of the authors of this study has the reputation of being a very experienced surgeon with extensive experience in neurosurgery. This presented technique, which requires passing through the anterior neurovascular structures, might be associated with a higher number of complications when used by an average surgeon. Therefore, it should be mentioned that this technique might have "dangers" associated with it, depending on the experience of the surgeon.

Considering that many other less risky techniques exist, such as open release through lateral or medial approaches or arthroscopic release, the described technique might be considered an outsider technique. Therefore, this study may only be of average interest.

A. G. Schneeberger, MD

Transfer of Pectoralis Major in Arthrogryposis to Restore Elbow Flexion: Deteriorating Results in the Long Term
Lahoti O, Bell MJ (Sheffield Children's Hosp, England)
J Bone Joint Surg Br 87-B:858-860, 2005   7–18

Background.—Two patterns of involvement of the upper limb in arthrogryposis multiplex congenita have been described. Type I is the most common type and presents with adduction and internal rotation at the shoulder, extension of the elbow, pronation of the forearm, and a flexion deformity of the wrist, suggesting involvement of the C5/6 neural segments. Type II is less common and shows adduction and internal rotation at the shoulder, a flexion deformity of the elbow, and flexion and deviation of the wrist, suggesting partial involvement of C5, complete involvement of C6, and partial involvement of C7. The inability to flex the elbow in arthrogryposis has a major adverse effect on function, as the most basic activities of daily life, including feeding and toilet hygiene, require assistance. Many tendon transfer procedures have been described to restore flexion. Long-term outcomes of pectoralis major transfer to restore elbow flexion in arthrogryposis were described.

Methods.—A clinical examination and review of the medical records of 7 patients (10 procedures) who had undergone a modified pectoralis transfer were performed. Three patients underwent simultaneous tricepsplasty to improve the arc of flexion. Four patients had a tricepsplasty 2 to 3 months before pectoralis major transfer. The age of the patients at operation ranged from 2.5 to 14 years. Staged bilateral procedures were performed in three patients. Follow-up ranged from 7 to 19 years.

Results.—The early results were encouraging in all patients. All patients but one retained useful power in the transferred pectoralis major muscle and maintained the arc of flexion after tricepsplasty. However, over time a gradual and progressive increase in flexion deformity and decrease in the arc of flexion were observed in 8 of 10 elbows. In all cases the deformity was 90° or more.

Conclusions.—The early encouraging results of transfer of pectoralis major for treatment of an extension contracture of the elbow in arthrogryposis deteriorate over time with development of a recalcitrant flexion deformity of the elbow. The procedure is recommended on one side only in cases of bilateral involvement.

▶ Seven patients with arthrogryposis who underwent transfer of pectoralis major to the elbow flexor had poorer function at follow-up that ranged from 7 to 19 years. All of the patients had fresh tricepsplasty—four within the 3 months prior to surgery, and three at the same procedure. The age range at the time of surgery was also quite wide—from 2.5 to 14 years.

This report stresses the need to regain passive range of motion before attempting flexorplasty and the importance of preserving active elbow extension.

M. Ezaki, MD

Effects of Elbow Flexion and Forearm Rotation on Valgus Laxity of the Elbow

Safran MR, McGarry MH, Shin S, et al (Univ of California, Irvine, Long Beach)
J Bone Joint Surg Am 87-A:2065-2074, 2005   7–19

Background.—Clinical evaluation of valgus elbow laxity is difficult. The optimum position of elbow flexion and forearm rotation with which to identify valgus laxity in a patient with an injury of the ulnar collateral ligament of the elbow has not been determined. The purpose of the present study was to determine the effect of forearm rotation and elbow flexion on valgus elbow laxity.

Methods.—Twelve intact cadaveric upper extremities were studied with a custom elbow-testing device. Laxity was measured with the forearm in pronation, supination, and neutral rotation at 30°, 50°, and 70° of elbow flexion with use of 2 Nm of valgus torque. Testing was conducted with the ulnar collateral ligament intact, with the joint vented, after cutting of the anterior half (six specimens) or posterior half (six specimens) of the anterior oblique ligament of the ulnar collateral ligament, and after complete sectioning of the anterior oblique ligament. Laxity was measured in degrees of valgus angulation in different positions of elbow flexion and forearm rotation.

Results.—There were no significant differences in valgus laxity with respect to elbow flexion within each condition. Overall, for both groups of specimens (i.e., specimens in which the anterior or posterior half of the anterior oblique ligament was cut), neutral forearm rotation resulted in greater valgus laxity than pronation or supination did ($p < 0.05$). Transection of the anterior half of the anterior oblique ligament did not significantly increase valgus laxity; however, transection of the posterior half resulted in increased valgus laxity in some positions. Full transection of the anterior oblique ligament significantly increased valgus laxity in all positions ($p < 0.05$).

Conclusions.—The results of this in vitro cadaveric study demonstrated that forearm rotation had a significant effect on varus-valgus laxity. Laxity was always greatest in neutral forearm rotation throughout the ranges of elbow flexion and the various surgical conditions.

▶ Conflicting reports are in the literature cocerning the effect of forearm rotation on valgus laxity testing of the elbow. This study finds that a neutral position results in the greatest degree of valgus laxity and may be the best position for physical examination. Intuitively, it makes sense that supination would provide passive stretch of the flexor pronator mass and this could contribute to stability and give the examiner a false sense of stability. The importance of the overlying muscle has also recently been discussed with respect to an examination for lateral elbow stability. The effect of pronation is less clear to me. It would appear that with pronation, one would take all of the passive stretch out of the pronator so that it would not contribute to valgus resistance, but the authors believe this may provide some increase in osseous stability as a result of proximal migration of the radius. Further study is needed to assess the impact of forearm rotation on graft tension and fixation during reconstruction.

T. R. McAdams, MD

Management of Cubitus Varus and Valgus
Kim HT, Lee JS, Yoo CI (Pusan Natl Univ, Korea)
J Bone Joint Surg Am 87-A:771-780, 2005   7–20

Background.—Many types of osteotomy have been proposed for the treatment of cubitus varus and valgus, but they have limitations, such as poor internal fixation, residual protrusion of the lateral or medial condyle, technical difficulty, the need for long-term immobilization, a risk of neurovascular injury, and patient discomfort. We reviewed the results of a simple step-cut translation osteotomy that overcomes these limitations.

Methods.—Between 1993 and 2002, we treated nineteen cases of cubitus varus and thirteen cases of cubitus valgus with use of a simple step-cut translation osteotomy and fixation with a Y-shaped humeral plate. After surgery, the patients were observed closely for more than one year. We compared preoperative and postoperative humerus-elbow-wrist angles, ranges of motion, and lateral or medial prominence indices for all patients. The results were evaluated according to the modified criteria of Oppenheim et al. The presence of tardy ulnar nerve palsy and its duration, and postoperative lazy-s deformity or unsightly scarring, were also noted.

Results.—There were twenty-six excellent and six good results. In the nineteen patients with cubitus varus, the average amount of correction of the humerus-elbow-wrist angle was 26.0°, to a mean postoperative angle of 8.6°, and the average increase in the lateral prominence index was 8.2%. In the thirteen patients with cubitus valgus, the average correction in the humerus-elbow-wrist angle was 27.6°, resulting in a final angle of 9.1°, and the average increase in the medial prominence index was 11.9%. In all patients, the desired range of motion, good alignment, and complete union of the bone were achieved.

Conclusions.—Step-cut translation osteotomy, with a wedge-shaped osteotomized surface, fixed with a Y-shaped humeral plate is a relatively simple procedure resulting in very firm fixation that allows early movement of the joint with good clinical results.

▶ This article provides an excellent description of the preoperative planning and surgical techniques for osteotomy in the management of both cubitus varus and valgus. The authors even discussed how to use the Adobe Photoshop software program for this application. I do have concerns over their type of Y plate, which is bent to match the contour of the bone, and about the rigidity of this plate, especially from 1 plane. However, all of their patients healed within 12 weeks, and they did not have any plate failures or nonunions. Anyone involved in the care of corrective osteotomies for cubitus varus and valgus deformities should review this important article.

T. R. McAdams, MD

The Fat Pad Sign Following Elbow Trauma in Adults: Its Usefulness and Reliability in Suspecting Occult Fracture

O'Dwyer H, O'Sullivan P, Fitzgerald D, et al (Beaumont Hosp, Dublin)
J Comput Assist Tomogr 28:562-565, 2004   7–21

Objective.—An elbow joint effusion with no fracture seen on radiographs after acute trauma has become synonymous with occult fracture. This study evaluates the incidence of fracture in such cases as determined by MR imaging and the predictive value of an elbow joint effusion.

Methods.—Twenty consecutive patients whose posttrauma elbow radiographs showed an effusion but no fracture and who were suitable for MR imaging were recruited. The elbow effusion size, represented by anterior and posterior fat pad displacement, was measured from the initial lateral elbow radiograph. Suitable candidates underwent MR imaging using a bone marrow sensitive sequence. The time between injury and MR imaging ranged from 0 to 12 days (mean 4 days).

Results.—Seventy-five percent of the 20 patients who underwent MR imaging had radiographically occult fractures identified. Some (86.6%) of these fractures were located in the radial head, 6.7% were in the lateral epicondyle, and 6.7% were in the olecranon. Ninety percent had evidence of bone marrow edema. Fifteen percent had collateral ligament disruption identified on MR imaging, and 5% had a loose body. There was no change in patient management as a result of the additional imaging. The anterior fat pad displacement ranged from 5 to 15 mm (mean 9.25), and the posterior fat pad was elevated from 1 to 6 mm (mean 3.2).

Conclusion.—Our data using MR imaging suggests that fat pad elevation in the presence of recent trauma is frequently associated with a fracture. The size of the effusion, anterior/posterior fat pad elevation, or a combination of both does not correspond to the likelihood of an underlying fracture. MR imaging reveals a broad spectrum of bone and soft tissue injury beyond that recognizable on plain radiographs as demonstrated by all patients in this study.

▶ This is a straightforward study documenting what has long been an assumption without proof, that is, that the presence of a visible fat pad sign at the elbow is a sensitive indicator of an occult fracture after trauma. In this study, 23 consecutive patients seen with acute elbow trauma were evaluated with standard radiographic imaging of the elbow. None had radiographically visible fractures, but all had elbow effusion, as defined by elevation of the fat pad anteriorly or posteriorly. Twenty of these patients went on to have MRI examination of the elbow (3 were unable to undergo MRI). Seventy-five percent of the patients had radiographically occult fractures, and 20% had no fracture (1 patient had nondiagnostic images). Twenty percent of the patients with fractures had significant soft tissue injuries detected at MRI. Ninety-five percent of patients undergoing MRI had bone injures, including 15 with fractures and 4 with bone contusions. Only 1 patient had no bone injuries and elbow effusion. The authors conclude that the presence of joint effusion after trauma, even when no fracture can be visualized radiographically, is a sensitive and specific indicator of underlying bone trauma.

K. K. Amrami, MD

The Detection of Loose Bodies in the Elbow: The Value of MRI and CT Arthrography
Dubberley JH, Faber KJ, Patterson SD, et al (Univ of Western Ontario, London, Canada)
J Bone Joint Surg Br 87-B:684-686, 2005   7–22

Our aim was to determine the clinical value of MRI and CT arthrography in predicting the presence of loose bodies in the elbow.

A series of 26 patients with mechanical symptoms in the elbow had plain radiography, MRI and CT arthrography, followed by routine arthroscopy of the elbow. The location and number of loose bodies determined by MRI and

CT arthrography were recorded. Pre-operative plain radiography, MRI and CT arthrography were compared with arthroscopy.

Both MRI and CT arthrography had excellent sensitivity (92% to 100%) but low to moderate specificity (15% to 77%) in identifying posteriorly-based loose bodies. Neither MRI nor CT arthrography was consistently sensitive (46% to 91%) or specific (13% to 73%) in predicting the presence or absence of loose bodies anteriorly. The overall sensitivity for the detection of loose bodies in either compartment was 88% to 100% and the specificity 20% to 70%. Pre-operative radiography had a similar sensitivity and specificity of 84% and 71%, respectively.

Our results suggest that neither CT arthrography nor MRI is reliable or accurate enough to be any more effective than plain radiography alone in patients presenting with mechanical symptoms in the elbow.

▶ The authors showed that neither MRI nor CT arthrography could outscore conventional radiography in detecting loose bodies in the elbow joint or determining where exactly the loose bodies were situated. So there is no need for more advanced imaging studies according to this study. Plain MRI and CT arthrography with double contrast medium is not worthwhile in detecting loose bodies. Nowadays, arthro-MRI probably will do better, but this technique has yet not been evaluated scientifically.

S. Lichtenberg, MD

8 Elbow: Arthroplasty

Thermal Tissue Damage Caused by Ultrasonic Cement Removal From the Humerus
Goldberg SH, Cohen MS, Yound M, et al (Rush Univ Med Ctr, Chicago)
J Bone Joint Surg Am 87-A:583-591, 2005   8–1

Background.—US technology has been used to selectively remove cement and preserve host bone in revision total hip arthroplasty, but cases have not documented its use in revision total elbow procedures. A patient underwent such a revision technique with US and sustained thermal necrosis of bone, the triceps muscle, and the radial nerve. The effect of US on the temperature of the humerus and surrounding soft tissue envelope during tissue removal was then evaluated in cadavers. From this arose strategies to minimize thermal injury.

Case Report.—Woman, 69, had a fracture-dislocation of the right elbow initially managed with open reduction, radial head replacement, and use of a hinged external fixator. She required a semiconstrained total elbow arthroplasty with cement 1 year later. An infection soon after this surgery was managed with serial debridement and chronic suppressive antibiotics, but 2 years later she needed an implant and cement removal from both humeral and ulnar canals. A 7-cm cement plug proximal to the tip of the humeral component was removed by using an US device. During the surgery, a tourniquet was maintained at the site for 2 hours. The lateral cortex was perforated during ulnar cement removal; soft tissue trauma was minimal, but the patient had a complete proximal radial nerve palsy. After 2 weeks, she sustained a pathologic spiral fracture of the humerus; surgery revealed widespread muscle necrosis. There was no evidence of canal perforation during cement removal, but the radial nerve had attenuated and thinned in the area along the posterior humeral cortex. Pathologic sections showed complete necrosis of muscle, cortical bone, and nerve tissue.

Methods.—Six cadaveric limb specimens from shoulder to midforearm were used to measure the temperature elevations occurring when cement is removed with the use of a US device, with and without irrigation. Temperature readings were obtained from bone and surrounding soft tissue.

Results.—The temperature increases during cement polymerization were moderate, with the highest found in the humeral cortex, then the radial nerve and triceps muscle. Those for the bone and radial nerve were significant. The temperature increases occurring with cement removal using a rapid and constant ultrasonic application were marked for all tissues. The average maximum temperatures were 62.8°C in bone, 51.7°C in the radial nerve, and 38.0°C in the triceps muscle. Temperatures increased first in bone, then in the nerve, and then in the triceps. The increases in the bone and radial nerve temperatures were significant. The use of chilled irrigation and a bulb syringe between each US pass minimized heat generation and transmission in all the tissues. With these strategies, the maximum bone, radial nerve, and triceps muscle temperatures were 51.0°C, 38.0°C, and 42.0°C, respectively.

Conclusions.—Potentially dangerous temperatures can be produced when US technology is used to remove cement in revision total elbow arthroplasty. Damage can occur to the humerus, triceps, and radial nerve. Intermittent cold irrigation of the canal between instrument passes, avoiding use of a tourniquet, and educating surgeons about ways to limit heat generation are appropriate precautions to take.

▶ This is an important warning article for those who perform revision elbow arthroplasty. The authors describe a case of complete radial nerve, bone, and triceps necrosis with the use of an ultrasonic cement removal device. The authors performed a follow-up study in cadavers with temperature probes during a simulated cement removal procedure. With the use of no irrigation fluid, temperatures went above the level needed to allow for bone and nerve necrosis. The authors recommend that cold irrigation be used during ultrasonic pulses and that the tourniquet not be inflated to allow for better heat dissipation. Ultimately, the lesson to be learned here is to use a cement restrictor when implanting a humeral component during total elbow arthroplasty. It was while removing an unnecessary 7-cm proximal plug of cement that the thermal injury occurred.

S. P. Steinmann, MD

Survivorship of the Souter-Strathclyde Elbow Replacement in the Young Inflammatory Arthritis Elbow
Talwalkar SC, Givissis PK, Trail IA, et al (Wrightington Wigan and Leigh NHS Trust, England)
J Bone Joint Surg Br 87-B:946-949, 2005   8–2

Background.—There has been an improvement in the last few decades in the results of total elbow arthroplasty. This improvement may be a result of superior prosthetic design or technical changes such as better cementation. However, these procedures are usually performed only in older patients with a lower demand because of the perceived risk of early loosening in young active patients. Several studies of the Souter-Strathclyde elbow replacement have reported predictable relief from pain, good to excellent function, and a survivorship of 77.4% to 85% at 10 years. The survivorship of the Souter-Strathclyde elbow replacement in patients under 50 years of age with survivorship in older patients was compared.

Methods.—A group of 309 patients with an inflammatory arthritis who had undergone primary elbow replacement using the Souter-Strathclyde implant were divided into two groups according to their age. The mean follow up in the older group (mean age 64 years) was 7.3 years; in the younger patients (mean age 42 years) the mean follow up was 12 years. Survivorship in both points was compared for three different failure end-points: revision, revision because of aseptic loosening of the humeral component, and gross loosening of the humeral implant.

Results.—There was no significant difference in the incidence of loosening when young rheumatoid patients were compared with the older group. However, when the risk of having gross loosening of the H implant for both age groups is considered, patients >50 years of age had a probability of survival of 29% at 16 years, compared with 79% in patients under 50 years of age. This apparently large difference is misleading, however, because the calculation depends on the number of subjects under investigation at any given time. A comparison of the distribution of the number of terminal events at distinct times for the two survival curves and the log-rank statistic showed that this difference was insignificant.

Conclusions.—A comparison of long-term survivorship of the Souter-Strathclyde elbow replacement in patients under 50 years of age and those over 50 years of age found no significant difference.

▶ This retrospective nonrandomized study reviews the charts and radiographs of 309 patients after Souter-Strathclyde total elbow replacement. Group I included patients younger than 50 years (46 cases, all radiological follow-up, 26 patients with 31 cases also clinical follow-up), while Group II was comprised of patients older than 50 years (only radiological analysis of 263 cases).

The study shows follow-up of up to 16 years (mainly radiological) with patients treated mainly for rheumatoid arthritis with one implant (using short or long humeral stems). The authors compared the survival curves of the 2 groups and the study shows the survival curves of this implant. This is the great contribution of the study.

The topic of total elbow replacement is interesting for the orthopaedic surgeon, especially when dealing with young patients. However, the design of the study is somewhat confusing: Group I had a clinical assessment (for only 31 of 46 cases); Group II had only a radiological review. In addition, the survival curves for patients over 50 years was always inferior to those for patients younger than 50 years, but the differences were not statistically significant due to the low number of patients with long-term follow-up. The conclusion of the authors that there is no difference in the survivorship of the 2 groups is probably doubtful, and a larger number of patients would probably show differences.

Overall, due to the survival curves, this study is an interesting contribution despite its methodological weakness.

A. G. Schneeberger, MD

Total Elbow Arthroplasty After Previous Resection of the Radial Head and Synovectomy
Whaley A, Morrey BF, Adams R (Mayo Clinic, Rochester, Minn)
J Bone Joint Surg Br 87-B:47-53, 2005   8–3

We examined the effects of previous resection of the radial head and synovectomy on the outcome of subsequent total elbow arthroplasty in patients with rheumatoid arthritis.

Fifteen elbows with a history of resection and synovectomy were compared with a control group of patients who had elbow arthroplasty with an implant of the same design. The mean age in both groups was 63 years. In the study group, resection of the radial head and synovectomy had been undertaken at a mean of 8.9 years before arthroplasty. The mean radiological follow-up for the 13 available patients in the study group was 5.89 years (0.3 to 11.0) and in the control group was 6.6 years (22 to 12.6). There were no revisions in either group. The mean Mayo elbow performance score improved from 29 to 96 in the study group, with similar improvement in the control group (28 to 87). The study group had excellent results in 13 elbows and good results in two. The control group had excellent results in seven and good results in six.

Our experience indicates that previous resection of the radial head and synovectomy are not associated with an increased rate of revision following subsequent arthroplasty of the elbow. However, there was a higher rate of complication in the study group compared with the control group.

▶ This study, published by a center well-known for high volume and excellence in elbow surgery, did not find a significant difference in outcome between patients with rheumatoid arthritis following total elbow arthroplasty, who had a previous radial head resection and synovectomy, and patients who had no prior surgery. There were slightly better results using the Mayo elbow performance score in the study group. The reason for this is unclear, and the groups were too small to identify contributing factors. There was a higher rate of complications in the study group compared to the control group; however, these were complications that are not uncommon following this type of surgery in rheumatoid patients in general. I don't believe these complications can be linked specifically to either group.

K. J. Renfree, MD

Polyethylene Wear After Total Elbow Arthroplasty

Lee BP, Adams RA, Morrey BF (Mayo Clinic, Rochester, Minn)
J Bone Joint Surg Am 87-A:1080-1087, 2005   8–4

Background.—Articular wear is considered to be a possible long-term complication of the use of stemmed, coupled elbow replacements with the capacity to correct deformity and restore function. There have been no reports on this topic, to our knowledge.

Methods.—A review of the results of 919 replacements with the semi-constrained linked Coonrad-Morrey total elbow implant, performed between 1981 and 2000, revealed that twelve patients (1.3%) had undergone an isolated exchange of the articular bushings as a result of polyethylene wear. The status of these patients was assessed clinically and radiographically.

Results.—The mean age of the twelve patients at the time of the initial total elbow replacement was forty-four years compared with a mean age of sixty-two years in the overall group (p < 0.001). Seven of the twelve patients had posttraumatic arthritis, and five had rheumatoid arthritis. Nine patients had extensive deformity. The group consisted of seven women and five men,

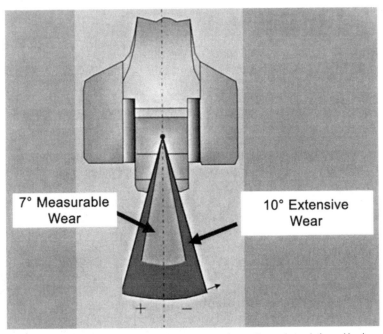

FIGURE 1.—Wear of the polyethylene bushing is measured according to the angle formed by the articulating portion of the ulnar component and the medial or lateral aspect of the humeral articular yoke. Angles in excess of 7° indicate displacement greater than allowed by the design tolerances. When this angle is 10°, mild-to-moderate wear is considered to be present and the patient is considered to be a candidate for surgery. (Courtesy of Lee BP, Adams RA, Morrey BF: Polyethylene wear after total elbow arthroplasty. *J Bone Joint Surg Am* 87-A:1080-1087, 2005. Reproduced with permission of the Journal of Bone and Joint Surgery, Inc. Reproduced by permission of the publisher via Copyright Clearance Center, Inc.)

and ten patients had involvement of the right dominant elbow. The mean age at the bushing revision was fifty-two years, and the bushings were revised at an average of 7.9 years after implantation. All twelve patients reported pain, and five reported crepitus or a squeaking sound. None had extensive osteolysis. The mean duration of follow-up after the bushing exchange was sixty-five months. The mean arc of motion improved from 89 degrees before the surgery to 109 degrees after it. Three of the twelve patients underwent an additional articular revision at fifty-three, fifty-four, and 136 months after the initial bushing exchange. At the time of final follow-up, all twelve patients had functioning elbows.

Conclusions.—Isolated bushing exchange can be a successful revision procedure in patients with a semi-constrained linked total elbow prosthesis. Younger patients with a posttraumatic condition and/or severe pre-existing deformity are at greater risk for the development of excessive bushing wear. Patients should be cautioned against exceeding the recommended activity and lifting restrictions (Fig 1).

▶ The use of total elbow arthroplasty in the treatment of elbow deformity and loss of function has increased significantly in recent years, with excellent success. Polyethylene wear of the articulating bushings is an uncommon cause of revision.

The authors present a retrospective review of 919 total elbow arthroplasties and their experience with isolated bushing wear. Twelve of 919 patients (1.3%) required surgical revision for isolated bushing exchange. The key radiographic feature that suggests bushing wear is greater than 7° of angulation measured from a line drawn parallel to the humeral yoke and 1 drawn parallel to the ulnar component.

Predisposing factors leading to revision include young age, severe preoperative deformity, component malalignment, and posttraumatic arthritis as the cause for the index procedure. The mean age of the patients requiring revision at the time of the index procedure was 44 years (62 years for the overall group). The mean period between the index procedure and the isolated bushing exchange was 7.9 years. The patients were followed for an average of 65 months, and although 3 required a second bushing exchange, all 12 of the patients had functional elbow arthroplasties at the time of final follow-up. Also, unlike implants for other joints, the presence of wear debris alone does not appear to lead to fixation-compromising osteolysis in total elbow arthroplasty.

The authors of this study report on their large series of total elbow arthroplasties and help define the predisposing factors, diagnostic features, surgical technique, and the results of revision surgery to correct a previously undocumented complication, isolated bushing wear. Revision arthroplasty for this entity is not an extensive procedure and has been shown to be successful. This information is useful, given the increasing use of total elbow arthroplasty in the treatment of the deformed, arthritic, or unstable elbow.

J. Yao, MD

Primary Semi-constrained Arthroplasty for Chronic Fracture-Dislocations of the Elbow

Mighell MA, Dunham RC, Rommel EA, et al (Florida Orthopaedic Institute, Temple Terrace, Fla)
J Bone Joint Surg Br 87:191-195, 2005   8–5

Background.—Both ligament repair and reconstruction are appropriate approaches to recurrent elbow instability. Patients age 17 to 70 years with complex posterior dislocations of the elbow have had successful results using primary open reduction and internal fixation (ORIF). However, the complication rate of ORIF is high, with nerve injury (usually transient) affecting up to 40% of patients. Dislocations lasting 1 month to 2 years have undergone open reduction with release of the contracture and pinning of the ulnohumeral joint, but less than half achieve an arc of movement exceeding 90°. Elbow arthroplasty after trauma or nonunion is an accepted technique, but is seldom employed for chronic dislocation. The medium-term outcomes for older patients having primary semiconstrained total elbow arthroplasty for chronic dislocation of the elbow and posttraumatic arthritis were reported.

Methods.—Six consecutive patients were studied. All cases were reviewed retrospectively, noting indications for the primary semiconstrained total elbow procedure, age factors, injury patterns, and pathologic changes. Factors indicating a need for surgery included pain, age, bone quality, level of activity, history of rheumatoid arthritis, and failed reduction or fixation approaches. The six women ranged in age from 51 to 76 years (mean 65 years), which is older than is usually recommended for reconstruction. Coronoid fracture, radial head fracture, and posterior dislocation of the elbow (the "terrible triad") caused chronic instability in four patients. One had nonunion of a distal humeral fracture. Pathologic conditions present at surgery included triceps contracture, capsular thickening and contracture, foreshortening of the collateral ligaments, and arthritis of the ulnohumeral joint. All patients were assessed using the American Shoulder and Elbow Surgeons scale (ASES).

Results.—Patients' mean ASES pain score was three times better at final follow-up than preoperatively, and mean ASES functional score was 5.2 times better. The mean total range of motion score was 33° preoperatively and 121° postoperatively ($p < 0.001$). Radiographs revealed that three patients developed eccentric polyethylene wear, the most common complication. One patient with both eccentric wear and radiolucency also developed asymptomatic fibrous union of the olecranon process. Revision was recommended but refused by one patient with polyethylene wear.

Conclusions.—Primary elbow arthroplasty lessened pain and dramatically increased function and range of motion. Such results complement those showing elderly patients also benefit from primary elbow arthroplasty done for other indications (eg, failed ORIF, nonunion, acute fracture-dislocation, or distal humeral fracture). A linked implant is strongly recommended to compensate for incompetent collateral ligaments caused by chronic dislocation. Polyethylene wear results when absent collateral ligaments permit translation of varus and valgus forces, producing misalignment of the joint and concentrating increased bearing forces on the small contact areas of the bushings. Rather than sacrifice collateral ligaments to gain exposure when the triceps is subluxed laterally, the triceps tendon is now split in the midline and soft tissues released from bone as continuous sleeves of tissue. The repair of these soft-tissue sleeves in toto back to bone after implantation should permit the collateral ligaments to reattach and protect the polyethylene material.

▶ The authors of this paper present a retrospective study of six patients with chronic dislocations of the elbow that were treated by primary semiconstrained total elbow arthroplasty. The age range of these patients was from 51 to 76 years of age, and they were all females. Other studies have been performed on instability as well as unreduced posterior dislocations; however, this is the first one to really focus in on this more senior age group. In younger patients, previous studies such as that by Ring et al have advocated open treatment. However, total elbow arthroplasty is a well-established procedure and is frequently used in trauma and posttraumatic situations, especially in the more elderly population. The authors found that the ASES scores were 5.2 times better and the mean total range of motion increased from 31° to 121°. These were statistically significant at a p value of less than 0.001 for both variables. Three of their patients did develop polyethylene wear and one required revision for a periprosthetic fracture with another one requiring a bushing exchange. The results of this midterm study show that primary elbow arthroplasty results in a significant improvement for the patient by both decreasing the pain and dramatically increasing the function and range of motion. This option for reconstruction should be considered for any patient, but more likely will be reserved for those over the age of 50. The authors' results were quite encouraging.

S. F. M. Duncan, MD, MPH

Impaction Grafting in Revision Total Elbow Arthroplasty
Loebenberg MI, Adams R, O'Driscoll SW, et al (Mayo Clinic and Mayo Found, Rochester, Minn)
J Bone Joint Surg Am 87:99-106, 2005   8–6

Background.—Patients with severe osteolysis of both the distal humerus and the proximal ulna may need revision total elbow arthroplasty. The patient satisfaction and prosthesis longevity associated with this procedure in patients with rheumatoid arthritis now approach those obtained with lower-extremity arthroplasty. To handle bone loss, impaction grafting has been added. The results for 12 patients were reviewed.

Methods.—Retrospective review of medical records identified patients who had revision total elbow arthroplasty with cement and impacted allograft bone performed between 1993 and 1997. The mean age of the eight women and four men was 57 years, and follow-up was reported for at least 2

A

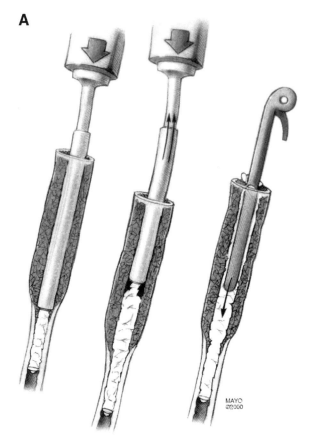

FIGURE 2A.—The smaller, inner tube is inserted farther than the outer tube, to a depth necessary for component fixation. (By permission of the Mayo Foundation.) (Courtesy of Loebenberg MI, Adams R, O'Driscoll SW, et al: Impaction grafting in revision total elbow arthroplasty. *J Bone Joint Surg Am* 87:99-106, 2005. Republished with permission of the Journal of Bone and Joint Surgery, Inc. Reproduced by permission of the publisher via Copyright Clearance Center, Inc.)

years and an average of 72 months (range 25 to 113 months). Rheumatoid arthritis was diagnosed in seven and posttraumatic arthritis in five patients. Aseptic loosening was the indication for revision arthroplasty in all cases. Two elbows were painless but had radiographic evidence of loosening of the humeral or ulnar component; 10 had pain and radiographic signs of loosening; and one of the 10 also had a periprosthetic fracture. Nine patients had at least one previous revision without impaction grafting, while three were having their initial revision procedure. Eight patients had ulnar and humeral component revision; one needed only humeral component replacement. Five patients required placement of six allograft struts to bridge structural defects; seven needed no strut graft augmentation. For 10 patients the linked semiconstrained Coonrad-Morrey prosthesis was used. Its humeral component has an anterior flange distally that resists posterior displacement and torsional stress when incorporated with bone graft. The procedure used a straight posterior skin incision unless the viability of later skin bridges required the use of previous incisions. The impaction grafting technique used a double-tube apparatus (Fig 2A).

Results.—At the latest follow-up evaluation, eight elbow prostheses were intact, two had been revised to address loosening, and one was revised because the ulnar component fractured. Infection complicated one patient's course, prompting resection arthroplasty; this patient had moderate instability. The average arc of elbow flexion improved from 86° before to 99° after the procedure. Preoperative range of motion was 29° in extension (range −15° to 60°) to 114° in flexion (range 70° to 145°). Postoperatively patients averaged 25° in extension to 123° in flexion. No functional range of motion was obtained in two patients. Functional scores based on ability to perform five tasks of daily function averaged 11 points before and 20 points after surgery (maximum possible score, 25 points). An average of 58 months (range 25 to 84 months) after impaction grafting, radiographs showed improvement in loosening and markedly better bone quality in the impact graft region of the eight patients with intact prostheses. Complications developed in six patients and required surgery in five. Included were infection (after 27 months), triceps rupture (repaired after 4 months), periprosthetic ulnar rupture (repaired after 9 months), symptomatic ulnar neuropathy, and radial nerve palsy.

Conclusions.—Revision arthroplasty is usually done for prosthetic loosening, which is often accompanied by substantial periprosthetic osteolysis. The 12 patients had impaction grafting with revision total elbow arthroplasty to treat osteolysis. Complications developed in several patients and required more surgery. The impaction technique employed differed. Three patients treated with one technique had a solidly fixed implant on later exploration. Intraoperative and perioperative complications did not exceed those reported in other reviews.

▶ This important study looks at the results of impaction grafting and revision total elbow arthroplasty. This was performed in patients who had osteolysis and bone resorption and was either a revision procedure or a re-revision procedure. The patients were of both genders and had mixed diagnoses including rheumatoid, osteoarthritic, and posttraumatic. The authors utilized the Coonrad-Morrey prosthesis in 10 patients. Others required custom components. The article nicely discussed the operative technique and included diagrams on the technique as well. Anyone considering performing an impaction grafting in a revision total elbow should definitely review this article the night prior to surgery to refresh them on some of the technique pointers. The authors did utilize the Mayo Elbow Performance Score, and the score was 55 points preoperatively and 83 points postoperatively. Patients improved from 23 points in pain to 36 points postoperatively at their last visit. Arc of range of motion improved from 86° to 99° after surgery. Two of their patients did not obtain functional range of motion. One patient did undergo a resection arthroplasty after deep infection developed. The ability to perform five tasks of daily living was scored; preoperatively this was 11 points compared with 20 points postoperatively. Six of the 12 patients did have complications; surgery was required for five of them. Two patients developed symptoms and radiographic signs of loosening. Deep infection developed in one patient, requiring implant removal. Another patient had a triceps rupture, which was repaired four months after the surgery, as well as a periprosthetic fracture of the ulna. Symptomatic ulnar neuropathy developed in one patient, and one patient had radial nerve palsy. These other complications resolved without further intervention. Prosthetic loosening remains the most common reason for revision arthroplasty. Overall, an impaction grafting offers a nice technique to try and salvage the total elbow with significant osteolysis and other bone loss. In their series, strut grafting was also utilized, which probably enhanced their results.

S. F. M. Duncan, MD, MPH

9　Elbow: Cubital Tunnel Syndrome and Ulnar Nerve

The Position of Crossing Branches of the Medial Antebrachial Cutaneous Nerve During Cubital Tunnel Surgery in Humans
Lowe JB III, Maggi SP, Mackinnon SE (Washington Univ, St Louis)
Plast Reconstr Surg 114:692-696, 2004　　　　　　　　　　　　　　9–1

Abstract.—The posterior branch of the medial antebrachial cutaneous nerve courses in proximity to the cubital tunnel and is particularly prone to injury during ulnar nerve release at the elbow. Inadvertent injury to medial antebrachial cutaneous nerve branches during surgery can result in the formation of painful neuromas that can be misdiagnosed as recurrent disease. It is important to understand the relevant anatomy of the medial antebrachial cutaneous nerve branches during cubital tunnel surgery to avoid significant postoperative morbidity. This prospective observational anatomic study examined the position of the posterior branch of the medial antebrachial cutaneous nerve in relationship to a standard approach to the cubital tunnel in a randomly selected group of 97 patients undergoing primary surgery over a 3-year period. Medial antebrachial cutaneous nerve branches were noted to cross at or proximal to the medial humeral epicondyle 61 percent of the time at an average proximal distance of 1.8 cm. Medial antebrachial cutaneous nerve branches were noted to cross distal to the medial humeral epicondyle 100 percent of the time at an average distal distance of 3.1 cm. Understanding the general position of crossing medial antebrachial cutaneous nerve branches during ulnar nerve release at the elbow may help to prevent iatrogenic injury to this cutaneous nerve.

▶ Injury to branches of the medial antebrachial cutaneous nerve with ulnar nerve decompression is very troublesome to patients. Protecting this nerve in cubital tunnel surgery is critical. The authors studied 97 consecutive cubital tunnel patients through an 8-cm typical exposure and documented the number and position of cubital tunnel branches intraoperatively. On average, patients had 1.9 branches crossing over the ulnar nerve. A proximal branch was, on average, 1.8 cm from the medial epicondyle, while a distal branch was, on average, 3.1 cm distal to the medial epicondyle. One hundred percent of patients had medial antebrachial cutaneous nerve branches crossing over or in the proximity of the wound. In other words, branches are potentially numerous, always present, and subject to iatrogenic injury. This study reinforces the need for careful intraoperative dissection in cubital tunnel surgery to avoid injury to this nerve and its branches.

R. Buntic, MD

Painful Neuroma of the Posterior Cutaneous Nerve of the Forearm After Surgery for Lateral Humeral Epicondylitis
Dellon AL, Kim J, Ducic I (Johns Hopkins Univ, Baltimore, Md; Univ of Arizona, Tucson; Keio Univ, Seoul, Korea; et al)
J Hand Surg [Am] 29:387-390, 2004   9–2

Background.—Failure of extensor tendon origin release to relieve the symptoms of lateral humeral epicondylitis is usually attributed to radial nerve entrapment, but painful neuroma presents an alternative explanation. The diagnostic and therapeutic approach to these patients was described.

Methods.—The charts of nine patients who had pain after lateral humeral epicondylitis surgery were evaluated retrospectively. Measures noted included pain history, surgical findings during exploration of the lateral elbow scar, and outcome of the operation. None of the patients had pain from radial tunnel syndrome as evidenced by lack of pain referred to the lateral humeral epicondyle with resisted middle finger extension.

Results.—All nine patients had a neuroma of the posterior cutaneous nerve of the forearm (PCNF) in the scar from the original surgery. Each neuroma was resected and the proximal end of the nerve was then implanted into the brachioradialis muscle proximal to the elbow joint. From 1.0 to 2.6 years (mean 1.4 years) after surgery, eight of the nine patients had excellent pain relief. The ninth patient had a good response. Repeat surgery was not needed, nor were there any complications postoperatively.

Conclusions.—When performing surgery in the region of the lateral humeral epicondyle or over the extensor mass or surgery to explore or decompress the radial nerve or its posterior interosseous branch, it is necessary to account for the PCNF to avoid inadvertent injury. Its location places it at risk for injury during surgery. It is best to identify the nerve immediately after making the skin incision. If injury does occur, treatment involving resection and implantation of the proximal nerve end into the brachioradialis muscle proximal to the elbow joint is highly successful.

▶ The combination of painful neuroma and lateral epicondylitis is indeed a frightening consideration. Recurrent pain following lateral epicondylitis surgery is frustrating for surgeon and patient alike, particularly when the condition has endured for long periods. The proximity of the PCNF to the lateral epicondyle should call in to question, as illustrated in this study of 9 patients, the possibility that previously documented failures from lateral epicondyle surgery could be related to painful PCNF neuromas. Perhaps PCNF should also be considered a primary source of lateral elbow pain. It would be interesting to know if any of these 9 patients had preoperative corticosteroid injections in the region of the PCNF, as this could also cause neuroma formation. On the basis of the anatomy of the PCNF and the findings of this study, it would seem appropriate to alter the location of the incision for lateral epicondylitis surgery.

P. M. Murray, MD

Ulnar Neuropathy at the Elbow: Follow-Up and Prognostic Factors Determining Outcome
Beekman R, Wokke JHJ, Schoemaker MC, et al (Atrium Med Ctr, Heerlen, The Netherlands; Univ Med Ctr, Utrecht, The Netherlands; St Elisabeth Hosp, Tilburg, The Netherlands; et al)
Neurology 63:1675-1680, 2004   9–3

Objective.—To determine the outcome in patients with ulnar neuropathy at the elbow (UNE) treated surgically or conservatively, and the prognostic value of clinical, sonographic, and electrophysiologic features.

Methods.—After a median follow-up of 14 months, 69 of 84 patients initially included in a prospective blinded study on the diagnostic value of sonography in UNE were re-evaluated. The patients underwent renewed systematic clinical and sonographic examination. Patients were scored as having a poor (stable or progressive symptoms) or favorable (complete remission of symptoms or improvement) outcome.

Results.—Of the 74 initially affected arms, 12 (16%) had a complete remission, 21 (28%) improved, 25 (34%) remained stable, and 16 (22%) had progression. Surgically treated patients (28 arms) had a more favorable outcome than those treated conservatively ($p = 0.03$). After surgery, the mean ulnar nerve diameter decreased from 3.2 to 2.9 mm ($p = 0.03$), while this was not seen after conservative treatment. Multiple logistic regression analysis showed that more outspoken nerve enlargement found during sonography at the time of the diagnosis was associated with a poor outcome (OR: 2.9, $p = 0.009$). Furthermore, the presence of a motor conduction block (OR: 0.2, $p = 0.03$) and motor velocity slowing across the elbow (OR: 0.1, $p = 0.01$) were associated with a favorable outcome.

Conclusion.—More pronounced ulnar nerve thickening at the time of the diagnosis is associated with poor outcome at follow-up, especially in conservatively treated cases, while electrodiagnostic signs of demyelination on testing indicate favorable outcome.

▶ This is a prospective study to evaluate treatment outcomes for UNE. The information derived from this article can be useful in counseling patients regarding surgical and conservative treatments for UNE. The interesting part of this study is the use of ultrasonography in delineating the extent of UNE.

Ultrasonography is rarely used to evaluate nerve compression syndrome. However, advancements in ultrasonography may yield more accurate visualization of nerve structures in the upper extremity. The ulnar nerve lies in a subcutaneous plane that is amendable to ultrasonographic examination. Perhaps ultrasonography will play an important role in diagnosing ulnar nerve entrapment syndrome at the elbow.

K. C. Chung, MD, MS

Outcomes of Cubital Tunnel Surgery Among Patients With Absent Sensory Nerve Conduction

Taha A, Galarza M, Zuccarello M, et al (American Univ of Beirut, Lebanon; VA Med Ctr, Cincinnati, Ohio; Kettering Med Ctr, Dayton, Ohio)
Neurosurgery 54:891-896, 2004   9–4

Objective.—To report the outcomes of cubital tunnel surgery for patients with absent ulnar sensory nerve conduction.

Methods.—The charts of 34 patients who exhibited clinical symptoms of ulnar nerve entrapment at the elbow and who had electromyography-confirmed prolonged motor nerve conduction across the cubital tunnel in association with absent sensory nerve conduction were reviewed. The mean age was 63 years, and the mean symptom duration was 17 months. Four patients had bilateral symptoms. Surgery was performed for 38 limbs, i.e., neurolysis for 21 limbs and subcutaneous transposition for 17 limbs. Fifteen limbs demonstrated associated ulnar nerve-related motor weakness. The mean postoperative follow-up period was 4 years (range, 3 mo to 11 yr).

Results.—Sensory symptoms (i.e., pain, paresthesia, and two-point discrimination) improved in 20 limbs (53%), and muscle strength improved in 2 limbs (13%). Improvements in sensory symptoms were not related to patient age, symptom duration, cause, severity of prolonged motor nerve conduction, select psychological factors, associated medical diseases, associated cervical pathological conditions, or type of surgery. Improvements in sensory symptoms were significantly decreased among patients who had experienced cervical disease for more than 1 year and patients with bilateral symptoms.

Conclusion.—Patients with cubital tunnel syndrome who have absent sensory nerve conduction seem to experience less improvement of sensory symptoms after surgery, compared with all patients with cubital tunnel syndrome described in the literature. Bilateral symptoms and delayed surgery secondary to associated cervical spine disease seem to be significant negative factors for postoperative improvement of sensory symptoms. Sensory symptoms improved similarly among patients who underwent neurolysis or subcutaneous transposition.

▶ Surgery for ulnar nerve entrapment at the elbow has worse outcomes than carpal tunnel release. Despite adequate decompression of the ulnar nerve at the elbow, patients continue to complain of sensory and motor dysfunction.

This retrospective study presented a limited number of patients with sensory conduction block who underwent ulnar nerve transposition at the elbow. Predictably, the authors found poor outcomes for this group of patients. The take-home message is simply that more severe nerve pathology will result in worse surgical outcomes.

K. C. Chung, MD, MS

Treatment of Cubital Tunnel Syndrome by Frontal Partial Medial Epicondylectomy. A Retrospective Series of 55 Cases
Popa M, Dubert Th (Clinique la Francilienne, Pontault-Combault, France)
J Hand Surg [Br] 29B:563-567, 2004   9–5

The outcomes of 55 cases of cubital tunnel syndrome treated by a partial frontal epicondylectomy are presented at a mean follow-up of 38 months. According to McGowan classification, 25 cases were grade I (45%), 12 grade II (22%) and 18 grade III (33%). The results (Wilson and Krout classification) were excellent or good in 41 patients (75%), fair in nine patients and unchanged in five, without any worsening or recurrence. Total relief was reported in 80% of grade I, 75% of grade II and 66% of grade III patients. Seven painful scars and one persistent 15° elbow extension deficit were the only complications. The satisfaction rate was 93%. This technique preserves bony protection, the blood supply and gliding tissues for the nerve and nerve recovery were comparable to other surgical procedures. Residual pain at the osteotomy site was not a serious problem (Figs 1 and 2).

▶ Primary surgical management of cubital tunnel syndrome produces good to excellent results in over 90% of patients. Often the choice of surgical procedures is based on the surgeon's previous experience and acceptance of the potential risks associated with each surgical procedure. Medial epicondylectomy with external neurolysis is one potential surgical intervention. Critics report that the morbidity of this procedure includes bone site pain and medial sided elbow instability. To address these critiques, modifications of the medial epicondylectomy include the subtotal medial epicondylectomy.

The authors of this article have provided a new modification of the medial epicondylectomy with the frontal partial medial epicondylectomy. In this series, there was no evidence of valgus instability or nerve subluxation. Furthermore, there was only mild local pain in 7 of the 55 elbows in the series. However, one must be cautious in interpreting the data and determining the efficacy of this procedure as (1) the outcome measures that were used had limited objective parameters and (2) a significant number of the patients in this series also had a concomitant carpal tunnel or Guyon's canal release.

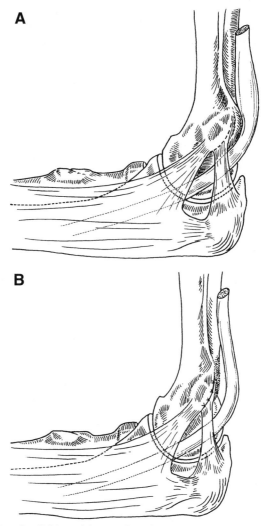

FIGURE 1.—Frontal medial epicondylectomy allows slight anterior translation of the ulnar nerve. In order to preserve the gliding and vascularization tissues around the ulnar nerve, the fibrous aponeurotic band is first detached from the medial epicondyle, allowing exposure to its posterior side. This structure is later reattached. (a) Pre-operative and (b) postoperative lateral view. (Reprinted from Popa M, Dubert Th: Treatment of cubital tunnel syndrome by frontal partial medial epicondylectomy: A retrospective series of 55 cases. *J Hand Surg [Br]* 29B:563-567. Copyright 2004, with permission from The British Society for Surgery of the Hand.)

Nevertheless, this series provides further evidence that a subtotal medial epicondylectomy is an effective surgical method of treating cubital tunnel syndrome without the risk of devascularizing the ulnar nerve. Surgeons should consider this procedure as a potential option for management of cubital tunnel syndrome in the appropriate patient.

R. Gupta, MD

FIGURE 2.

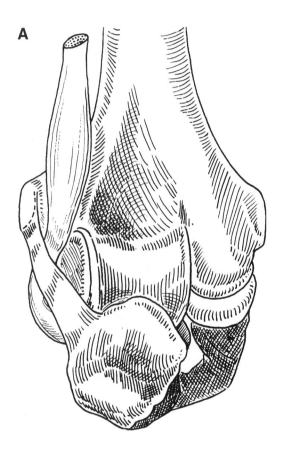

(Continued)

FIGURE 2 (cont.)

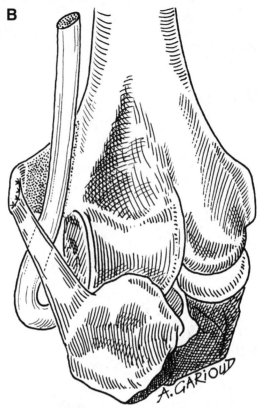

FIGURE 2.—Same as in Fig 1: (a) Pre-operative and (b) Postoperative frontal posterior view. (Reprinted from Popa M, Dubert Th: Treatment of cubital tunnel syndrome by frontal partial medial epicondylectomy: A retrospective series of 55 cases. *J Hand Surg [Br]* 29B:563-567. Copyright 2004, with permission from The British Society for Surgery of the Hand.)

Functional Outcomes in Young, Active Duty, Military Personnel After Submuscular Ulnar Nerve Transposition

Fitzgerald BT, Dao KD, Shin AY (Naval Med Ctr San Diego, Calif; Westminster, Calif; Mayo Clinic, Rochester, Minn)
J Hand Surg [Am] 29A:619-624, 2004   9–6

Purpose.—The purpose of this study was to report on the results of submuscular ulnar nerve transposition (SMUNT) for treatment of cubital tunnel syndrome in a young, active duty, military population.

Methods.—Twenty patients (20 extremities) were evaluated retrospectively a minimum of 12 months after surgery. Outcome analyses were performed using the Disability of the Arm, Shoulder, and Hand (DASH) questionnaire and the Bishop-Kleinman rating scales, physical examination, return-to-work analysis, evaluation of complication rate, and overall patient satisfaction.

Results.—At an average follow-up evaluation of 24 months (range, 12–38 mo), 19 patients had returned to full military active duty work status. The average duration of limited work capacity after surgery was 4.8 months (range, 3–7 mo). The DASH scores improved from an average of 32.5 points before surgery to 6.2 points after surgery. In 19 patients the functional outcome evaluated with the Bishop-Kleinman rating system was excellent. There were no poor outcomes using this rating score. Statistically significant improvements in both key pinch and grip strength were noted. Complications included one permanent and 2 transient neuropraxias of the medial antebrachial cutaneous nerve. Overall 19 of 20 patients were satisfied with the procedure and would have the surgery again if required.

Conclusions.—Submuscular ulnar nerve transposition for cubital tunnel syndrome provides a reliable rate of return to full active duty work in military personnel with good patient satisfaction and minimal complications.

▶ Twenty active duty military patients underwent SMUNT for cubital tunnel syndrome. This retrospective review demonstrates functional improvement in the 19 patients who underwent evaluation. Overall, a 95% satisfaction rate was found. The study demonstrates that this operation is effective and supports the existing literature. It would be interesting to compare these results with any other surgical techniques that the same authors may have utilized to add further understanding as to which operation may best treat cubital tunnel syndrome, as they are treating a healthy and motivated group of patients.

C. Carroll IV, MD

The V-Sling: A Modified Medial Intermuscular Septal Sling for Anterior Transposition of the Ulnar Nerve
Tan V, Pope J, Daluiski A, et al (Univ of Medicine and Dentistry of New Jersey, Newark; Hosp for Special Surgery, New York)
J Hand Surg [Am] 29:325-327, 2004   9–7

Background.—Surgery for cubital tunnel syndrome is designed to relieve pressure on the nerve at the elbow and includes various techniques. A modification of the method developed by Pribyl and Robinson was developed in which a second limb to the sling is developed to permit a gentler transition of the ulnar nerve on entry into the flexor carpi ulnaris muscle belly.

> *Technique.*—Elevate the arm and apply a tourniquet for exsanguination. Abduct and externally rotate the shoulder, then flex the elbow. Center a 10-cm long medial curvilinear skin incision over the cubital tunnel. Carry the dissection down through the subcutaneous levels to the deep fascia over the triceps and flexor-pronator mass, taking care to avoid any cutaneous nerves. Identify the ulnar nerve,

which should be located proximal to the tunnel and posterior to the medial intermuscular septum. Free it along its entire course from the proximal end of the incision to the proximal muscle belly of the flexor carpi ulnaris. Preserve the inferior ulnar collateral vessels if possible. Divide the medial intermuscular septum about 8 cm proximal to where it attaches to the medial epicondyle. Dissect a longitudinal strip of the septum until only the medial epicondylar attachment remains. Transpose the ulnar nerve anterior to the medial epicondyle. Create an inverted V of the free distal end of the intermuscular septum, then suture its midpoint onto the flexor-pronator fascia or subcutaneous tissue. This keeps the ulnar nerve from subluxating posteriorly. Attach the distal limb of the fascial sling about 1 to 1.5 cm distal to the proximal attachment, permitting a gentler course and avoiding perching the ulnar nerve on top of the medial epicondyle. Check the nerve again once the sling is sutured in place, releasing any compression under the fascial sling. Ensure that the nerve does not become kinked when the elbow is flexed or extended. Close the arm wound and wrap it in cast padding, then apply a compressive bandage over the cotton. Leave the compressive dressing in place for 10 to 14 days, but do not restrict the patient's activities except by the presence of the dressing. Full activity is resumed once the dressing and sutures are removed.

Conclusions.—Use of the V-sling technique may prove advantageous for patients with cubital tunnel syndrome not responding to 6 weeks of elbow splinting and anti-inflammatory medications; for patients whose ulnar nerve symptoms develop after elbow contracture release; and for patients who suffer fractures about the elbow requiring fixation hardware that could impinge on the ulnar nerve. Patients who have had previous medial elbow surgery may not be helped if the septum is not available.

▶ The technique described by the authors is a modification of a previous anterior subcutaneous ulnar nerve transposition technique described by Pribyl and Robinson.[1] The original technique, which is similar to the flexor/pronator muscle facial sling technique described by Black et al, describes harvesting a proximally based sling of intermuscular septum to act as a barrier to posterior subluxation of the anteriorly transposed ulnar nerve. The V-sling technique employs an additional limb to the construct based on the notion that two limbs of the intermuscular septum creates a "more gentle transition" for the ulnar nerve as it is mobilized anterior to the medial epicondyle. In comparing the intraoperative pictures from this article with the articles by Pribyl and Robinson as well as Black et al,[2] it is difficult to detect if a there is a clear advantage from the use of any of these three techniques. However, it does appear that the use of medial intermuscular septum for the creation of an ulnar nerve anterior transposition stabilizing sling is technically easier and may result in a more predictable construct. The potential for ulnar constriction or kinking after subcutaneous anterior transposition of the ulnar nerve seems less likely when broader contact exists between some form of subdermal sling, irrespective of technique.

P. M. Murray, MD

References

1. Pribyl CR, Robinson B: Use of the medial intermuscular septum as a fascial sling during anterior transposition of the ulnar nerve. *J Hand Surg [Am]* 23:500-504, 1998.
2. Black BT, Barron OA, Townsend PF, et al: Stabilized subcutaneous ulnar nerve transposition with immediate range of motion: Long-term follow-up. *J Bone Joint Surg Am* 82:1544-1551, 2000.

Revision Anterior Submuscular Transposition of the Ulnar Nerve for Failed Subcutaneous Transposition
Vogel RB, Nossaman BC, Rayan GM (Univ of Oklahoma, Oklahoma City)
Br J Plast Surg 57:311-316, 2004   9–8

Summary.—We evaluated the results of revision surgery for persistent cubital tunnel syndrome after failed surgical treatment. Eighteen patients were evaluated with an average age of 44 years. The majority of the primary procedures were subcutaneous transpositions (15 patients). The average follow-up time was 34 months. All patients were treated with a submuscular transposition of the ulnar nerve and Z-lengthening of the flexor-pronator origin. The most common operative findings were perineural scarring (16), retained medial intermuscular septum (10) and common flexor aponeurosis (9). Pre-operative and post-operative data were compared. The majority of patients improved their postoperative grade and their ability to do daily activities or work and stated that the surgery met some or all of their expectations. Most patients had partial relief of their pain and the satisfaction rate was 78%. Our study suggests that although these results are less favorable than those for the primary procedure, submuscular transposition is a useful technique for revision of failed cubital tunnel syndrome surgery.

▶ These authors review their experience with reoperation after cubital tunnel release. There are several important points presented. The first important point is the distinction between recurrent and persistent symptoms. The latter implies either incomplete release of the ulnar nerve or the creation (after transfer) of a new site of compression. Neither of these scenarios would be particularly related to the transposition method. The former implies an ongoing process, perhaps with perineural scarring creating new compression after an initial successful decompression.

Unfortunately, when evaluating this work, the reader is unable to review the electrodiagnostic studies. The authors mention that 9 (50%) of the patients had positive electromyelograms, but it is not clear whether this was before or after the original surgery. Certainly, all of the patients that presented for reoperation had electrodiagnostic studies done prior to re-release. It would have been helpful to compare these with their initial preoperative electrodiagnostic findings.

Intraoperative findings at re-operation were interesting: 89% had perineural scarring; 27% had an intact arcade of Struthers, 55% had an intact/retained medial intermuscular septum, and 50% had an intact common flexor aponeurosis. These data illustrate the following:

1. Perineural scarring occurred in all groups, regardless of type of transposition performed. Although it is difficult to say from these data whether this scarring had a significant role in the recurrence of symptoms, it does seem to support the observation that the technique of ulnar nerve transposition does not appear to impact the degree of perineural scarring.
2. Perhaps the most important component of this operation is adequate release of the ulnar nerve. The most compelling and frequent finding at re-operation was some residual anatomical point that had not been adequately released at the initial operation.

M. Concannon, MD

Missile-Caused Ulnar Nerve Injuries: Outcomes of 128 Repairs
Roganovic Z (Military Med Academy, Belgrade, Serbia)
Neurosurgery 55:1120-1129, 2004   9–9

Objective.—This prospective study presents repair results after missile-caused ulnar nerve ruptures as well as factors influencing the outcomes.

Methods.—Between 1991 and 1994, 128 casualties with missile-caused complete ulnar nerve injury were managed surgically in the Neurosurgical Department of the Belgrade Military Medical Academy. At least 4 years after surgery, we scored sensorimotor recovery, neurophysiological recovery, and patient judgment of the outcome. On the basis of the total score, we defined the final outcome as poor, insufficient, good, or excellent. The last two outcomes were considered to be successful.

Results.—A successful outcome was obtained in 0% of high-level, 33.8% of intermediate-level, and 77.3% of low-level repairs ($P < 0.001$). On average, the nerve defect, preoperative interval, and patient age were lower for patients with a successful outcome than for those with an unsuccessful outcome ($P = 0.004$, $P = 0.032$, and $P = 0.003$, respectively). Worsening of the outcome was related to nerve defect longer than 4.5 cm, preoperative interval longer than 5.5 months, and age older than 23 years ($P = 0.002$, $P = 0.034$, and $P = 0.023$, respectively). A successful outcome occurred in 48.8% of patients repaired with direct suture and in 41.2% of patients repaired with a nerve graft ($P > 0.05$). A successful outcome also occurred in 22.2% of combined ulnar-median nerve repairs and in 49.5% of isolated ulnar nerve repairs ($P = 0.011$). Repair level ($P < 0.001$), preoperative interval ($P = 0.001$), length of the nerve defect ($P < 0.001$), and associated median nerve rupture ($P = 0.028$) were independent predictors of a successful outcome.

Conclusion.—The outcome of ulnar nerve repair depends significantly on the repair level, preoperative interval, associated median nerve injury, length of the nerve defect, and age of the patient. High-level ulnar nerve repair is probably useless if performed in the classic manner.

▶ Ulnar nerve repair after high-velocity penetrating trauma can have mixed results. While repair can often be achieved with nerve transposition and release of tension with wrist and elbow flexion, nerve grafting may be necessary. In this group of 128 war-wounded ulnar nerve injury patients requiring surgical repair, the authors very carefully document postoperative results with a unique classification system. A total of 43 patients had end-to-end nerve repair, while 85 required nerve grafting. The authors conclude that the following factors negatively influenced outcome: high level of injury (above the elbow), long duration to repair (>5 months), associated median nerve rupture, and increasing patient age. The series is large, and the results are well documented and reinforce our general understanding of severe ulnar nerve injury and repair. Although the classification system used is not directly comparable to other sources in the literature, the authors break down results in enough detail that sensory and motor recovery as measured by the British Medical Research Council classification is present and comparable to that in other studies.

R. Buntic, MD

Endoscopic Release of the Ulnar Nerve at the Elbow Using the Agee Device: A Cadaveric Study
Bain GI, Bajhau A (Modbury Public Hosp, Adelaide, Australia; Univ of Adelaide, Australia)
Arthroscopy 21:691-695, 2005   9–10

Background.—Ulnar nerve compression occurs most often at the arcade of Struthers, the cubital tunnel, and the fascia of the flexor carpi ulnaris. Performing ulnar nerve release around the elbow can be accomplished by using either an open or an endoscopic method. The safety and efficacy of the Agee endoscopic system for the release of the ulnar nerve at the elbow were evaluated.

Methods.—In 6 cadaveric specimens, the ulnar nerve was identified through a 3-cm longitudinal incision between the medial epicondyle and olecranon. Ulnar nerve release was then performed by using the Agee device under endoscopic guidance. Loupe magnification was used to evaluate the ulnar nerve, its branching, and the structures that had been divided.

Results.—Complete division of the arcade of Struthers, cubital tunnel retinaculum, and flexor carpi ulnaris aponeurosis was achieved in all cases. The intermuscular septum and flexor-pronator aponeurosis around the ulnar nerve were dilated. The ulnar nerve sustained no injuries, and the motor and sensory branches were intact. From 2 to 4 motor branches were found in each elbow and were located between 9 mm proximal and 31 mm distal to the medial epicondyle. Thirteen of the 18 motor branches (72%) were radial. All the capsular branches were also intact. These were found between 15 mm proximal and 4 mm distal to the medial epicondyle. Eight were radial, and most (88%) were identified proximal to the medial epicondyle.

Conclusions.—No injury to the ulnar nerve was incurred in any of the specimens. An average of 3 motor branches and 1 to 2 sensory branches of the ulnar nerve were found at each elbow. Seventy-two percent of the motor and 88% of the sensory branches arose from the radial side of the nerve. The endoscopic Agee system was found to be safe and effective in addressing ulnar nerve decompression in these cadaveric specimens.

▶ The use of the endoscope/arthroscope has revolutionized the surgical treatment of many conditions. However, the use of the endoscope to release peripheral nerves has been met with significant controversy. Early reports of nerve injury and incomplete release have led many to avoid or abandon these procedures. Others (including myself) believe that endoscopic techniques can lead to diminished postoperative patient discomfort, earlier recovery, and possibly improved outcomes. Recent prospective human studies have shown endoscopic carpal tunnel release to be a safe and effective procedure. This cadaver study demonstrates the possibility that endoscopic ulnar nerve decompression can be a safe and effective procedure. However, more study is needed before recommending this as a good alternative to open treatment. I am particularly concerned about the small diameter of the cubital tunnel compared with the carpal tunnel, especially in patients undergoing surgery who likely have constriction of the cubital tunnel. In addition, if this procedure proves to be safe and effective, we must heed the lessons of endoscopic carpal tunnel release and mandate adequate training of surgeons before performing this procedure in clinical practice.

D. I. Ilan, MD

10 Distal Radius

Biomechanics in Uniaxial Compression of Three Distal Radius Volar Plates
Osada D, Sujita S, Tamai K, et al (Dokkyo Univ, Tochigi, Japan)
J Hand Surg [Am] 29A:446-451, 2004   10–1

Purpose.—A new fixed-angle volar plate for a dorsally displaced distal radius fracture was designed with the aim of avoiding soft tissue problems due to dorsal plating. The purpose of this study was to compare the biomechanical properties of this new plate with 2 existing volar plates in a cadaver model.

Methods.—Three different plates were applied on surgically simulated unstable extra-articular distal radius fractures in formalin-fixed cadaver radiuses. Group 1 (volarly placed AO titanium Distal Radius plates [Synthes Ltd, Paoli, PA]; n = 6), group 2 (volarly placed titanium Symmetry plates [DePuy ACE Co, El Segundo, CA]; n = 6), and group 3 (volarly placed newly designed titanium plates; n = 6) were tested to failure under axial compression with a materials testing machine. Specimens of all 3 groups had similar bone mineral density.

Results.—Group 3 specimens had significantly greater elastic limit and ultimate strength than the other 2 groups. Specimens of group 3 had the greatest rigidity, although this was statistically insignificant compared with the other 2 groups. All plates (groups 1, 2, 3) failed in apex volar angulation.

Conclusions.—The newly designed plate fixation system is the strongest of the systems tested and may offer adequate stability for the treatment of a distal radius fracture in which the dorsal and/or volar metaphyseal cortex is comminuted severely.

▶ This is a cadaver study that investigates the ability of 3 volarly placed internal fixation plates used in distal radius fractures to resist displacement of the fracture fragments. The 3 systems tested were the volar AO titanium Distal Radius plates designed by Synthes, the Symmetry plates designed by DePuy, and newly designed locking plates designed and available in Japan. The plates designed in Japan were found to have the greatest strength. Analysis of the data reveals the presumed reason for their strength is that this new design combines a thicker plate with locking screws. The results of this study may help when choosing an internal fixation system for the distal radius, although multiple other factors should be considered.

W. Short, MD

A Cadaver Model to Evaluate the Accuracy and Reproducibility of Plain Radiograph Step and Gap Measurements for Intra-Articular Fracture of the Distal Radius
McCallister WV, Smith JM, Knight J, et al (Univ of Washington, Seattle; Central Illinois Orthopaedic Ctr, Decatur)
J Hand Surg [Am] 29A:841-847, 2004   10–2

Purpose.—The purpose of this study was to determine the accuracy and reproducibility of intra-articular step-off and gap displacements measured on plain radiographs using a standard cadaver model.

Methods.—Twenty-two physicians, in a blinded randomized fashion using a standard technique, examined the radiographs of 12 unique combinations of step and gap displacement created by a 3-part intra-articular osteotomy of the distal radius. Observer accuracy, inter- and intraobserver agreement, and tolerance limits were calculated.

Results.—The results of this study suggest that observers, independent of skill level, may measure step-off and gap displacements accurately to within .62 ± .53 mm (95% confidence interval = .59–65). The accuracy of measurement was influenced by the quality of the radiograph. Intraclass correlation coefficient scores showed "substantial" (.78) to "almost perfect" (.81) inter- and intraobserver agreement.

Conclusions.—These data can aid in the interpretation of clinical studies of acute distal radius fractures that are based on plain radiography.

▶ Post-traumatic degenerative joint disease is one of the potential sequelae of a displaced intra-articular distal radius fracture. The literature suggests that displacement of the articular surface of the distal radius of 2 mm or greater increases the risk of postfracture arthritis. McCallister et al questioned the ability to accurately and reliably measure intra-articular fracture displacement of less than 2 mm on plain radiographs. They utilized a cadaver model to create intra-articular fractures of the distal radius. Twelve unique combinations of step and gap displacement were created and evaluated. Accuracy and reproducibility of intra- and inter-observer measurements were assessed. Twenty-two physicians with varied levels of experience in evaluation and treatment of distal radius fractures examined the radiographs in a blinded, randomized fashion. Radiographic technique was standardized to control for magnification. Inter-observer reliability was substantial for step-off and almost perfect for gap measurements. Intra-observer reliability was almost perfect for step-off and gap measurements. The authors conclude that observers may accurately and reliably measure step-off and gap displacement of less than 1 mm using plain radiographs. The results were independent of observer skill level and were influenced by quality of radiographs. The study supports use of radiographic step-off and gap displacement measurements on plain radiography when assessing alignment of the distal radial articular surface post fracture.

S. H. Berner, MD

Displaced Fracture of the Distal Radius in Children: Factors Responsible for Redisplacement After Closed Reduction

Zamzam MM, Khoshhal KI (King Khalid Univ, Riyadh, Saudi Arabia)

J Bone Joint Surg Br 87-B:841-843, 2005   10–3

Background.—Fractures of the distal forearm are among the most common fractures in children. Healing is rapid, and functional recovery is excellent after closed reduction and casting. It has been reported that up to 34% of fractures of the distal radius can redisplace early after reduction. The factors responsible for redisplacement after an initially acceptable closed reduction have not been clearly defined. The risk factors for redisplacement of a displaced fracture of the distal radius in children after closed reduction were identified.

Methods.—A retrospective review was conducted of 183 children with simple fractures of the distal radius, with or without fractures of the ulna, treated by closed reduction and cast immobilization. The patients included 144 boys and 39 girls (mean age, 8 years; range, 3-16 years). Hospital charts were reviewed for the following data: age, sex, level of the treating physician, type of anesthesia used for the initial closed reduction, time at which the redisplacement was diagnosed, management of the redisplacement, duration of follow-up, and the final outcome. Radiographs were reviewed for initial displacement, the presence of an ipsilateral distal ulnar fracture, the acceptability of the initial closed reduction, criteria for diagnosing redisplacement, and the final radiographic outcome.

Results.—Redisplacement occurred in 46 patients (25%), of whom 35 (76%) had an associated fracture of the distal ulna. Redisplacement was diagnosed in the first 14 days after the initial closed reduction.

Conclusions.—Children who initially have a completely displaced fracture of the distal radius should be manipulated under general anesthesia. It is also recommended that percutaneous K-wire fixation be used to ensure stabilization and avoid redisplacement, even in patients in whom perfect closed reductions have been achieved.

▶ This study from Saudi Arabia retrospectively examined children younger than 16 years with displaced radius fractures, from 1998 to 2003. The authors found that a completely displaced fracture was the single greatest predictor for redisplacement. The accompanying risk factors (involvement of the ulnar column and inadequate anesthesia) correlated with the severity of injury, which is a finding similar to that in the adult population. The authors reported that age was not a significant factor. This is surprising, given the changes in bone elasticity and periosteal thickness that occur in children corresponding to variable incidence and fracture patterns. I suspect a prospective study would better evaluate the effect of a child's age. The authors recommend percutaneous fixation under general anesthesia for a completely displaced fracture. They do not, however, comment on clinical long-term results in these redisplaced fractures, along with the associated remodeling, which is a factor that is largely age dependent. They also do not comment on the clinical results and complications of patients who have undergone pin fixation, which is the authors' current method of treatment. As a result, they are advocating anatomical reduction without addressing outcomes. The remodeling potential unique to the pediatric population warrants further evaluation.

A. L. Ladd, MD

Nonbridging External Fixation for Fractures of the Distal Radius
Bednar DA, Al-Harran H (McMaster Univ, Hamilton, Ont, Canada)
Can J Surg 47:426-430, 2004   10–4

Objective.—To assess the feasibility of using standard components from the small AO external fixator set to support fractures of the distal radius with a construct incorporating distal fixation in the periarticular radius fragment that would allow for primary mobilization of the wrist joint during fracture healing.

Methods.—In a prospective pilot study of a nonbridging external fixator in early 2001, 6 consecutive cases of fracture in the distal radius presenting at a tertiary care centre, the Hamilton General Division of Hamilton Health Sciences, were compared with 6 historical controls treated with a standard bridging construct immobilizing the wrist. Both groups were or had been treated with closed reduction and external fixation of the distal radius under fluoroscopic control. Fracture alignment was measured on radiographs after healing and removal of the fixation devices; additional (secondary) outcome measures were pin-tract sepsis and implant loosening (treatment failure).

Results.—Compared radiographically with controls, alignments after fracture healing were improved (and virtually anatomic) with use of the nonbridging external fixator. The incidence of pin-tract sepsis was similar in the 2 groups, neither of which included any treatment failures.

Conclusions.—Nonbridging external fixation of comminuted distal radius fractures can be accomplished safely and effectively. The results of this pilot study suggest that improved radiographic alignment may be achieved with this technique.

▶ This study reports the authors' experience with 6 consecutive cases of comminuted and displaced distal radius fractures without volar displacement treated with nonbridging external fixation. This treatment group was compared with 6 consecutive similar fractures treated with radiocarpal joint bridging external fixation constructs. Comparison of radial height and radial inclination was similar between the 2 groups; however, the nonbridging group had better restoration of volar tilt.

The shortcomings of this study include the statistical limitations of a small sample size, lack of randomization, fairly short long-term follow-up (mean, 21 weeks), and the absence of functional outcome evaluations. Furthermore, there is no mention of surgery time or the restoration of articular step-offs.

Despite its limitations, this pilot study confirmed the feasibility of distal radius fracture treatment with nonbridging external fixation. Compared with the radiocarpal joint bridging fixators, this technique provides the potential benefit of early wrist rehabilitation by allowing active wrist mobilization with the fixator in situ.

K. Azari, MD

Augmented External Fixation Versus Percutaneous Pinning and Casting for Unstable Fractures of the Distal Radius: A Prospective Randomized Trial
Harley BJ, Scharfenberger A, Beaupre LA, et al (Upstate Med Univ, Syracuse, NY; Univ of Alberta, Edmonton, Canada)
J Hand Surg [Am] 29A:815-824, 2004   10–5

Purpose.—Many outcome studies of various surgical techniques for unstable fractures of the distal radius have been published but applicability of the results remains limited because the majority of these trials were not done in a prospective and/or randomized manner. In this study we evaluated 2 common surgical techniques used in the treatment of unstable distal radius fractures in a randomized prospective fashion with a 1-year radiographic and clinical follow-up period. Our hypothesis was that external fixation with augmentation would provide superior results compared with percutaneous pinning and casting.

Methods.—Fifty patients younger than 65 years of age with unstable fractures of the distal radius were randomized into 1 of 2 surgical treatment groups: percutaneous pins with casting or augmented external fixation. All surgery was performed by 1 of 3 surgeons within 10 days of injury. Over 80% of the fractures were classified as AO-ASIF C2 or C3 and there was a similar distribution of fracture types in each group.

Results.—The use of augmented external fixation did not improve the mean radiographic parameters of radial length, radial angulation, or volar tilt. Restoration of volar tilt of highly comminuted fractures was difficult to achieve regardless of the technique. Improved articular surface reduction was realized with the use of an external fixator but overall only 3 patients were noted to have steps or gaps greater than 2 mm. No significant differences in mean Disabilities of the Arm, Shoulder, and Hand scores, total range of motion, grip strength, or health-related quality of life were observed between the groups. All 3 patients diagnosed with sympathetic dystrophy had had external fixation.

Conclusions.—Although augmented external fixation represents a popular first line treatment for unstable fractures of the distal radius this study suggests that for fractures with minimal articular displacement similar clinical results can be obtained with percutaneous pinning and casting.

▶ The optimal choice of fixation for unstable distal radius fractures is controversial and ever-changing based on available technology, the surgeon's experience, and outcomes data. The use of K-wires and supplemental external fixation is an old technique but still quite useful for many fracture patterns. This study questions the utility of external fixation used in addition to percutaneous pinning for unstable distal radius fractures in patients younger than 65 years. Overall, the use of an external fixator did not result in any clinical or radiographic statistical advantage over pins alone other than apparent maintenance of articular alignment. However, the conclusion of improved articular alignment is suspect considering previous studies that have shown poor interobserver reliability related to plain radiographic analysis of articular congruency.

In addition, within each group of 25 patients, over 30% required open reduction with internal fixation and some with bone grafting, leaving at most, 17 patients in each group treated purely percutaneously. Statistical analysis was not included, and there appeared to be insufficient power for definitive conclusions. A 12% rate of reflex sympathetic dystrophy in the group treated with external fixation is also worrisome. Despite these shortcomings, there is little evidence that a supplemental external fixator provides a significant advantage over pins alone in younger patients with healthy bone stock. Larger future studies may help clarify any benefit.

R. Goitz, MD

External Fixation With or Without Supplementary Intramedullary Kirschner Wires in the Treatment of Distal Radial Fractures
Lin C, Sun J-S, Hou S-M (Natl Taiwan Univ, Taipei, Republic of Chine; Natl Yang Ming Univ, Taipei, Taiwan, Republic of China; Taipei Municipal Yang Ming Hosp, Taiwan, Republic of China)
Can J Surg 47:431-437, 2004   10-6

Objectives.—To determine radiographic outcomes in the fracture of distal radius treated by close reduction and external fixation, with or without supplementary intramedullary Kirschner wires.

Methods.—At the Orthopedic Department of National Taiwan University Hospital, we carried out a retrospective study of distal radial fractures treated with close reduction and external fixation. A consecutive series of 20 fractures were treated (from March 1995 to June 1998) with external fixation only; later (from January 1999 to December 2001), 36 distal radius fractures were treated with external fixation supplemented with intramedullary wires. The fractures were evaluated via good-quality posteroanterior and lateral radiographs. In both groups, the radial height, radial inclination and volar tilting were measured on initial (preoperative) and immediate postoperative radiographs and on others taken immediately after the removal of external fixation. Overall results were based on objective radio-

TABLE 4.—Functional Evaluation of Distal Radial Fractures
Treated by External Fixation Alone (EFA) or
With imK Augmentation

	Treatment: Mean (and SD)		
Measurement	EFA Group	imK Group	p Value
Extension,°	14.1 (13.0)	35.3 (17.9)	<0.0001
Flexion,°	19.1 (13.7)	41.5 (17.9)	<0.0001
Pronation,°	29.4 (19.4)	64.3 (27.6)	<0.0001
Supination,°	62.0 (13.4)	82.8 (31.1)	<0.0005
Radial deviation,°	13.3 (4.6)	15.6 (2.8)	0.0236
Ulnar deviation,°	16.9 (6.5)	20.2 (3.3)	0.0192
Grip power, % of contralateral	49.5 (21.4)	75.8 (18.0)	<0.0001

imK = intramedullary Kirchner wires; SD = standard deviation
(Reprinted from Lin C, Sun J-S, Hou S-M: External fixation with or without supplementary intramedullary Kirschner wires in the treatment of distal radial fractures, by permission of the publisher, *CJS*, Vol. 47, No. 6, December, 2004, Canadian Medical Association.)

graphic and functional data as well as on subjective assessments with demerit-point scoring. Data were analyzed with a 2-tailed *t* test.

Results.—Radial height and radial inclination improved significantly immediately after surgery, but volar tilting of distal-radius deformity was little improved by treatment with external fixation alone. When external fixation was supplemented with intramedullary Kirschner wires, improvement in all 3 measurements was statistically significant. Clinical examination likewise found significantly better functional results in patients treated with the Kirschner wires.

Conclusion.—External fixation is a popular method to reduce osseous deformity of the distal radius, but can not assure maintenance of the reduction. Supplementing external fixation with intramedullary Kirschner wires can improve retention of fracture reduction during healing, resulting in better functional results (Table 4).

▶ This is a retrospective review of patients treated for displaced fractures of the distal radius using 1 of 2 methods: either external fixation alone (EFA) or external fixation with supplementary K-wire fixation (imK). Results of treating 20 patients between 1995 and 1998 with EFA alone were compared to results of treating 36 patients between 1999 and 2001 with imK. The authors concluded the supplementary K-wires maintained palmar tilt of the radius better and that, in turn, correlated with improved outcomes as judged by wrist range of motion and grip strength.

One of the weaknesses of this study is that the 2 groups of patients were treated during different periods of 1 surgeon's career rather than at the same time in a prospective comparison manner. The groups may not be comparable because there were 4 times the number of male patients and 1.5 times the number of total patients in the second group (imK) versus the first group (EFA). Nonetheless, the data, as reported, support the contention that use of supplemental K-wires can improve maintenance of fracture reduction during healing, resulting in better functional outcome.

Many authors previously have highlighted the importance of obtaining and maintaining fracture alignment as closely as possible to normal anatomy and the correlation between radiographic and functional outcomes as related to radius fractures. If the current trend of treating distal radius fractures with internal fixation and locking plates continues, it will be interesting to see if there is incremental improvement in functional outcomes or if the added surgical trauma results in improved radiographs without increase in clinical function.

R. R. Slater, Jr, MD

Editor's Note: A different comment on the same abstract can be found on page 135 (Abstract 10–10).

Unstable Extra-articular Fractures of the Distal Radius: A Prospective, Randomised Study of Immobilisation in a Cast *Versus* Supplementary Percutaneous Pinning
Azzopardi T, Ehrendorfer S, Coulton T, et al (Wishaw Gen Hosp, Scotland)
J Bone Joint Surg Br 87-B:837-840, 2005   10–7

Abstract.—We performed a prospective, randomised study on 57 patients older than 60 years of age with unstable, extra-articular fractures of the distal radius to compare the outcome of immobilisation in a cast alone with that using supplementary, percutaneous pinning.

Patients treated by percutaneous wires had a statistically significant improvement in dorsal angulation (mean 7°), radial length (mean 3 mm) and radial inclination (mean 3 mm) at one year. However, there was no significant difference in functional outcome in terms of pain, range of movement, grip strength, activities of daily living and the SF-36 score except for an improved range of movement in ulnar deviation in the percutaneous wire group. One patient developed a pin-track infection which required removal of the wires at two weeks.

We conclude that percutaneous pinning of unstable, extra-articular fractures of the distal radius provides only a marginal improvement in the radiological parameters compared with immobilisation in a cast alone. This does not correlate with an improved functional outcome in a low-demand, elderly population.

▶ This article supports what we have seen in our practice—that percutaneous pins do not provide sufficient support for unstable extra-articular distal radius fractures. We have learned that the prereduction films are often the best predictor of likelihood for displacement. This report gives support to fixation of significantly displaced fractures with options more rigid than percutaneous wires. Volar fixed-angle plates have revolutionized our approach to these extra-articular fractures in the elderly, which are certain to settle to some degree. The fixed-angle plating will help prevent settling and will maintain distal radial ulnar joint congruity along with proper tilt and radial height. Percutaneous pinning may be best suited for the younger patient with better bone quality. Additional studies are needed to compare these techniques to the volar fixed-angle plating in this elderly population.

T. R. McAdams, MD

Two Procedures for Kirschner Wire Osteosynthesis of Distal Radial Fractures: A Randomized Trial
Strohm PC, Müller CA, Boll T, et al (Städtisches Klinikum Karlsruhe, Germany)
J Bone Joint Surg Am 86-A:2621-2628, 2004   10–8

Background.—The treatment of displaced Colles-type fractures of the distal part of the radius remains a challenge. Two procedures for closed reduction and Kirschner wire osteosynthesis of these fractures were compared in a prospective randomized study.

Methods.—One hundred consecutive patients with a Colles fracture of the distal part of the radius (AO classification 23-A2, 23-A3, or 23-C1) were treated over an eighteen-month period. One group was managed with the conventional method, described by Willenegger and Guggenbuhl in 1959, in which two Kirschner wires are introduced into the styloid process of the radius (Fig 1, C and D). The other group was treated with the Kapandji method, as modified by Fritz et al., in which two Kirschner wires are inserted into the fracture gap and a third is placed through the styloid process (Fig 2, C and D). Postoperative care was standardized for both groups and carried out according to a strict procedure. Forty patients who had been operated on according to the modified Kapandji method and forty-one treated with the

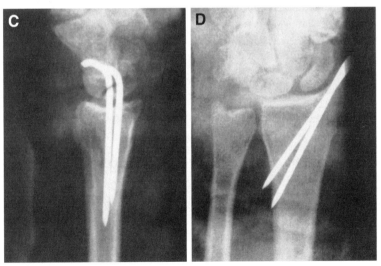

FIGURE 1.—Radiographs made after Kirschner wire osteosynthesis with the Willenegger technique. (Courtesy of Strohm PC, Müller CA, Boll T, et al: Two procedures for Kirschner wire osteosynthesis of distal radial fractures: A randomized trial. *J Bone Joint Surg Am* 86-A:2621-2628, 2004. Republished with permission of the Journal of Bone and Joint Surgery, Inc. Reproduced by permission of the publisher via Copyright Clearance Center, Inc.)

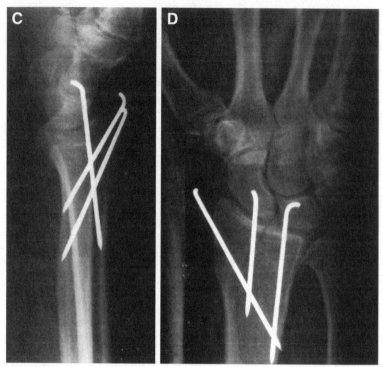

FIGURE 2.—Postoperative radiographs made after Kirschner wire osteosynthesis with the modified Kapandji technique. (Courtesy of Strohm PC, Müller CA, Boll T, et al: Two procedures for Kirschner wire osteosynthesis of distal radial fractures: A randomized trial. *J Bone Joint Surg Am* 86-A:2621-2628, 2004. Republished with permission of the Journal of Bone and Joint Surgery, Inc. Reproduced by permission of the publisher via Copyright Clearance Center, Inc.)

Willenegger technique were available for follow-up, for a follow-up rate of 81%. The follow-up assessment was performed with a modified version of the Martini score.

Results.—The median time to follow-up was ten months (range, six to twenty months). The results as assessed with the Martini score were, on the average, good to very good for the patients treated with the Kapandji method and satisfactory to good for the patients treated with the conventional Kirschner wire fixation. The duration of radiographic exposure was significantly shorter with the Kapandji method than with the Willenegger technique.

Conclusions.—Conventional Kirschner wire fixation remains a good method of osteosynthesis for the treatment of displaced fractures of the distal part of the radius. We found both the functional and radiographic outcomes of the Kapandji method to be significantly better than those of the Willenegger technique.

▶ The authors provide a randomized controlled trial on the treatment of 100 consecutive patients with distal radius fractures using 2 techniques of Kirschner wire osteosynthesis. The Willenegger technique, originally described in 1959, entailed inserting 2 uniplanar Kirschner wires through the radial styloid and into the opposite cortex. The technique described by Kapandji in 1976 and modified by Fritz entailed the use of "intrafocal" Kirschner wires inserted dorsally into the fracture site in addition to the radial styloid wire, thereby providing biplanar fixation and a dorsal buttress that resists the tendency of the distal fragment to dorsally angulate.

Kirschner wire osteosynthesis using the Kapandji technique required less imaging time, allowed earlier rehabilitation, and provided significantly better radiographic and functional outcomes in the patients treated in this study, as measured using a modified Martini score. There was no significant difference in the number of complications between the 2 techniques.

It is my preference to use the Kapandji technique in most extra-articular fractures of the distal radius with mild to moderate comminution, and in select intra-articular fractures where the articular surface is readily reducible. With increasing recent interest in the newer volar plating systems for the treatment of distal radius fractures, this study is useful to reconfirm that excellent results may be achieved in the treatment of a certain subset of fractures using less invasive, less costly means.

J. Yao, MD

Use of a Distraction Plate for Distal Radial Fractures With Metaphyseal and Diaphyseal Comminution
Ruch DS, Ginn TA, Yang CC, et al (Wake Forest Univ, Winston-Salem, NC)
J Bone Joint Surg Am 87-A:945-954, 2005   10–9

Background.—Distal radial fractures with extensive comminution involving the metaphyseal-diaphyseal junction present a major treatment dilemma. Of particular difficulty are those fractures involving the articular surface. One approach is to apply a dorsal 3.5-mm plate extra-articularly from the radius to the third metacarpal, stabilizing the diaphysis and maintaining distraction across the radiocarpal joint.

Methods.—Twenty-two patients treated with a distraction plate for a comminuted distal radial fracture were included in the study. With use of three limited incisions, a 3.5-mm ASIF plate was applied in distraction dorsally from the radial diaphysis, bypassing the comminuted segment, to the long-finger metacarpal, where it was fixed distally. The articular surface was anatomically reduced and was secured with Kirschner wires or screws. Eleven of the twenty-two fractures were treated with bone-grafting. The plate was removed after fracture consolidation (at an average of 124 days), and wrist motion was initiated. All patients were followed prospectively with use of radiographs, physical examination, and DASH (Disabilities of the Arm, Shoulder and Hand) scores.

Results.—All fractures united by an average of 110 days. Radiographs showed an average palmar tilt of 4.6° and an average ulnar variance of neutral (0°), whereas loss of radial length averaged 2 mm. Flexion and extension averaged 57° and 65°, respectively, and pronation and supination averaged 77° and 76°, respectively. The average DASH scores were 34 points at six months, 15 points at one year, and 11.5 points at the time of final follow-up (at an average of 24.8 months). According to the Gartland-Werley rating system, fourteen patients had an excellent result, six had a good result, and two had a fair result. Grip strength and the range of motion of the wrist at one year correlated inversely with the proximal extent of fracture comminution into the diaphysis. The duration of plate immobilization did not correlate with the range of motion of the wrist or with the DASH score at one year.

Conclusions.—The use of a distraction plate combined with reduction of the articular surface and bone-grafting when needed can be an effective technique for treatment of fractures of the distal end of the radius with extensive metaphyseal and diaphyseal comminution. A functional range of motion with minimal disability can be achieved despite a prolonged period of fixation with a distraction plate across the wrist joint.

▶ This is a prospective clinical study to evaluate the use of a long internal fixation plate to span and distract severely comminuted distal radius fractures. A 12- to 16-hole 3.5-mm ASIF compression plate is used with a limited incision. Screws are placed in the 2nd metacarpal and in the radius proximal to the fracture while the fracture is being distracted. The fracture itself is fixed with screws, K-wires, and allograft bone. Results show this technique produces excellent results according to the DASH scores. Range of motion is relatively well maintained with an average follow-up of 2 years. This technique should be considered when severely comminuted intra-articular fractures of the distal radius are being treated, and gives the surgeon one more option when more conventional methods of internal fixation are impractical or impossible.

W. Short, MD

External Fixation With or Without Supplementary Intramedullary Kirschner Wires in the Treatment of Distal Radial Fractures
Lin C, Sun J-S, Hou S-M (Natl Taiwan Univ, Taipei Republic of China; Natl Yang Ming Univ, Taipei, Taiwan Republic of China; Taipei Municipal Yang Ming Hosp, Taiwan Republic of China)
Can J Surg 47:431-436, 2004   10–10

Objectives.—To determine radiographic outcomes in the fracture of distal radius treated by close reduction and external fixation, with or without supplementary intramedullary Kirschner wires.

Methods.—At the Orthopedic Department of National Taiwan University Hospital, we carried out a retrospective study of distal radial fractures treated with close reduction and external fixation. A consecutive series of 20 fractures were treated (from March 1995 to June 1998) with external fixation only; later (from January 1999 to December 2001), 36 distal radius fractures were treated with external fixation supplemented with intramedullary wires. The fractures were evaluated via good-quality posteroanterior and lateral radiographs. In both groups, the radial height, radial inclination and volar tilting were measured on initial (preoperative) and immediate postoperative radiographs and on others taken immediately after the removal of external fixation. Overall results were based on objective radiographic and functional data as well as on subjective assessments with demerit-point scoring. Data were analyzed with a 2-tailed *t* test.

Results.—Radial height and radial inclination improved significantly immediately after surgery, but volar tilting of distal-radius deformity was little improved by treatment with external fixation alone. When external fixation was supplemented with intramedullary Kirschner wires, improvement in all 3 measurements was statistically significant. Clinical examination likewise found significantly better functional results in patients treated with the Kirschner wires.

Conclusion.—External fixation is a popular method to reduce osseous deformity of the distal radius, but can not assure maintenance of the reduction Supplementing external fixation with intramedullary Kirschner wires can improve retention of fracture reduction during healing, resulting in better functional results.

▶ External fixation continues to be one of the appropriate techniques that can be chosen by a surgeon faced with an unstable and displaced distal radius fracture. Although internal fixation of these fractures is presently popular, the external fixator maintains a prominent place in the selection of fixation techniques for this fracture. The authors demonstrate that the use of Kirschner wires can improve retention of the reduction of the fracture during the healing phase. The retention of the fracture reduction results in better clinical outcomes. Careful placement of the wires is necessary to prevent complications. Use of properly placed Kirschner wires should be considered when the surgeon performs external fixation of the distal radius fracture.

C. Carroll IV, MD

Editor's Note: A different comment on the same abstract can be found on pages 129 and 130 (Abstract 10–6).

Loss of Fixation of the Volar Lunate Facet Fragment in Fractures of the Distal Part of the Radius

Harness NG, Jupiter JB, Orbay JL, et al (Massachusetts Gen Hosp, Boston; Miami Hand Ctr, Fla; New York Univ; et al)
J Bone Joint Surg Am 86-A:1900-1908, 2004   10–11

Background.—The purpose of the present study is to report on a cohort of patients with a volar shearing fracture of the distal end of the radius in whom the unique anatomy of the distal cortical rim of the radius led to failure of support of a volar ulnar lunate facet fracture fragment.

Methods.—Seven patients with a volar shearing fracture of the distal part of the radius who lost fixation of a volar lunate facet fragment with subsequent carpal displacement after open reduction and internal fixation were evaluated at an average of twenty-four months after surgery. One fracture was classified as B3.2 and six were classified as B3.3 according to the AO comprehensive classification system. All seven fractures initially were deemed to have an adequate reduction and internal fixation. Four patients required repeat open reduction and internal fixation, and one underwent a radiocarpal arthrodesis. At the time of the final follow-up, all patients were assessed with regard to their self-reported level of functioning and with use of Sarmiento's modification of the system of Gartland and Werley.

Results.—At a mean of two years after the injury, six patients had returned to their previous level of function. The result was considered to be excellent for one patient, good for four, and fair for two. The average wrist extension was 48°, or 75% of that of the uninjured extremity. The average wrist flexion was 37°, or 64% of that of the uninjured extremity. The one patient who underwent radiocarpal arthrodesis had achievement of a solid union. The four patients who underwent repeat internal fixation had maintenance of reduction of the lunate facet fragment. The two patients who declined additional operative intervention had persistent dislocation of the carpus with the volar lunate facet fragment.

Conclusions.—The stability of comminuted fractures of the distal part of the radius with volar fragmentation is determined not only by the reduction of the major fragments but also by the reduction of the small volar lunate fragment. The unique anatomy of this region may prevent standard fixation devices for distal radial fractures from supporting the entire volar surface effectively. It is preferable to recognize the complexity of the injury prior to the initial surgical intervention and to plan accordingly.

▶ The authors report on a not uncommon complication of distal radius fractures: the displaced or unstable volar lunate facet fragment (also known as the volar marginal fragment). In particular, they underscore the importance of preoperative evaluation and identification of this fracture and emphasize that particular attention must be paid to this small fragment as it may not be captured by some of the more common volar plates because of the distal location of this small fragment.

Their study reported good results for those 4 patients who underwent revision fixation for the late displaced volar fragment. The other 2 had continued dislocation of the lunate with the displaced fragment.

This study highlights the need for appropriate preoperative and intraoperative evaluation of the fracture, the reduction, the fixation, and the stability of the construct.

The authors report on cases that were all associated with volar subluxation of the carpus, but this is not always apparent initially and may develop after initial cast treatment of an otherwise benign-appearing distal radius fracture.

CT imaging is very helpful when there is a suspicion of this injury because it can delineate the size of the fragment and direct the surgical plan. Larger fragments may be stabilized with current plates or implants; however, others may be so small that they require suture anchor fixation of the volar carpal ligaments to the volar distal radius. Small fragments that are not controlled by volar plates require additional fixation or stability, as the authors have discussed (eg, a tension band, K-wires, adjuvant external fixation, etc).

After reduction and fixation, it is also necessary to assess the stability of the construct. Volar–dorsal translation and flexion–extension of the carpus, as well as pronation and supination, should be checked to be certain that stable fixation has occurred. Palpation and visualization, as well as fluoroscopy, are used to ensure stability.

In summary, the authors have reported on the outcomes of these frequently troublesome fractures. Early identification of the problem and appropriate reduction with stable fixation is associated with good outcomes.

D. G. Dennison, MD

Indirect Reduction and Percutaneous Fixation *Versus* Open Reduction and Internal Fixation for Displaced Intra-articular Fractures of the Distal Radius: A Randomised, Controlled Trial
Kreder HJ, Hanel DP, Agel J, et al (Univ of Toronto; Univ of Washington, Seattle)
J Bone Joint Surg Br 87-B:829-836, 2005   10–12

Background.—The management of patients with distal radius fractures depends on the unique characteristics of each case, with the options varying widely from immediate functional bracing to open reduction and internal fixation. The efficacy of indirect reduction and primary external fixation compared with open reduction and internal fixation was investigated in patients with a severely comminuted distal radius fracture with joint incongruity.

Methods.—Random assignment placed 88 patients in a group receiving indirect percutaneous reduction and external fixation. Ninety-one patients were randomly assigned to treatment with open reduction and internal fixation. Patients having indirect reduction had percutaneous Kirschner wires or a small elevator inserted through a small incision to manage fracture fragments, and did not have arthrotomy. Patients having open reduction generally underwent arthrotomy. Results were compared based on upper limb musculoskeletal function assessment score, SF-36 bodily pain subscale score, overall Jebsen score, and pinch and grip strength values. Follow-up assessments were done after 6 weeks, 6 months, 1 year, and 2 years.

Results.—At baseline, the groups had statistically significant differences in bone grafting (used for 50% of the open reduction group but only 13% of the indirect reduction group) and work-related injury (trend toward more in the indirect reduction group). Eight patients assigned to indirect reduction eventually needed open reduction and internal fixation. Overall function was better for indirect reduction patients than open reduction patients. Indirect reduction patients had better function test scores and overall pain scores; the difference in pain level did not reach statistical significance. Both groups improved significantly in upper limb function and degree of pain with time. At 6 weeks, both groups had considerable pain and markedly impaired upper limb function. Bodily pain level was significantly greater for indirect reduction patients only at 6 weeks. Upper limb function test results were significantly better for indirect reduction patients than open reduction patients until 6 months, with no significant differences thereafter. For both groups, Jebsen score and pad, chuck, and pinch test results improved over time. At all assessments, grip strength results favored the indirect group. Range of motion (ROM) improvements were comparable in the 2 groups, with all but 4 patients with reflex sympathetic dystrophy regaining finger ROM by 6 weeks. Mean wrist flexion on the injured side was nearly 20° less than on the normal side in both groups after 6 months. Forearm ROM was regained within 6 months. Radiologic studies showed all fractures united by 6 months. Complications included superficial pin-track infections and wound infections, pin-track infections requiring operative intervention, broken fixator pin, tears of the triangular fibrocartilage complex requiring arthroscopic repair, and reflex sympathetic dystrophy. These occurred with similar frequency in both groups.

Conclusions.—Indirect reduction and percutaneous fixation provided patients a more rapid return to function and a better functional outcome than open reduction and internal fixation over the course of 2 years. Better results depended on minimizing any intra-articular step and gap deformities. Both treatments yielded similar functional outcomes after 1 year that tended to be stable.

▶ In this multicenter, randomized, prospective, controlled trial, distal radius fractures were randomly assigned to treatment with indirect reduction and percutaneous fixation with or without supplemental K-wires, or to treatment with open reduction and internal fixation. Inclusion criteria included adult patients with intra-articular distal radius fractures who had a minimum of 2 mm of step off or gap. Of the 179 patients enrolled into the study, 88 underwent external fixation with indirect percutaneous reduction, and 91 underwent open reduction and internal fixation.

The indirect reduction technique was performed using percutaneous K-wires or through a limited incision. A small incision was used to manipulate the fragments, and arthrotomy was not performed. Bone grafting was carried out per the discretion of the treating surgeons, and fixation was limited to K-wires, cannulated or regular type screws, and external fixation using an AO fixator. The authors defined a successful reduction as a step deformity of 2 mm or less, a neutral palmar tilt or better, and a radial shortening of less than 5 mm compared with the opposite side. The fixator and percutaneous pins were removed between 6 and 8 weeks after surgery.

For the open reduction group, the operation was performed using a volar extended carpal tunnel approach or a dorsal approach to the wrist, and typically involved an arthrotomy. Fixation was performed by smaller mini-fragment plates and screws and was supplemented with K-wires or an external fixator.

The primary outcome measure was a Musculoskeletal Functional Assessment (MFA) questionnaire in addition to the SF-36. Secondary outcome measures included the Jebson test, grip strength, pinch strength, and 3-chuck pinch. ROM was obtained, and preoperative and postoperative radiographs were compared. Statistical analysis was performed. Both groups were similar with the exceptions that there was a statistically significant higher usage of bone grafts in the open reduction and internal fixation group, and more patients had work-related injuries in the indirect reduction group.

The overall primary functional outcome demonstrated that patients receiving indirect reduction and external fixation had better function overall and better scores on the MFA test, compared with those who received open reduction and internal fixation. The pain scores were also better overall in the indirect reduction group, although the results just fell below statistical significance ($P = .052$). With regard to secondary outcomes, the grip strength showed statistically significant less deficit after indirect than after open reduction and internal fixation; however, 6 months after surgery there was essentially no difference. There were no statistical differences between the 2 groups with respect to the Jebson score and the different methods of grip testing. There was no statistical difference in ROM between the 2 groups tested. Five superficial pin-track infections (6%) occurred in the indirect reduction group compared with 2 (2%) in the open group. There were 2 superficial wound infections (2%) in the indirect group requiring local care, and 1 (1%) in the open group. Radiologically, all fractures healed. Fourteen percent of patients had an intra-articular deformity after indirect reduction, compared with 14% after open reduction and internal fixation. With respect to the development of arthritis, the authors were unable to demonstrate a statistically significant association between function and method of fixation.

Overall, the authors conclude that displaced intra-articular fractures of the distal radius can be treated by indirect reduction and percutaneous fixation with a rapid return to function and superior functional outcome within 2 years of the injury, compared with open reduction and internal fixation, provided the intra-articular step and gap deformity is minimized. The authors recommend that despite their results, it is important to restore the anatomy with the least amount of dissection, which results in the quickest return of function.

This is an important and interesting article. It should be kept in mind for the different techniques that exist in fixation of distal radius fractures, especially in light of the high popularity of volar open reduction and internal fixation using fixed angle plates.

A. Y. Shin, MD

Combined Dorsal and Volar Plate Fixation of Complex Fractures of the Distal Part of the Radius

Ring D, Prommersberger K, Jupiter JB (Klinik fur Handchirurgie, Bad Neustadt, Germany; Massachusetts Gen Hosp, Boston)
J Bone Joint Surg Am 86-A:1646-1652, 2004 10–13

Background.—Fractures of the distal part of the radius that are associated with complex comminution of both the articular surface and the metaphysis (subgroup C3.2 according to the Comprehensive Classification of Fractures) are a challenge for surgeons using standard operative techniques.

Methods.—Twenty-five patients with subgroup-C3.2 fractures that had been treated with combined dorsal and volar plate fixation were evaluated at an average of twenty-six months after the injury. Subsequent procedures included implant removal in twenty-one patients and reconstruction of a ruptured tendon in two patients.

Results.—An average of 54° of extension, 51° of flexion, 79° of pronation, and 74° of supination were achieved. The grip strength in the involved limb was an average of 78% of that in the contralateral limb. The average radiographic measurements were 2° of dorsal angulation, 21° of ulnar inclination, 0.8 mm of positive ulnar variance, and 0.7 mm of articular incongruity. Seven patients had radiographic signs of arthrosis during the follow-up period. A good or excellent functional result was achieved for twenty-four patients (96%) according to the rating system of Gartland and Werley and for ten patients (40%) according to the more stringent modified system of Green and O'Brien.

Conclusions.—Combined dorsal and volar plate fixation of the distal part of the radius can achieve a stable, mobile wrist in patients with very complex fractures. The results are limited by the severity of the injury and may deteriorate with longer follow-up. A second operation for implant removal is common, and there is a small risk of tendon-related complications.

▶ Distal radius fractures with complex comminution of both the articular surface and metaphysis are difficult to treat. As demonstrated by the article, the outcomes of these fractures are often poor even when the anatomy is restored surgically. Patients must be counseled preoperatively about this information. However, most hand surgeons would agree that adequate reduction of distal radius fractures gives patients the best chance of a good outcome.

There is no consensus on the optimal way to surgically treat even simple distal radius fractures. Recently, many have advocated the use of locked, volar, fixed-angle plating, although external fixation and pinning remain in common use. To date, no study has demonstrated clear superiority of any surgical technique. The authors demonstrate that "double plating" of the distal radius can result in a stable and mobile wrist. Certainly, this technique should be in the "war chest" of every surgeon treating these complex fractures. The recent trend toward volar fixed-angle fixation has greatly reduced the need for dorsal treatment of distal radius fractures; however, certain cases are likely best treated with the addition of a dorsal approach with or without plating or bone grafting.

D. I. Ilan, MD

Corrective Osteotomy of Malunited Distal Radius Fractures Using Carbonated Hydroxyapatite as an Alternative to Autogenous Bone Grafting
Luchetti R (Univ of Ancona, Italy)
J Hand Surg [Am] 29-A:825-834, 2004   10–14

Purpose.—The purpose of the present study was to report on the author's experience using carbonated hydroxyapatite as a bony substitute in distal radius corrective osteotomies.

Methods.—Six patients had a corrective osteotomy for a malunited distal radius fracture using carbonated hydroxyapatite as an alternative to an autogenous bone graft. Internal fixation of the osteotomy was achieved by using 2 or 3 K-wires.

Results.—At an average follow-up evaluation of 33 months (range, 22–45 mo) all the osteotomies united. Wrist flexion-extension motion improved

FIGURE 8.

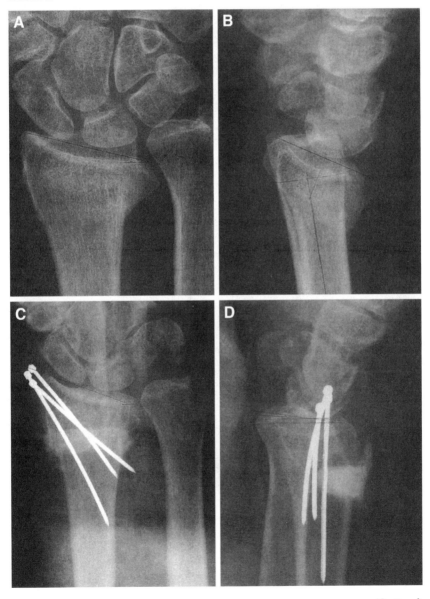

(Continued)

FIGURE 8 (cont.)

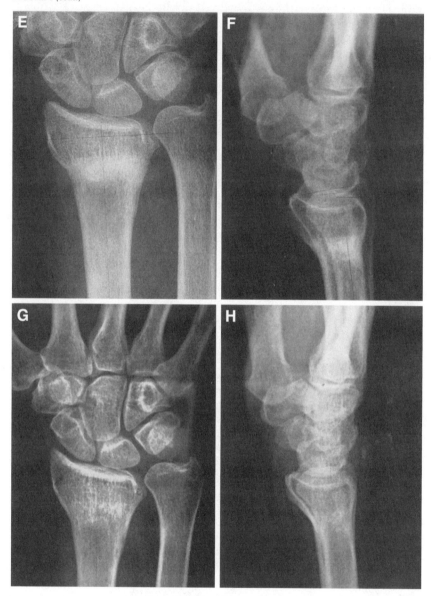

(Continued)

from 75° to 110°, forearm rotation increased from 116° to 157°, and grip strength had an average increase of 140% at the time of the final follow-up evaluation. All patients were satisfied and there were no reports of persistent pain. Radiographic evaluation showed an average volar tilt improvement from a preoperative dorsal angulation shifting into a neutral position in the sagittal plane; radial lengthening improved from an average of 4 mm (range, 2–6 mm) before surgery to 7 mm (range, 5–9 mm) after surgery; and ulnar plus deformity improved by 5 mm. Radiographically the carbonated hydroxyapatite material was integrated completely into the bone tissue with evidence of progressive re-absorption and bony calcification over time. The Mayo wrist score system, according to Cooney and Krimmer modifications, improved by an average of 88 and 98 points (0–100 points), respectively.

Conclusions.—On the basis of this preliminary experience it is reasonable to consider carbonated hydroxyapatite as a viable alternative to bone grafting in conjunction with surgical correction of a distal radius malunion. It must be augmented, however, with internal fixation (Fig 8).

▶ I have spent many years studying synthetic bone graft substitutes, and I presented the clinical results of the multicenter trial using Norian calcium phosphate cement to the Food and Drug Administration in 1998.[1] As a result, I have tested the clinical utility of many of the calcium-based substitutes and can appreciate the author's use of calcium phosphate for osteotomy.

Technically, the material is calcium phosphate with a carbonated apatite, not "carbonated hydroxyapatite" as described in the article. The carbonated component adds what is believed to be osteoclastic activity and thus bony remodeling at the surface of the cement mass in areas of maximal loading according to Wolff's Law. Remodeling is a unique feature of the calcium phosphate cements as compared to calcium sulfate (which resorbs by dissolution). The author or editors did not identify this nuance in nomenclature, although it is probably irrelevant for purposes of this review.

The author describes a wide exposure but uses Kirschner wires, which seems counterproductive to me. Why not use more structurally advantageous hardware, or consider a smaller incision? I have used different formulations of calcium phosphate cement in radius osteotomy, with different configurations:

FIGURE 8.—A 64-year-old woman with right distal radius malunion after conservative treatment for Colles' type fracture. The patient had surgery 4 months later. Preoperative clinical evaluation: flexion, 20°; extension, 35°; pronation, 80°; supination, 80°; radial deviation, 30°; ulnar deviation, 20°; grip strength, 8 kg (54% of the opposite unaffected side); Cooney and Krimmer modified Mayo wrist score, 20 and 30 points, respectively. (A, B) Preoperative x-rays showed volar tilt, −30°; radial inclination, 16°; ulnar plus, 10 mm; radial length, 5 mm; and presence of DISI deformity. (C, D) Immediate postoperative corrections of radius deformities: volar tilt, −2°; radial inclination, 20°; radial length, 8 mm; ulnar plus, 6 mm; absence of DISI deformity. (E, F) Radiographic results at final follow-up evaluation (42 mo): volar tilt, −6°; radial inclination, 18°; radial length, 8 mm; and ulnar plus, 7 mm. Carbonated hydroxyapatite appeared to diminish over time. (G, H) Biomaterial completely disappeared at 42 months at the level of the osteotomy without clinical consequence. Final clinical result: flexion, 45°; extension, 60°; pronation and supination, 85°; radial deviation, 30°; ulnar deviation, 25°; grip strength, 21.5 kg (123% of the opposite unaffected side); Cooney and Krimmer modified Mayo wrist score, 90 and 100 points, respectively. (Courtesy of Luchetti R: Corrective osteotomy of malunited distal radius fractures using carbonated hydroxyapatite as an alternative to autogenous bone grafting. *J Hand Surg [Am]* 29-A:825-834. Copyright 2004, with permission from The American Society for Surgery of the Hand.)

dorsal plates; volar plates; fragment-specific fixation using wireforms, some-times with adjunctive Kirschner wires; and various combinations of the above.

In summary, calcium phosphate cement is useful as a synthetic graft for ra-dius osteotomy, with the following caveats. It "subsides" radiographically if not supported with plate fixation, and it is shown in this article: The final follow-up radiographic measurements are not as good as the postoperative measure-ments. I believe this is from constant remodeling and local osteoporosis—stress shielding, if you will—from the dense, strong mass of cement in the local environment of metaphyseal bone. This slight loss of height does not cor-respond to a loss of reduction.

Also, I have found calcium phosphate is least useful in nascent malunions with displaced intra-articular components, as supported by fragment-specific hardware. I have revised several of these within a year of surgery, and I have found the cement has not remodeled sufficiently. Nonetheless, for extra-articular or simple intra-articular malunions, I almost exclusively use calcium phosphate cement as graft, with hardware fixation, and I believe it to be a sig-nificant advancement to eliminate the morbidity of a large trapezoidal iliac crest harvest.

A. L. Ladd, MD

Reference

1. Cassidy C, Jupiter JB, Cohen M, et al: Norian SRS cement compared with con-ventional fixation in distal radial fractures: A randomized study. *J Bone Joint Surg [Am]* 85-A:2127-2137, 2003.

Delayed Union and Nonunion Following Closed Treatment of Diaphyseal Pediatric Forearm Fractures
Adamczyk MJ, Riley PM (Children's Hosp Med Ctr of Akron, Ohio; Akron Gen Med Ctr, Ohio)
J Pediatr Orthop 25:51-55, 2005   10–15

Abstract.—Delayed unions and nonunions of diaphyseal pediatric fore-arm fractures are exceedingly uncommon. In the past they generally have been reported in conjunction with open fracture or initial operative manage-ment of these fractures. The authors report six cases that occurred in low-energy, closed fractures initially managed with casting. The cases all oc-curred in teenage patients from age 13 to 16, and all cases involved the ulna. The mid-diaphysis was the most common location, and this may represent a watershed zone of perfusion with a relatively poor intraosseous blood sup-ply. All of these patients were managed with compression plating with or without bone grafting. Three of these patients had rapid healing in an aver-age of 2 months, while one had an inadequate radiographic record and an-other was lost to follow-up. The other patient had a more prolonged course to healing after surgery.

▶ The authors report on 6 ulnar malunions occurring after closed, diaphyseal fractures. The patients were all healthy and between 13 and 16 years of age. The definition of nonunion used by the authors was lack of radiographic fracture bridging and continued pain at 2 months after injury. This group was .3% of all diaphyseal forearm fractures. The authors' algorithm for treatment for these fractures is initial closed treatment for 2 months, adding a stimulator at this point if there is no evidence of healing, and compression plating if there is still no healing at 4 months. Bone graft was used except in the case of a hypertrophic nonunion.

J. A. Katarincic, MD

11 Carpus: Trauma

Results of Arthroscopic Reduction and Percutaneous Fixation for Acute Displaced Scaphoid Fractures
Shih J-T, Lee H-M, Hou Y-T, et al (Armed Forces Taoyuan Gen Hosp, Long-Tan, Taiwan)
Arthroscopy 21:620-626, 2005   11–1

Purpose.—This study used percutaneous techniques augmented by simultaneous wrist arthroscopy to visualize the fracture and thus confirm the fracture alignment and reduction and also to assesses the concurrent associated ligament injuries.

Type of Study.—Retrospective study.

Methods.—Arthroscopy was used to help to reduce scaphoid fractures and assess soft-tissue injuries in 15 acute cases (13 male and 2 female patients). The fractures were treated by reduction under arthroscopic control and percutaneous fixation with the cannulated interosseous compression screw. Soft-tissue lesions were also treated at the same time using debridement, suture repair, or K-wire transfixation. The average age of the patients was 29.2 years (range, 19 to 48 years).

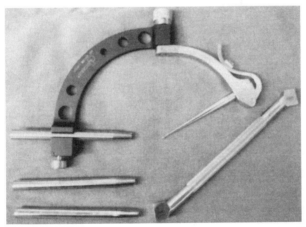

FIGURE 2.—The microvector drill guide system. (Courtesy of Shih J-T, Lee H-M, Hou Y-T, et al: Results of arthroscopic reduction and percutaneous fixation for acute displaced scaphoid fractures. *Arthroscopy* 21:620-626. Copyright 2005, with permission from The Arthroscopy Association of North America.)

Results.—Two patients (13.3%) had scapholunate (SL) ligament injuries, and both exhibited partial tear of the SL ligament. Four patients (26.7%) suffered lunotriquetral (LT) ligament injuries and received ligament debridement, K-wire fixation of the LT joint, and splinting. Six patients (40%) had chondral fractures. Additionally, the triangular fibrocartilage complex (TFCC) was torn in 5 patients (33%). Finally, 5 patients (33%) suffered radioscaphocapitate ligament or long radiolunate ligament injuries. All fractures healed without malunion or nonunion and, at follow-up of 24 to 28 months, 11 patients had excellent results and 4 had good results based on Mayo Modified Wrist Scores.

Conclusions.—We believe that arthroscopic reduction may be considered for scaphoid fractures because this approach can use a single procedure to achieve acceptable restoration of fractures as well as assessment and management of soft-tissue lesions (Fig 2).

▶ A retrospective review is presented of 15 patients (13 males, ages 19-48 years) who were treated for displaced scaphoid fractures with wrist arthroscopy and cannulated screw fixation. Intra-articular soft tissue injuries noted at the time of surgery were treated simultaneously and dictated the time of cast immobilization postoperatively. At an average follow-up of 26 months, patients were evaluated using the Mayo wrist score, and the results were excellent in 11 cases and good in 4.

Astonishingly, the authors report the wrist motion was "equal to that of the contralateral wrist" at last follow-up. Such excellent results have never before been reported in any series of scaphoid fractures or wrist trauma and, if true, may warrant consideration of the methods employed in this study.

The authors admit that arthroscopic reduction and screw fixation of displaced scaphoid fractures is technically demanding. A special alignment guide system was used, but no information is provided about its cost or whether or not the authors have any financial interest in its success. There is no comparison group of patients treated with percutaneous screw fixation alone without arthroscopy or via a more traditional open approach with scaphoid fixation to know how much the arthroscopy helped, if at all.

Surprisingly, the authors found associated soft tissue lesions in only 73% of cases. One might imagine all wrists would have soft tissue injuries if there had been enough trauma to cause a displaced scaphoid fracture in a young male. The real question is whether or not those associated lesions require additional treatment.

R. R. Slater, Jr, MD

Vascularised Bone Graft From the Base of the Second Metacarpal for Refractory Nonunion of the Scaphoid

Sawaizumi T, Nanno M, Nanbu A, et al (Nippon Med School, Tokyo)
J Bone Joint Surg Br 86-B:1007-1012, 2004   11–2

Abstract.—A vascularised bone-graft procedure from the base of the second metacarpal was performed in 14 patients with nonunion of the scaphoid. There were 11 men and three women with a mean age of 22 years. In eight patients, who had dorsiflexed intercalated segment instability (DISI), an open wedge was formed at the site of nonunion, and the vascular pedicle was grafted from the volar side. In the six patients without DISI, transplantation was carried out through the same dorsal skin incision.

Complete bony union was obtained in all patients after a mean postoperative period of 10.2 weeks, and DISI was corrected in all affected patients. According to Cooney's clinical scoring system, the results were excellent in five, good in six, and fair in three patients. Because of its technical simplicity and the limited dissection needed, the procedure should be considered for the primary surgical treatment of patients with nonunion of the scaphoid.

▶ The authors present their experience with 14 patients who had refractory scaphoid nonunion treated with vascularized bone grafts from the second metacarpal. The grafts were fixed with K-wires or Herbert screws and were postoperatively immobilized for an average of 7.5 weeks. Complete bony union was achieved in all patients. In cases where DISI was present preoperatively, correction was obtained.

▶ According to the authors, this technique has many advantages including ease of dissection because of the large 1 mm in diameter vessel; good cancellous bone stock that can be elevated en bloc with the graft; requirement for a relatively small skin incision that does not traverse the wrist joint (predisposing to kinking); and the ability to apply the graft dorsally or volarly. Because of its technical simplicity and limited dissection, this procedure should be added to the hand surgeon's armamentarium of vascularized grafts for the treatment of scaphoid nonunion.

K. Azari, MD

B. Wilhelmi, MD

A Survey of the Surgical Management of Acute and Chronic Scapholunate Instability

Zarkadas PC, Gropper PT, White NJ, et al (Univ of British Columbia, Vancouver, Canada)
J Hand Surg [Am] 29A:848-857, 2004   11–3

Purpose.—Scapholunate instability is a challenging problem and controversy persists among hand surgeons with respect to treatment choice. The purpose of this study was to evaluate the pattern of practice among specialized hand surgeons in the management of both acute and chronic scapholunate instability.

Methods.—A mailed survey study was sent to the 1,628 members of the American and Canadian Societies for Surgery of the Hand. Hand surgeons were asked to complete a comprehensive management questionnaire that examined a surgeon's treatment algorithm in the clinical case of acute and chronic scapholunate instability. The algorithm included the choices of further investigation, timing of surgery, surgical approach, surgical procedure, fixation, and predicted outcome.

Results.—Of the 468 hand surgeons who responded to the survey the vast majority elected to perform surgery when confronted with a case of scapholunate instability. Early surgical intervention within 6 weeks of injury using an open dorsal approach was favored in both acute and chronic cases. The preferred surgical procedure in the acute case was scapholunate repair combined with a capsulodesis followed by scapholunate ligament repair alone. Favored management of the chronic case included Blatt capsulodesis alone, capsulodesis combined with a scapholunate ligament repair, or scaphotrapezium-trapezoid arthrodesis. A majority of surgeons used K-wire fixation, especially of the scapholunate and scaphocapitate in both acute and chronic cases.

Conclusions.—This survey confirms a consensus for the early soft tissue surgical management of acute scapholunate instability using a scapholunate ligament repair with or without a capsulodesis. The management of chronic scapholunate instability is highly variable among respondents and the choice of either a soft tissue or bony procedure may depend to a large extent on intraoperative findings.

▶ This is an interesting article that basically shows practice patterns in a relatively broad spectrum of hand surgeons through a written survey. It is acknowledged that this does not represent a statement of quality of treatment or send a message advising one procedure over another. The results are not entirely unexpected, although there does seem to be substantial emphasis on the timing of surgical intervention, which I found confusing. It found that the majority of respondents preferred to treat the cases within 6 weeks of the time of injury in both acute and chronic situations, but I would have thought that the term chronic would have denoted a period much longer than 6 weeks from the time of initial injury. With that in mind, this certainly provides an interesting comparison for individuals to see how they are treating scapholunate dissociation relative to some of their peers. Of course, the principal determinant of the technique one particular surgeon would choose to use should be based upon their personal results, unless there is some mandate from a validated outcome study that convinces them otherwise.

R. A. Berger, MD, PhD

Dorsal Wrist Ligament Insertions Stabilize the Scapholunate Interval: Cadaver Study

Elsaidi GA, Ruch DS, Kuzma GR, et al (Wake Forest Univ, Winston-Salem, NC)
Clin Orthop 425:152-157, 2004   11–4

Abstract.—This study examined sequential arthroscopic sectioning of volar, interosseous, and dorsal ligaments about the scapholunate complex in cadaver wrists. We attempted to clarify the contributions of the dorsal ligamentous complex to scapholunate instability and carpal collapse. We found that after sequential sectioning of volar ligaments and the scapholunate interosseous ligament, no scapholunate diastasis or excessive scaphoid flexion occurred. After dividing the dorsal intercarpal ligament, scapholunate instability occurred without carpal collapse. With sectioning of the dorsal radiocarpal ligament from the lunate, a dorsal intercalated scapholunate instability deformity ensued. This information may be of value in comprehending the pathogenesis of scapholunate instability and carpal collapse and in devising the rationales for conservative measures and surgical intervention.

▶ Scapholunate ligament instability is a common problem with multiple treatments recommended based on incomplete biomechanical outcomes data. Many authors have suggested the use of the dorsal intercarpal ligament for reconstruction of this complex instability pattern. This study further advances our knowledge of the contributions to intercarpal stability by more precisely sequentially sectioning ligaments arthroscopically. However, the authors did not vary the order of ligament sectioning and, therefore, it is uncertain whether there is a critical ligament or ligaments that are responsible for scaphoid and lunate instability. This study does confirm the importance of the dorsal intercarpal ligament in stabilizing the scaphoid and the dorsal radiolunotriquetral ligament in stabilizing the lunate, thereby supporting reconstruction of a dorsally based capsuloligamentous tether.

R. Goitz, MD

Pre-osteotomy Plate Application Technique for Ulnar Shortening

Chennagiri R, Burge P (Nuffield Orthopaedic Centre, Headington, Oxford, England)
J Hand Surg [Br] 29B:453-457, 2004   11–5

The self-compressing mode of the AO/ASIF LC-DC plate can be harnessed to close and compress modest osteotomy gaps that are created after provisional application of the plate with two screw holes on either side of the osteotomy. The oblique osteotomy cuts are made through 70% of the bone diameter and the actual osteotomy width is measured. After provisional plate application and removal, the cuts are completed and the plate is reapplied. Eccentric drilling of up to five holes of a 6-hole plate using the 3.5 mm universal drill guide allows closure and compression of osteotomy gaps of up to 4 mm. An interfragmentary screw is placed across the oblique oste-

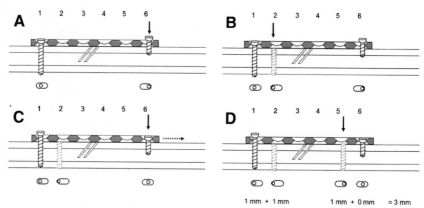

FIGURE 2.—(a) After making a double incomplete osteotomy and measuring the width in the axis of the bone, screw 1 (neutral) and screw 6 (eccentric, short) are inserted. (b) Eccentric hole is drilled at position 2. (c) Screw 1 is loosened and screw 6 is tightened, thus moving the plate 1 mm to the right. (d) Hole 5 is drilled eccentrically and the plate is removed. (Reprinted from Chennagiri R, Burge P: Pre-osteotomy plate application technique for ulnar shortening. *J Hand Surg [Br]* 29B:453-457. Copyright 2004, with permission from The British Society for Surgery of the Hand.)

otomy through the remaining hole. The technique is simple but requires careful planning and execution (Figs 2, 3, and 4).

▶ Utilizing a standard dynamic compression plate, the authors describe a sequence of screw insertion that can produce up to 4 mm of compression after

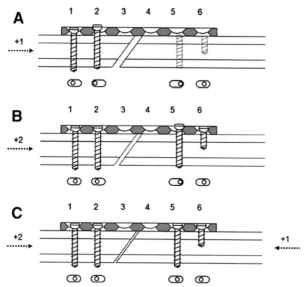

FIGURE 3.—The osteotomy is completed and the plate reapplied. As screw 1 is tightened, the gap is narrowed by 1 mm (a) and by a further 1 mm as screw 2 is tightened (b). Screw 6 (neutral) and screw 5 are inserted and 1 mm of gap closure results from tightening screw 5 (c). (Reprinted from Chennagiri R, Burge P: Pre-osteotomy plate application technique for ulnar shortening. *J Hand Surg [Br]* 29B:453-457. Copyright 2004, with permission from The British Society for Surgery of the Hand.)

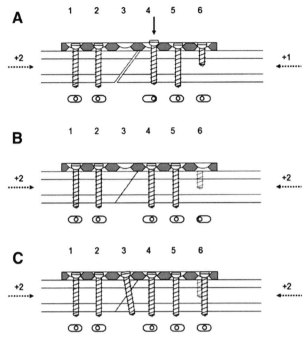

FIGURE 4.—A further 1 mm closure is obtained, if necessary, by an eccentric screw at position 4 (a), but before it is tightened screw 6 must be removed (b). The far cortex of hole 6 is drilled and a full length neutral screw is inserted. The osteotomy is compressed by a lag screw at position 3 (c) (Reprinted from Chennagiri R, Burge P: Pre-osteotomy plate application technique for ulnar shortening. *J Hand Surg [Br]* 29B:453-457. Copyright 2004, with permission from The British Society for Surgery of the Hand.)

an oblique ulnar shortening osteotomy. The technique does not require specialized jigs, compression devices, or equipment. The materials necessary for this technique should be available in any hospital or outpatient surgery center that performs routine orthopedic trauma care. The technique does require careful planning and attention to detail.

S. H. Berner, MD

12 Carpus: Kienböck's Disease

Scaphotrapeziotrapezoid (STT)-Arthrodesis in Kienböck's Disease
Meier R, van Griensven M, Krimmer H (Clinic for Handsurgery, Bad Neustadt ad Saale, Germany)
J Hand Surg [Br] 29B:580-584, 2004   12–1

Abstract.—This study reviews the results of 59 of 84 patients with severe Kienböck's disease who were treated with STT fusion.
The average follow-up period was 4 (ranges: 2-8 years). The average arc of wrist extension and flexion was 67° (60% of the contralateral side, 81% of pre-operative range) and that of ulnar and radial deviation was 31° (52% of the contralateral side, 56% of pre-operative range). Pre-operative pain values (VAS) were 56 (non-stress) and 87 (stress) and were significantly higher than the postoperative values of 12 (non-stress) and 41 (stress). Grip strength improved from 45 kPa pre-operatively to 52 kPa postoperatively. The mean modified Mayo wrist score was 63 points. The patients reported low disability in the DASH scores, with an average of 28 points.
Our data show that STT fusion is a reliable and effective treatment for pain relief and offers a good functional result in advanced stages of Kienböck's disease. However the long-term effect of this procedure on radioscaphoid and other intercarpal joints is yet to be determined.

▶ Multiple treatments have been proposed for Kienböck's disease, often without a comparative group or long-term follow-up data, making the optimal choice of treatment difficult. The use of STT fusion has long been advocated for Kienböck's disease, but has fallen out of favor for other disorders such as scapholunate advanced collapse (SLAC) wrist because of its reported high nonunion rate and long-term development of degenerative changes. This study provided confirmatory data consistent with other intermediate follow-up studies that STT fusion is a possible treatment option in the short- to intermediate-term follow-up of patients with advanced Kienböck's disease. However, this study confirms a 15% nonunion rate and the development of radioscaphoid arthritis in over 22% at an average follow-up of only 4 years.

Long-term follow-up data would be needed before one can counsel patients about this alternative.

R. Goitz, MD

The Use of the 4 + 5 Extensor Compartmental Vascularized Bone Graft for the Treatment of Kienböck's Disease
Moran SL, Cooney WP, Berger RA, et al (Mayo Clinic, Rochester, Minn)
J Hand Surg [Am] 30A:50-58, 2005   12–2

Purpose.—The use of vascularized bone grafts for the treatment of Kienböck's disease may prevent ongoing lunate collapse and provide relief of wrist symptomatology. This study examines our experience with the use of the 4 + 5 extensor compartmental artery (ECA) bone graft for the treatment of Kienböck's disease.

Methods.—A retrospective review was performed of all patients having pedicled vascularized bone grafts for Kienböck's disease between 1991 and 2002. Only those patients who had reconstruction with a 4 + 5 ECA graft were included in the study. Presurgical and postsurgical measurements included range of motion, grip strength, and pain evaluation. Measurements of the radiolunate angle, radioscaphoid angle, Ståhl's index, and carpal height ratio were taken from presurgical and final follow-up radiographs. Postsurgical magnetic resonance imaging scans were also examined to verify revascularization of the lunate. Statistical analysis was performed using Student's t test. A chi-square test was used to evaluate the effects of lunate revascularization on radiographic progression of disease. Twenty-six 4 + 5 ECA vascularized bone grafts were performed as treatment for Kienböock's disease (Figs 1, 2, 3, 4, 5, 6, and 7). The average patient age was 32 years. At the time of surgery 12 patients were graded as stage II, 10 as IIIA, and 4 as IIIB. Mean follow-up time was 31 months.

Results.—At a mean follow-up of 3 months, motion improved from 68% to 71% of the unaffected side, grip strength improved from 50% to 89% of the unaffected side, and 92% of patients had significant improvement in their pain. Satisfactory results were seen in 85% of patients based on the Lichtman outcome score. Seventy-seven percent of patients showed no further collapse on postsurgical radiographs. Sixty-five percent of patients had follow-up magnetic resonance imaging scans at a mean of 20 months after surgery. Seventy-one percent of patients showed evidence of revascularization with improvement in the T2 and/or T1 signal.

Conclusions.—The 4 + 5 ECA bone graft provides a reliable alternative for the treatment of Kienböck's disease and may aid in lunate revascularization.

► This elegant operation has been clearly described and illustrated in the article. This article should be read and kept as a technique review for all surgeons who perform vascularized bone grafts. This procedure is effective as delineated by the authors. The technique compares well to other procedures such

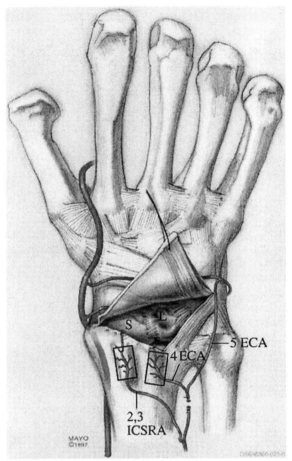

FIGURE 1.—Location of the 2,3 extensor compartmental artery (*2,3 ECA*), fourth ECA (*4 ECA*), and fifth ECA (*5 ECA*) pedicles in relation to the radiocarpal joint. The 4 + 5 ECA graft allows for capsulotomy without injury to the vascular pedicle. *Abbreviations: L,* Lunate; *S,* scaphoid; *ICSRA,* intercompartmental supraretinacular artery. (Reprinted from Moran SL, Cooney WP, Berger RA, et al: The use of the 4 + 5 extensor compartmental vascularized bone graft for the treatment of Kienböck's disease. *J Hand Surg [Am]* 30A:50-58. Copyright 2005, with permission from The American Society for Surgery of the Hand.)

as radial shortening osteotomy. Future prospective, randomized, and controlled studies will answer the question as to which operation is the best for avascular necrosis of the lunate, since a variety of different operations appear to be effective as of this time.

C. Carroll IV, MD

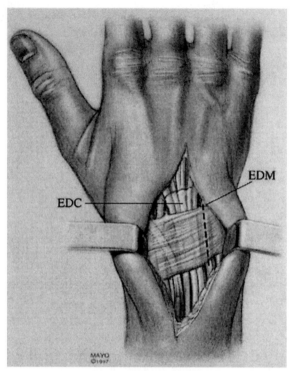

FIGURE 2.—Harvesting the fourth extensor compartmental artery (ECA) + fifth ECA graft requires identification of the fifth ECA by opening of the fifth dorsal extensor compartment. *Abbreviations: EDC,* Extensor digitorum communis; *EDM,* extensor digiti minimi. (Reprinted from Moran SL, Cooney WP, Berger RA, et al: The use of the 4 + 5 extensor compartmental vascularized bone graft for the treatment of Kienböck's disease. *J Hand Surg [Am]* 30A:50-58. Copyright 2005, with permission from The American Society for Surgery of the Hand.)

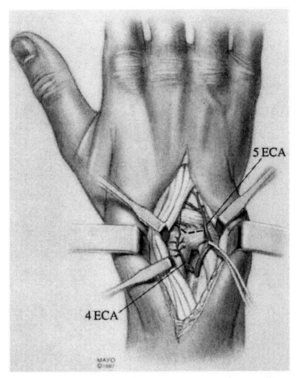

FIGURE 3.—The fifth extensor compartmental artery (*5 ECA*) is traced proximally to its origin from the anterior interosseous artery where the fourth ECA (*4 ECA*) also is identified and distally traced. (Reprinted from Moran SL, Cooney WP, Berger RA, et al: The use of the 4 + 5 extensor compartmental vascularized bone graft for the treatment of Kienböck's disease. *J Hand Surg [Am]* 30A:50-58. Copyright 2005, with permission from The American Society for Surgery of the Hand.)

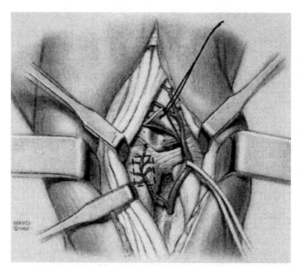

FIGURE 4.—A bone graft centered 11 mm proximal to the radiocarpal joint and overlying the fourth extensor compartmental artery (ECA) that includes the nutrient vessels is outlined. Once the graft is marked a capsulotomy is performed to expose the joint. (Reprinted from Moran SL, Cooney WP, Berger RA, et al: The use of the 4 + 5 extensor compartmental vascularized bone graft for the treatment of Kienböck's disease. *J Hand Surg [Am]* 30A:50-58. Copyright 2005, with permission from The American Society for Surgery of the Hand.)

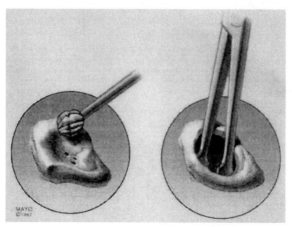

FIGURE 5.—Necrotic bone is removed with a burr or curettes, leaving a shell of intact cartilage and subchondral bone through a dorsal opening. The lunate is gently expanded to normal. (Reprinted from Moran SL, Cooney WP, Berger RA, et al: The use of the 4 + 5 extensor compartmental vascularized bone graft for the treatment of Kienböck's disease. *J Hand Surg [Am]* 30A:50-58. Copyright 2005, with permission from The American Society for Surgery of the Hand.)

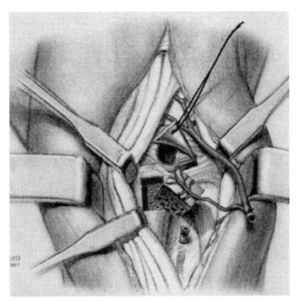

FIGURE 6.—The anterior interosseous artery is ligated proximal the fourth and fifth extensor compartmental arteries (ECAs). Graft elevation is completed and the tourniquet is deflated to verify blood flow to the graft. (Reprinted from Moran SL, Cooney WP, Berger RA, et al: The use of the 4 + 5 extensor compartmental vascularized bone graft for the treatment of Kienböck's disease. *J Hand Surg [Am]* 30A:50-58. Copyright 2005, with permission from The American Society for Surgery of the Hand.)

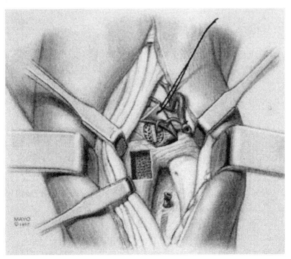

FIGURE 7.—Cancellous bone graft is packed into the lunate followed by insertion of the vascularized bone graft. (Reprinted from Moran SL, Cooney WP, Berger RA, et al: The use of the 4 + 5 extensor compartmental vascularized bone graft for the treatment of Kienböck's disease. *J Hand Surg [Am]* 30A:50-58. Copyright 2005, with permission from The American Society for Surgery of the Hand.)

13 Carpus: Imaging

Normal Sonographic Anatomy of the Wrist and Hand
Lee JC, Healy JC (Chelsea and Westminster Hosp, London)
Radiographics 25:1577-1590, 2005   13–1

The advent of ultra-high-frequency sonographic transducers has significantly enhanced our ability to image superficial structures. As a result, sonography now can be used to assess injuries of the tendons in the wrist and hand. A clear understanding of normal sonographic anatomy is required to prevent misdiagnosis and ensure optimal patient care. The anatomy of the wrist and hand is best described by considering the extensor and flexor surfaces separately. The carpal extensor retinaculum divides the dorsal extensor tendons into six separate synovial compartments, which are demarcated by the points of its attachment to the radius and ulna. The course of these tendons from the wrist to the sites of their insertion can be traced by using sonography. The intrinsic wrist ligaments, triangular fibrocartilage, and dorsal finger extensor hood also can be assessed sonographically. The anatomy of the flexor surface of the wrist is defined principally by the flexor retinaculum. The median nerve, which is located deep to the retinaculum in the carpal tunnel, and the ulnar nerve, which is superficial to the retinaculum in the Guyon canal, can be easily detected. The long flexor tendons in the wrist and hand

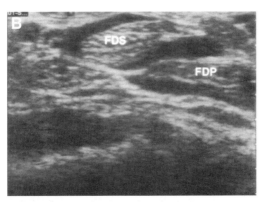

FIGURE 1.—Normal US appearance of tendons in the wrist. **B,** Transverse sonogram at the same level as a (see original article) shows the musculotendinous junctions of the flexor digitorum superficialis (*FDS*) and flexor digitorum profundus (*FDP*). The tendons appear as hypoechoic fibrils in echogenic fascicles surrounded by an echogenic epitendineum. (Courtesy of Lee JC, Healy JC: Normal sonographic anatomy of the wrist and hand. *Radiographics* 25:1577-1590, 2005.)

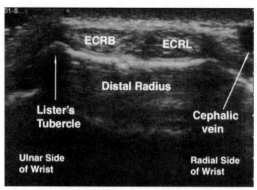

FIGURE 6.—Transverse sonogram shows the second extensor compartment, which contains the extensor carpi radialis brevis (*ECRB*) and longus (*ECRL*) tendons. (Courtesy of Lee JC, Healy JC: Normal sonographic anatomy of the wrist and hand. *Radiographics* 25:1577-1590, 2005.)

are also clearly depicted at sonography. The flexor annular pulley system is formed by five foci of thickening along the long flexor finger tendon synovial sheath, and the second and fourth annular pulleys can be identified sonographically in most patients. Sonography provides a rapid, cheap, noninvasive, and dynamic method for examination of the soft-tissue structures of the wrist and hand. Familiarity with the appearance of normal anatomic structures is a prerequisite for reliable interpretation of the resultant sonograms (Figs 1, 6, and 25).

▶ US is an attractive modality because of its relatively low cost (for equipment and to patients). Although acceptance of US has increased for musculoskeletal applications such as evaluating the rotator cuff and assessing ganglion cysts, its use in evaluating the hand and wrist has lagged behind. This excellent review shows the technique of high-resolution US for the hand and wrist with many examples of normal anatomy. While mostly a pictorial display, the article also has brief text that describes indications for the use of US in the hand and wrist and the appearance of some pathologic conditions such as the

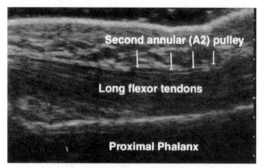

FIGURE 25.—Longitudinal sonogram of the finger at the level of the proximal phalanx shows the second annular pulley as a thin hyperechoic line (*arrows*) superficial to the long flexor tendons. (Courtesy of Lee JC, Healy JC: Normal sonographic anatomy of the wrist and hand. *Radiographics* 25:1577-1590, 2005.)

Stener lesion, which can be seen well at US in experienced hands. This article is a very complete beginning article showing normal anatomy and describing the US techniques required to visualize this degree of detail in the hand and wrist. Anyone considering using US for this purpose in their practice will find this article helpful.

K. K. Amrami, MD

MRI and Plain Radiography in the Assessment of Displaced Fractures of the Waist of the Carpal Scaphoid

Bhat M, McCarthy M, Davis TRC, et al (Univ Hosp, Nottingham, England)
J Bone Joint Surg Br 86-B:705-713, 2004   13–2

We treated 50 patients with fractures of the waist of the scaphoid in a below-elbow plaster cast for up to 13 weeks. Displacement of the fragments

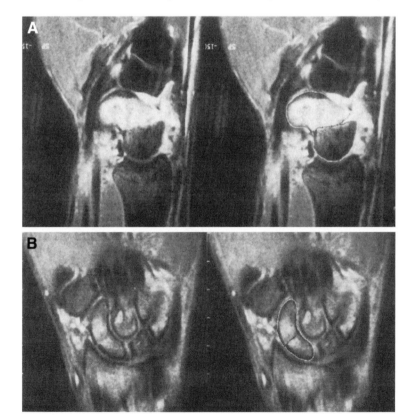

FIGURE 4.—MR scans of a moderately displaced fracture showing (**A**) the sagittal scan with and without the scaphoid and fracture outlined and (**B**) the coronal scan with and without the scaphoid and fracture outlined. (Courtesy of Bhat M, McCarthy M, Davis TRC, et al: MRI and plain radiography in the assessment of displaced fractures of the waist of the carpal scaphoid. *J Bone Joint Surg Br* 86-B:705-713, 2004.)

was assessed independently by two observers using MRI and radiographs performed within two weeks of injury.

The MRI assessments showed that only the measurement of sagittal translation of the fragments and an overall assessment of displacement had satisfactory inter- and intra-observer reproducibility and revealed that nine of the 50 fractures were displaced. Only three of the 49 fractures with adequate follow-up failed to unite, and all were displaced with more than 1 mm of translation in the sagittal plane. If the MRI assessment of displacement of the fracture was used as the measurement of choice, assessment of displacement on the initial scaphoid series of radiographs showed a sensitivity of between 33% and 47% and a positive predictive value of between 27% and 86%. Neither observer was able correctly to identify more than 33% to 47% of the displaced fractures from the plain radiographs. Although the overall assessment of displacement and gapping and translation in the coronal plane on the plain radiographs influenced the rate of union, none of these parameters identified all three fractures which failed to unite.

We conclude that the assessment of displacement of scaphoid fractures on MRI can probably be used to assess the likelihood of union although the small number of nonunions limits the power of the study. In contrast, the assessment of displacement on routine radiography is inaccurate and of less value in predicting union (Fig 4).

▶ This is a very nicely done study that shows the value of MRI in assessing displacement and alignment of the scaphoid after waist fractures. There has long been controversy regarding the value of MRI for this purpose, but in this study, the concordance and accuracy regarding translation and displacement was excellent (the *P* value of displacement between observers was 0.02). The reproducibility of specific measurements of intrascaphoid and dorsal cortical angles was poor, but this was possibly limited by the single slice in each plane available for reviewers; if the entire examination had been available, more optimal slices may have improved results for those measurements. All cases were treated conservatively, and only 3 fractures failed to unite: all 3 had displacement of greater than 1 mm in the sagittal plane. The authors note that the assessment of fracture union is more accurate on MRI than on radiography. CT, with its superior spatial resolution, remains the gold standard for evaluating scaphoid fracture comminution and displacement, but the authors of this study have shown that MRI is adequate for determining displacement, which has previously been cited as the most important predictor of nonunion. In addition, MRI provides information about other soft tissue and bone injuries and is more accurate than CT in identifying nondisplaced and radiographically occult fractures. With this study, clinicians can be confident making assessments of displacement on the basis of MRI examinations obtained for diagnosis. The authors recommend that CT or MRI be obtained in all cases of scaphoid fractures.

K. K. Amrami, MD

MRI in the Diagnosis of Cartilage Injury in the Wrist

Haims AH, Moore AE, Schweitzer ME, et al (Yale Univ, New Haven, Conn; Thomas Jefferson Univ, Philadelphia)
AJR 182:1267-1270, 2004   13–3

Objective.—Our purpose was to evaluate the accuracy of MRI in identifying articular cartilage abnormalities in the distal radius, scaphoid, lunate, and triquetrum of patients with wrist pain.

Materials and Methods.—Eighty-six MRI examinations of the wrist in 85 patients (41 indirect MR arthrograms and 45 unenhanced [nonarthrographic] MR images) were evaluated. The study population consisted of 47 male (54.7%) and 38 female (45.3%) patients with an average age of 37.5 years (range, 7–62 years). Three experienced musculoskeletal radiologists who were unaware of surgical findings retrospectively evaluated the MRI examinations for cartilage abnormalities in the distal radius, scaphoid, lunate, and triquetrum. All patients underwent arthroscopy of the radiocarpal joint with inspection of the articular surfaces of the distal radius, scaphoid, lunate, and triquetrum. The articular cartilage was evaluated on the basis of the 5-point scale of the Outerbridge classification system.

Results.—When at least two of the three radiologists had concordant interpretations, sensitivity for abnormalities in the distal radius was 27%; the scaphoid, 31%; the lunate, 41%; and the triquetrum, 18%. Specificity for the distal radius was 91%; the scaphoid, 90%; the lunate, 75%; and the triquetrum, 93%. Weighted kappa values among the three observers showed only fair agreement (0.279–0.360). High-grade more extensive cartilage lesions were no more accurately identified than low-grade lesions. Indirect MR arthrograms were not statistically more sensitive, specific, or accurate than unenhanced studies. No bone was more frequently or less frequently graded correctly or incorrectly with statistical significance. The variables of sex, age, and the presence of multiple bones with lesions did not affect accuracy.

Conclusion.—Our findings suggest that MRI of the wrist with the techniques described is not adequately sensitive or accurate for diagnosing cartilage defects in the distal radius, scaphoid, lunate, or triquetrum.

▶ This article looks at the accuracy of a qualitative assessment of cartilage comparing 2 unenhanced MRI sequences (T2 fast spin-echo with fat suppression and 3D T1-weighted gradient echo; 45 cases) and indirect gadolinium arthrography (41 cases) to arthroscopic evaluations of the cartilage of the distal radius, lunate, scaphoid, and triquetrum. The specificity is relatively good (except for the lunate), but the sensitivity was dismal, ranging from 18% to 41% (interestingly, slightly better for the lunate). This study suffers from several significant limitations related to the MRI techniques used in the study. The echo time of the T2-weighted sequences was 70 to 80 ms, which is far too long to effectively evaluate 2 changes in cartilage (the accepted range is about 20-45 ms), and the in-plane resolution on all sequences was low (the best was 0.4 mm, and the worst was 0.8 mm). Two different types of radiofrequency coils were used, of which only 1 was a dedicated wrist coil. The arthrograms were performed with the use of an indirect technique with IV gadolinium, which is suboptimal in terms of joint distension, and the T1 techniques with fat suppression show only cartilage defects and not subsurface abnormalities such as signal changes seen in grade 1 and 2 chondromalacia. This study understates the value that MRI can provide in prospective diagnosis of cartilage abnormalities of the wrist. Hopefully, a future study will use optimized sequences, resolution, and field strength to more accurately assess the value of this tool for carpal chondromalacia.

K. K. Amrami, MD

14 Hand: Congenital Differences

Brachioradialis Re-routing for the Restoration of Active Supination and Correction of Forearm Pronation Deformity in Cerebral Palsy
Ozkan T, Tuncer S, Aydin A, et al (Istanbul Univ, Turkey; American Hosp, Istanbul, Turkey)
J Hand Surg [Br] 29B:265-270, 2004   14–1

Background.—Pronation deformity of the forearm in association with a flexion contracture of the wrist is a common finding in patients with cerebral palsy. The ability to function is severely limited in patients with hemiplegia who are forced to use the dorsum of their hand or forearm for 2-handed tasks. The manipulation of small objects between the hands is difficult in these patients because the pronation contracture prevents the palms of the hands from facing each other. Several surgical procedures have been described to overcome this problem, including the flexor–pronator muscle slide, tendon transfers, and muscle releases. In this study, the re-routing of the brachioradialis tendon through the interosseous membrane is reported; the brachioradialis muscle then acts as a supinator of the forearm (Fig 1).

Methods.—The procedure was performed on 5 children with spastic hemiplegic cerebral palsy (mean age, 7 years; range, 4-14 years). After release and lengthening of the pronator quadratus and pronator teres muscles, respectively, the brachioradialis tendon was divided as a Z-plasty. The distal part of the tendon was then passed through the interosseous space in a dorsal to palmar direction and then sutured to its proximal end.

Results.—A loss of 10° to 30° of active pronation occurred in all patients because of the pronator release procedures, but this loss did not create any functional deficits. None of the patients had postoperative supination contracture. A slight increase in passive supination was seen in 3 patients, and passive supination was unchanged in the other 2 patients. The mean increase in active supination was 81° (range, 40° to 140°). The overall appearance and function of the upper limb after surgery was improved.

Conclusions.—Re-routing of the brachioradialis may be indicated in children with pronation contractures of the forearm when both pronators of the forearm are to be released or when active control of the pronator teres muscle is not possible, as determined clinically or electromyographically.

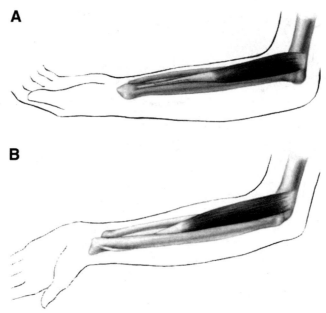

FIGURE 1.—The brachioradialis re-routing technique. (a) The tendon is cut in a Z fashion. (b) The distal tendon is passed between the radius and ulna in a dorsal to palmar direction and is sutured back to the proximal brachioradialis tendon. (Courtesy of Ozkan T, Tuncer S, Aydin A, et al: Brachioradialis re-routing for the restoration of active supination and correction of forearm pronation deformity in cerebral palsy. *J Hand Surg [Br]* 29B:265-270. Copyright 2004, with permission from the British Society for Surgery of the Hand.)

▶ The authors report their experience with 5 youngsters who lack supination as a consequence of cerebral palsy. In combination with pronator release and/ or lengthening, they rerouted the brachioradialis so that it acted as a better supinator. The children all gained some active supination but lost some pronation.

We have learned a great deal about the brachioradialis. It is a complex muscle. Although thought to be an accessory elbow flexor, it has additional attributes. It assists in supinating the forearm to neutral from the fully pronated position and assists in pronating the forearm from the fully supinated position. Thus re-education as a supinator may be an easier task. We have also learned that the position of the elbow has a large effect on the force-generating capacity of this muscle. Therefore, the position of the elbow at the time of transfer is critically important to the outcome. The authors do not state in what position the elbow is placed at the time of setting the tension of the transfer. If the elbow is fully extended, the muscle fiber length is set on the downslope of the length–tension curve and vice versa if the elbow is flexed at the time of transfer. A transfer made in one condition may perform well when the elbow is in extension, as in reaching for an object, but may become a poorer performer biomechanically as the elbow is flexed, as in bringing the object obtained toward the mouth. One may, therefore, wish to set the tension of the transfer differently for individual patients depending on patient desires.

The authors correctly stress that lack of supination is far less consequential than lack of pronation and emphasize that changing a pronation posture into one of supination is a real risk and a functional disaster. For this reason, they strive not to overlengthen the pronator teres or overtighten the rerouted brachioradialis. Personally, we discourage surgery for children who can stabilize the forearm in the neutral range and reserve surgery only for those with functionally more troublesome persistent pronation.

V. R. Hentz, MD

The Steindler Flexorplasty for the Arthrogrypotic Elbow
Goldfarb CA, Burke MS, Strecker WB, et al (Washington Univ, St Louis; Shriners Hosp for Children, St Louis)
J Hand Surg [Am] 29A:462-469, 2004   14–2

Purpose.—The arthrogrypotic elbow often lacks active flexion. If active elbow flexion can be provided by muscle transfer, patient independence increases and the patient can function in a less conspicuous manner by avoid-

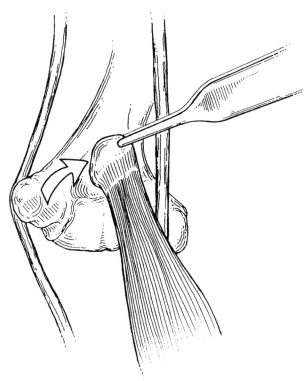

FIGURE 3.—Transferred flexor/pronator mass. (Courtesy of Goldfarb CA, Burke MS, Strecker WB, et al: The Steindler flexorplasty for the arthrogrypotic elbow. *J Hand Surg [Am]* 29A:462-469. Copyright 2004, with permission from The American Society for Surgery of the Hand.)

ing adaptive mechanisms. The purpose of this article is to review the outcome of patients with arthrogryposis treated with the Steindler flexorplasty to obtain active elbow flexion.

Methods.—Seventeen elbows in 10 patients with an average age of 7 years were treated surgically with the Steindler flexorplasty procedure. Before surgery none of the patients was able to flex actively the elbow against gravity. All of the patients had at least 70° of passive elbow flexion. Upper-extremity active and passive range of motion, strength of flexion, functional outcome, and patient satisfaction were assessed at an average of 5 years after surgery (range, 2–9 years).

Results.—After surgery all patients obtained active elbow flexion against gravity averaging 85 degrees (range, 30°–120°); patients were able to lift an average of 1 kg through their entire arc of elbow flexion. At last follow-up evaluation patients lost an average of 27° of elbow extension. Patients lost forearm rotation but did not lose wrist or finger range of motion. Subjectively, 9 of the 10 patients were satisfied with the outcome of the surgery and would recommend the surgery to others.

Conclusions.—The Steindler flexorplasty provides improved elbow flexion strength and patient function and should be considered for children with arthrogryposis (Fig 3).

▶ The authors describe their experience with the Steindler flexorplasty as a means of improving elbow flexion in children with arthrogryposis. The data indicate that, in their hands, the procedure is reliable in properly selected candidates. It does increase active elbow flexion and significantly so when one considers that none of these patients had any active elbow flexion preoperatively.

Some additional information would make this report more valuable for the clinician treating similar patients. It would be helpful to know if the outcomes of patients who had to have surgical release of elbow flexion contractures differed from those who had flexible elbows. Our past experience in other types of patients, such as those with obstetrical palsy or tetraplegia, is that patients with contracted elbows do much worse after transfer than those whose elbows have retained decent passive motion.

The level of function is a consequence of strength and arc of motion. The reader finally finds mention of the postoperative arc of motion on the penultimate page of the article. When analyzed, it is clear that a number of the patients achieved very little active motion. In fact, 7 out of the 10 patients achieved 40° or less. The mean was 58° but the median was only 35°, indicating that a few high performers skewed the mean. These data should be included in the abstract.

Finally, recent biomechanical studies indicate that the location of the transfer relative to the elbow flexion-extension axis is a more significant factor than most appreciate. Perhaps we are unnecessarily attaching this transfer too tightly for optimum outcomes.

V. R. Hentz, MD

Surgical Treatment of Type 0 Radial Longitudinal Deficiency
Mo JH, Manske PR (Washington Univ, St Louis)
J Hand Surg [Am] 29A:1002-1009, 2004   14–3

Purpose.—The purpose of this study was 2-fold: (1) to describe the surgical anatomy associated with type 0 radial longitudinal deficiency (radially deviated hand in the presence of a normal-length radius) and (2) to report the results of a surgical procedure designed to improve the alignment of the hand and forearm.

Methods.—Since 1986 there have been 6 cases of type 0 radial longitudinal deficiency in 5 children seen at the St. Louis Shriner's Hospital (Fig 1). These children were treated with a surgical procedure to release the radial

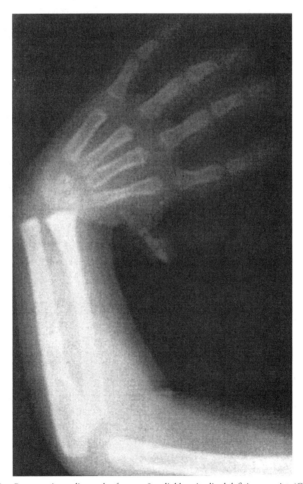

FIGURE 1.—Preoperative radiograph of a type 0 radial longitudinal deficiency wrist. (Courtesy of Mo JH, Manske PR: Surgical treatment of type 0 radial longitudinal deficiency. *J Hand Surg [Am]* 29A:1002-1009. Copyright 2004, with permission from The American Society for Surgery of the Hand.)

soft tissues and correct the alignment with tendon transfers. Age at surgery ranged from 12 to 40 months, with an average age of 21 months. The average follow-up period was 21 months. The tight radial wrist extensors were detached at their distal insertion and the tight radial wrist capsule was released dorsally and volarly, thus relieving the radial tether. The extensor carpi ulnaris (ECU) tendon also was detached just proximal to its insertion and sutured to the dorsal wrist capsule to augment wrist extension. The radial wrist extensor tendon was reattached to the ECU tendon at its insertion, converting it into an ulnar deviator.

Results.—In each case the radial wrist extensor was noted to be hypoplastic and the radial wrist capsule was noted to be tight, tethering the hand in radial deviation. In 4 cases there was only a single radial wrist extensor tendon. Average radial deviation at rest improved from 58° to 12°. Improvement in radial deviation at rest averaged 47°, ranging from 25° to 75°. Improvement in active wrist extension averaged 53° and improvement in passive wrist extension averaged 28°.

Conclusions.—For children with type 0 radial longitudinal deficiency a soft-tissue procedure that releases the radial tether and augments ulnar deviation and wrist extension by tendon transfer satisfactorily improves wrist alignment with minimal morbidity.

▶ The authors present 5 children (6 wrists) who underwent reconstruction of a type 0 radial longitudinal deficiency where the radial length was adequate and the deficiency was present in the carpus. The tendon transfer and release of the tight radial capsule allowed for satisfactory realignment before thumb reconstruction. Although follow-up was short, the article defines a technique that should be considered in the surgical reconstruction of these patients.

C. Carroll IV, MD

Correction of Madelung's Deformity by the Ilizarov Technique
Houshian S, Schrøder HA, Weeth R (Odense Univ, Denmark)
J Bone Joint Surg Br 86-B:536-540, 2004   14–4

We present our experience with correction of Madelung's deformity by the Ilizarov technique. Seven patients (eight deformities) were treated by osteotomy of the radius with subsequent lengthening and angular correction. They were reviewed at a mean of 30 months (1.5 to 5.5 years). At the time of operation their mean age was 19 years (9 to 44).

At follow-up all were free from pain and supination had improved by a mean of 34° and pronation by 9°. Flexion had increased in most cases with a median increase of 15°, but only one patient gained further extension. Radial and ulnar deviation were increased by a mean of 6° and 9°, respectively. Radiographic measurements showed that the mean volar angulation had been reduced from 25° to 11°, ulnar inclination from 45° to 30° and carpal malalignment (volar translation) from 7 to 2 mm. The mean lengthening of the radius was 12 mm (6 to 25). All the patients were satisfied with the functional and cosmetic results.

▶ The authors present their experience with correction of Madelung's deformity by the Ilizarov technique. The amount of correction of each component of the deformities was small, but enough correction was achieved, and all patients were satisfied with results after surgery. The mean distraction and consolidation time was reasonable at 53 days. The most unique point of this article may be that the authors have modified the configuration of the frame to avoid transfixation of the forearm bones or the radioulnar and radiocarpal joints. With this technique, near-normal anatomy of the wrist has been restored, and the mobility of the wrist and forearm has been improved in all directions.

For skeletally immature patients with Madelung's deformity, early resection of the ulnar zone of the epiphysis of the distal radius with an autologous fat graft, as reported by Vickers et al.,[1] gives good results. The procedure reported in this article may become a first-choice surgical treatment for Madelung's deformity in skeletally mature patients.

T. Ogino, MD

Reference

1. Vickers D, Nielsen G: Madelung deformity: Surgical prophylaxis (physiolysis) during the late growth period by resection of the dyschondrosteosis lesion. *J Hand Surg [Br]* 17:401-407, 1992.

Treatment of Traumatic Radial Clubhand Deformity With Bone Loss Using the Ilizarov Apparatus
Sabharwal S (New Jersey Med School–UMDNJ, Newark)
Clin Orthop 424:143-148, 2004   14–5

Abstract.—Radial clubhand deformity secondary to atrophic nonunion of an open distal radius fracture with bone loss is a challenging reconstructive problem. Two patients with this deformity had staged reconstruction using the Ilizarov apparatus. After gradual realignment of the distal radius metaphyseal fragment, a proximal to distal bone transport of the radial shaft was done. At completion of the bone transport, the docking site was augmented with autologous iliac crest bone graft. Both patients achieved radiographic union at the proximal and distal ends of the bone transport site and were satisfied with the outcome. At 3 years followup, full finger and elbow mobility were maintained. The wrist had improved appearance with limited painless mobility. Posttraumatic radial club hand deformities with associated bone loss can be treated successfully with staged reconstruction using the Ilizarov apparatus and methodology.

▶ The authors successfully treated 2 cases of nonunion of the distal radius with large bone loss with staged reconstruction, including gradual realignment of the distal radius metaphyseal fragments and proximal-to-distal bone transport of the radial shaft using the Ilizarov apparatus, followed by autologous iliac crest bone grafting. This same treatment concept has been applied to non-union with massive bone loss after open tibial and ulnar fractures. However, no similar report exists for distal radius fractures.

There are several potential benefits of this staged technique. There is the ability to safely distract the soft tissues through the atrophic nonunion site over several days, gradually restoring the length and alignment of the radius. Also, this innovation avoids problems with acute neurovascular stretching, flexor tendon contractures, and skin dehiscence.

T. Ogino, MD

Keloid Formation After Syndactyly Reconstruction: Associated Conditions, Prevalence, and Preliminary Report of a Treatment Method

Muzaffar AR, Rafols F, Masson J, et al (Texas Scottish Rite Hosp for Children, Dallas)
J Hand Surg [Am] 29A:201-208, 2004   14–6

Purpose.—The purpose of this study is 3-fold: to review our cases of keloid formation after syndactyly release, to report a clinical association between primary enlargement of the digits and risk of keloid formation, and to report treatment using low-dose, short-term methotrexate as an adjunct to revision surgery.

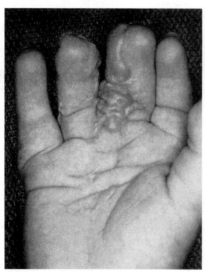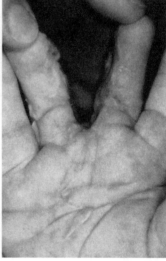

FIGURE 2.—Keloid formation after syndactyly reconstruction of the long and ring fingers in a patient with Proteus syndrome. **Left,** Appearance after syndactyly separation. **Right,** Result of keloid excision, full-thickness skin grafting, and methotrexate therapy. (Reprinted from Muzaffar AR, Rafols F, Masson J, et al: Keloid formation after syndactyly reconstruction: Associated conditions, prevalence, and preliminary report of a treatment method. *J Hand Surg [Am]* 29A:201-208. Copyright 2004, with permission from The American Society for Surgery of the Hand.)

Methods.—A retrospective review of patients identified with keloid formation after syndactyly reconstruction showed associated enlargement of the involved digits. A search of medical records for cases in which both syndactyly and digital enlargement occurred was carried out. Charts and images, where available, were reviewed for information about age, gender, involved site, associated conditions, and treatment.

Results.—Eight cases of keloids occurred in 1004 surgical procedures in 681 patients carried out during the 20-year period reviewed. Seven patients were white and 1 was Hispanic. Seven of the 8 had associated primary digital enlargement. Two patients who had enlarged syndactylized digits did not develop keloids after surgery. There was no family history in any case. Standard treatment (pressure, topical or intralesional corticosteroids, and re-excision) was unsuccessful in resolving the keloids. Two children treated with adjunctive methotrexate had successful treatment of their keloids and near-normal healing (Fig 2). Length of follow-up time after the last treatment ranged from 6 months to 11 years (average, 5.5 years).

Conclusions.—Primary digital enlargement is highly predictive of risk of keloid formation after syndactyly reconstruction. Very-low-dose, short-term methotrexate was successful as an adjunct to surgical treatment in 2 cases.

▶ Keloid formation on the hands and the feet is rare, but it may develop after release of simple syndactyly or polysyndactyly. In this retrospective review of patients with keloid formation after syndactyly, the authors reported that primary enlargement of the digits appeared to be a common finding. Careful attention to possible keloid formation is needed when performing release of syndactyly associated with digital enlargement. The authors also reported that 2 children treated with adjunctive methotrexate had successful treatment of their keloids and near-normal healing. This article provides us with an alternative treatment for severe keloid formation after syndactyly release. However, the only problem is that "the long-term risks of very-low-dose methotrexate in children are not known," as the authors mentioned.

There have been a few reports on the treatment of severe keloid formation after syndactyly release. There has been a report that tranilast, an allergy medication, has an inhibitory action on the excessive collagen biosynthesis of keloid fibroblasts.[1] This drug is clinically used to prevent keloid formation after surgery.

T. Ogino, MD

Reference

1. Shigeki S, Murakami T, Yata N, et al: Treatment of keloid and hypertrophic scars by iontophoretic transdermal delivery of tranilast. *Scand J Plast Reconstr Surg Hand Surg* 31:151-158, 1997.

A Unique Case of Total Foot-to-Hand Transfer in an Infant With Monodactyly

Hashem FK, Al-Qattan MM (King Faisal Specialist Hosp, Riyadh, Saudi Arabia)
J Hand Surg [Br] 30B:343-345, 2005   14–7

Background.—Congenital absence of the digits is frequently treated by toe-to-hand transfer. Reconstruction can be done using single or multiple toe-to-hand transfers, depending on the number of missing digits. A unique case was presented in which the entire foot, including the calcaneus, was transferred to the hand.

> *Case Report.*—Infant, 8 months, was born with congenital deformities involving all 4 limbs. The left upper limb was normal except for aplasia of the ulnar 2 fingers. The right shoulder had normal range of motion but the elbow and wrist had moderately restricted range of motion; the right hand was monodigital. Both lower limbs had identical deformities: the hips were normal but the knees had fixed flexion contractures of about 80°. Each leg had a tibia and no fibula, and the feet were grossly deformed and hypoplastic. The left foot was monodigital and the right foot had 2 synostosed digits.
>
> It was decided to perform bilateral through-knee amputations in order to fit the child with bilateral prosthesis and to initiate an early mobilization program. It was also decided to transfer the right foot to act as a post against the partially mobile single digit of the right hand. The foot-to-hand transfer was completed by arterial anastomosis end-to-side between the popliteal artery and the brachial artery in the lower arm. A venous anastomosis was then performed end-to-end between the popliteal vein and a large antecubital vein. The posterior tibial nerve was sutured end-to-side to the median nerve at the wrist after a partial neurectomy of about 15% of the substance of the median nerve. Bony fixation of the calcaneus to the shaft of the radius was performed using 2 K-wires.
>
> Postoperative recovery was uneventful. The K-wires were removed at 6 weeks. The parents were not satisfied with the appearance of the hand at the initial follow-up visit, and it was explained to them that function was the primary goal of the surgery. There were no further complaints. Recovery of sweating at 8 months after surgery indicated sensory recovery. At final follow-up at 18 months after surgery, the foot transfer was stable and acting as a post against which the partially mobile single digit pinched.

Conclusion.—Toe transfers in infants and young children are more demanding technically than transfers in older children. In addition to being unique because the whole foot was transferred, this case illustrates the concept of using "spare parts" from the foot in hand reconstruction for children with severe upper and lower limb congenital defects. Children undergoing toe-to-hand transfer should be reviewed with their parents and assessed for functional and psychosocial performance. The parents of this patient were not happy initially with the cosmetic appearance of the hand, despite their participation in several preoperative meetings.

▶ An 8-month-old infant with monodactyly due to ulnar deficiency of the right arm and 2 synostosed digits due to tibial deficiency of the right leg treated with total foot-to-hand transfer is described. It is not difficult to consider this type of foot-to-hand transfer for an infant with monodactyly. The article teaches us that we, as hand surgeons with microsurgical technique, should always think about reconstruction of the hand by using "spare parts" from the foot. The author succeeded in the operation; however, the timing of surgery is questioned. Complex microsurgery is safer after the age of 2 years.

T. Ogino, MD

15 Hand: Carpal Tunnel Syndrome

The Relationship of VEGF and PGE$_2$ Expression to Extracellular Matrix Remodelling of the Tenosynovium in the Carpal Tunnel Syndrome
Hirata H, Nagakura T, Tsujii M, et al (Mie Univ, Tsu City, Japan; Suzuka Kaisei Gen Hosp, Tsu City, Japan)
J Pathol 204:605-612, 2004   15–1

Abstract.—Tenosynovial thickening within the confined space of the carpal tunnel is thought to be the cause of the carpal tunnel syndrome (CTS). However, little is known about the pathological mechanism of tenosynovial thickening. In this study, the role of prostaglandin E$_2$ (PGE$_2$) and vascular endothelial growth factor (VEGF) (two representative molecules that can induce oedema by increasing vascular permeability) was analysed in CTS by using immunohistochemistry and enzyme-linked immunosorptive assay (ELISA). Expression of these molecules was compared with the patients' clinical histories and a temporary increase in production of these molecules was found in cells within the vessels and synovial lining during the intermediate phase of the syndrome when the histology of the tenosynovium changes from oedematous to fibrotic. Statistical analysis clearly demonstrated that there is a close correlation between the expression of PGE$_2$ and VEGF. Furthermore, immunohistochemical analysis with anti-proliferating cell nuclear antigen (PCNA) revealed that the area with distinct VEGF expression closely matched the area where endothelial cells, vascular smooth muscle cells, and synovial lining cells proliferate. In contrast, despite marked alteration in the extracellular matrix (ECM) component of the tenosynovium, the fibroblasts responsible for most ECM framework production do not proliferate during any phase of CTS. Histological analysis demonstrated that angiogenesis takes place only during the intermediate phase. Since clusters of capillaries and arterioles are often surrounded by type III collagen-rich, disorganized, degenerate connective tissue, which contains fewer fibroblasts than normal, angiogenesis appears to take place as a part of a regenerative reaction that results in fibrosis. These findings strongly indicate that both PGE$_2$ and VEGF are expressed in the tenosynovium in CTS during the intermediate phase and induce the histological changes seen in the tenosynovium.

▶ There is currently a limited understanding of the cellular and molecular changes to the median nerve secondary to CTS. As excisional biopsy of human median nerves would create significant morbidity, investigators often biopsy the surrounding tissue to gain greater insight to the pathogenesis of CTS.

The authors performed a histologic analysis of the tenosynovium to determine altered levels of VEGF and PGE_2. They confirmed previous reports in the literature that there is marked remodeling of the ECM with continued disease progression. They also performed an analysis of the effects of mechanical strain on the tenosynovial fibroblasts.

One may interpret these data as showing that there is a phenotypic change to these cells that produces the increased production of VEGF and PGE_2 secondary to mechanical strain. It is interesting to note that the increased expression of VEGF and PGE_2 does not correlate with the edema that is seen with CTS, but rather occurs later in the disease progression.

As such, this alteration in protein expression is likely a secondary response to the actual pathology of CTS. While this study provides new information about the pathogenesis of CTS, it also reaffirms that alternative methods of exploring this disease—such as animal models or in vitro modeling systems—are required to gain a better understanding and eventual improved treatment regimens for compression neuropathies.

R. Gupta, MD

Randomized Controlled Trial of Nocturnal Splinting for Active Workers With Symptoms of Carpal Tunnel Syndrome

Werner RA, Franzblau A, Gell N (Univ of Michigan, Ann Arbor)
Arch Phys Med Rehabil 86:1-7, 2005   15–2

Objectives.—To determine whether nocturnal splinting of workers identified through active surveillance with symptoms consistent with carpal tunnel syndrome (CTS) would improve symptoms and median nerve function as well as impact medical care.

Design.—Randomized controlled trial.

Setting.—A Midwestern auto assembly plant.

Participants.—Active workers with symptoms suggestive of CTS based on a hand diagram.

Intervention.—The treatment group received customized wrist splints, which were worn at night for 6 weeks; the control group received ergonomic education alone.

Main Outcome Measures.—Change in wrist, hand, and/or finger discomfort, carpal tunnel symptom severity index, median sensory nerve function, and the percentage of subjects who had carpal tunnel release surgery.

Results.—The splinted group, unlike the controls, had a significant reduction in wrist, hand, and/or finger discomfort and a similar trend in the Levine carpal tunnel symptom severity index, which was maintained at 12 months. A secondary analysis showed that more median nerve impairment at baseline was associated with less clinical improvement among controls but not among the splinted group.

Conclusions.—Workers identified with CTS symptoms in an active symptom surveillance tended to benefit from a 6-week nocturnal splinting trial, and the benefits were still evident at the 1-year follow-up. The splinted group improved in terms of hand discomfort regardless of the degree of median nerve impairment, whereas the controls showed improvement only among subjects with normal median nerve function. Results suggest that a short course of nocturnal splinting may reduce wrist, hand, and/or finger discomfort among active workers with symptoms consistent with CTS.

▶ This study showed the benefit of a 6-week trial of nocturnal splinting for employees/patients at risk for CTS. Additionally, this is the first randomized, controlled study of short-term night splinting for CTS. Although it would be impossible to blind this type of study, I agree with the authors that a greater number of subjects and longer follow-up would add more power to this study.

I use night wrist splinting in my hand therapy practice with CTS patients and have found it to be very helpful to the patient in terms of reducing overall discomfort, especially nocturnal pain and paresthesias. I prefer custom-fitted wrist splints (constructed with a light, breathable material) to prefabricated wrist splints because I have found improved patient compliance with night wear due to greater comfort. In today's fast-paced hand clinic environment, this is not always a feasible option due to restraints on the therapist's time. It is imperative, therefore, to research various prefabricated splinting options in order to determine which would provide the greatest comfort and, hence, improved compliance.

M. Outzen, MS, OTR/L

A Meta-Analysis of Randomized Controlled Trials Comparing Endoscopic and Open Carpal Tunnel Decompression
Thoma A, Veltri K, Haines T, et al (McMaster Univ, Hamilton, Ont, Canada)
Plast Reconstr Surg 114:1137-1146, 2004   15–3

Controversy exists regarding the benefit of endoscopic carpal tunnel release versus open carpal tunnel release in terms of grip/pinch strength, scar tenderness, pain, return to work, reversible/irreversible nerve damage, and adverse effects. Although a number of randomized controlled trials and systematic reviews have been published on the subject, to date, no large definitive randomized controlled trial or meta-analysis has been performed comparing endoscopic to open carpal tunnel release. This meta-analysis was undertaken to address the effectiveness of endoscopic carpal tunnel release relative to open carpal tunnel release. Key outcome measures from 13 randomized controlled trials were extracted and statistically combined. Heterogeneity was observed in three of the outcomes (i.e., grip strength, pain, and return to work), but the causes of heterogeneity could not be explained because of insufficient detail in the reported studies. Using the Jadad et al scale, nine of 13 studies were of low methodologic quality. The effect sizes were compared between the studies that were rated as high quality and the studies that were rated as low quality on the Jadad et al. scale. Similarly, the studies that were rated as high quality on the Gerritsen et al. scale were compared with those that were rated as low quality. No clinically significant difference in effect sizes was apparent between studies of high and low methodologic quality. This meta-analysis supports the conclusion that endoscopic carpal tunnel release is favored over the open carpal tunnel release in terms of a reduction in scar tenderness and increase in grip and pinch strength at a 12-week follow-up. With regard to symptom relief and return to work, the data are inconclusive. Irreversible nerve damage is uncommon in either technique; however, there is an increased susceptibility to reversible nerve injury that is three times as likely to occur with endoscopic carpal tunnel release than with open carpal tunnel release.

▶ This study represents a follow-up of a previous study by the same authors. The initial study was a systematic review of reviews comparing endoscopic and open carpal tunnel decompression. The authors concluded that meta-analysis would permit definitive conclusions about the relative effectiveness of endoscopic carpal tunnel release to open carpal tunnel release. In the current study a search of the literature was undertaken, and 13 randomized controlled trials comparing 2 techniques of carpal tunnel release were identified. The Jadad and Gerritsen scales were applied to each of the individual 13 studies, and the studies were rated based on methodological quality. The authors compared various outcome measures of clinical status, including relief of symptoms, grip strength, pinch strength, number of days until return to work or activities of daily living, reversible nerve damage, irreversible nerve damage, and reflex sympathetic dystrophy. The authors concluded that grip and pinch strength at 12 weeks were favored in the endoscopic group. However, only 3 of the 13 studies included appropriate criteria to permit appropriate statistical analysis. Scar tenderness was favored in the endoscopic group as well. There was a 3 times more likely incidence of reversible nerve damage in the endoscopic carpal tunnel release group. There were no significant differences between the groups with respect to pain and return to work. This may in part be due to the fact that there is a significant subjective component to pain measurement, and there are inherent biases with respect to return to work. The authors were unable to pool data regarding resolution of numbness and tingling. Irreversible nerve damage was exceedingly rare, and, therefore, data could not be appropriately pooled either. The authors do suggest further investigation. It may end up taking a large multi-center randomized controlled trial with a standardized methodology for assessment. Such a study would require a great number of patients but may ultimately address the controversy involving the efficacy of endoscopic carpal tunnel release as compared to open carpal tunnel release.

S. H. Berner, MD

Endoscopic Carpal Tunnel Release: Modification of Menon's Technique and Data From 191 Cases
Tuzuner S, Sherman M, Özkaynak S, et al (Akdeniz Univ, Antalya, Turkey; SUNY Upstate Med Univ, Syracuse)
Arthroscopy 20:721-727, 2004   15–4

Background.—Among the postoperative complications found with open carpal tunnel release are painful hypertrophic scars, persistent symptoms, infection, and median or ulnar nerve injuries. Even successful operations impose a lengthy perioperative disability and extended recovery time that can prove costly for the patient and employer. Endoscopic carpal tunnel release was developed to address many of these concerns and has been linked to less scarring, less postoperative pain, preservation of pinch and grip strength, and faster healing. Menon's technique is one of several variations of endoscopic carpal tunnel release. Patient satisfaction, changes in grip strength, time until work was resumed, and complications were documented for a series of patients undergoing Menon's technique for the treatment of carpal tunnel syndrome. Modifications to reduce complications and improve patient outcomes were undertaken, and the results were compared.

Methods.—One surgeon performed endoscopic carpal tunnel release on an outpatient basis for 227 hands of 191 patients. Patients were then surveyed for their degree of satisfaction with the outcome. Quantitative measurements were made of grip strength, time until return to work, and complications. The technique was modified after the first 50 hands (41 cases) were operated on. These changes resulted from difficulty maintaining the knife in the center of the cannula's slot and a relatively high rate of complications. For the modified method, use of a 2.7-mm 25° endoscope and triangular diamond-tipped knife permitted more room for the instruments and produced a safer technique.

Results.—At final evaluation, 91% of the patients reported satisfaction with the results. One hundred sixty-three patients (196 hands) had an improved grip strength postoperatively. By 12 weeks postoperatively, 81% of the patients obtained 75% to 100% or greater grip strength compared with preoperative levels. Patients were able to return to work an average of 18 days after surgery. Of the first 50 hands, which were operated on using the original technique, complications included wound healing (1 patient), needed reexploration of the carpal tunnel (2 patients), abnormal sensations (12 patients), and partial median nerve injury repaired during the initial surgery (1 patient). None of the patients who had the modified technique developed major complications. One patient had postoperative hypoesthesia along the long and ring fingers that improved over time.

Conclusions.—Patients with carpal tunnel syndrome can be effectively treated with the use of Menon's technique, but there is a risk of damage to the neurovascular structures. Modification of the technique as described lessened this risk, making it safer. Patients' subjective satisfaction with both of the procedures was high, with substantially improved grip strength and a return to work within 3 weeks.

▶ As an advocate and user of the open carpal tunnel release technique, I must admit my bias away from endoscopic releases. For a period of my career, I did perform endoscopic releases using another single portal technique, but my own experience led me to believe that there was no measurable difference in the outcomes of my patients between the 2 groups, and I felt that the addition of an endoscopic release added a level of technologic complexity that perhaps would not be worth it in my own practice balanced against the limited improvement in expectations. With this said, I continue to be concerned about the potential complications when we are dealing with structures that we cannot see directly. This was illustrated in the authors' own finding of a partial median nerve laceration using this technique. I am not saying at all that this cannot happen with an open technique, particularly given the variation of the location of both the ulnar nerve and the median nerve in the region that is being operated on. However, regardless of which technique is being used, one nerve laceration is one too many in my estimation. If there is a learning curve that is necessary with these procedures, I would hope that the majority of that learning curve is carried out on cadaveric practice sessions rather than patients. I for one will continue performing an open carpal tunnel release, and I advocate to those I train to do the same for precisely the same reasons that I have stated here.

R. A. Berger, MD, PhD

Functional Tests to Quantify Recovery Following Carpal Tunnel Release
Radwin RG, Sesto ME, Zachary SV (Univ of Wisconsin, Madison)
J Bone Joint Surg Am 86-A:2614-2635, 2004   15–5

Background.—An objective test is needed to evaluate outcome following carpal tunnel release. A method to evaluate sensory and motor function related to carpal tunnel syndrome was investigated.

Methods.—Thirty-six candidates for carpal tunnel surgical procedures underwent a physical examination and nerve-conduction studies and completed a survey regarding symptoms. A battery of psychomotor and sensory tests was administered bilaterally immediately before surgery and again six weeks after surgery. The outcome variables included dynamic sensory gap-detection thresholds and rapid pinch-and-release rates.

Results.—The average gap-detection threshold for the index finger in the surgical-treatment group demonstrated a 43% improvement, decreasing from 0.14 mm preoperatively to 0.08 mm at six weeks postoperatively (p < 0.01). The average gap-detection threshold for the index finger in the non-surgical-treatment group demonstrated no significant improvement, decreasing from 0.10 mm preoperatively to 0.08 mm postoperatively (p = 0.10). With the upper force level set at 10% of the maximum voluntary contraction, the average pinch rate in the surgical-treatment group demonstrated a 20% improvement, increasing from 6.65 pinches per second preoperatively to 7.96 pinches per second postoperatively (p < 0.001). The average pinch rate in the non-surgical-treatment group demonstrated a 7% improvement, increasing from 6.89 pinches per second preoperatively to 7.37 pinches per second at six weeks postoperatively (p < 0.05).

Conclusions.—Measurable and significantly greater improvement was observed when the surgical-treatment group was compared with the non-surgical-treatment group in terms of these two sensory and psychomotor functional testing outcomes at six weeks.

▶ The purpose of this article is to test the responsiveness of a computerized instrument entitled the "automated aesthesiometer" to measure sensory recovery after carpal tunnel release. Carpal tunnel surgery is one of the most effective procedures in hand surgery. While outcome questionnaires often demonstrate a marked improvement in symptom resolution, objective tools have not been developed to quantify these improvements.

The design of an automated instrument as described in this article is an interesting concept, but more testing is necessary before this instrument can be prescribed for general application. Although this instrument was touted as an objective functional measure after carpal tunnel release, the interpretation of the sensory input is still dependent on patients' responses. Therefore, similar to outcome questionnaires, there is an element of subjectivity that is influenced by patient factors.

K. C. Chung, MD, MS

Validity and Responsiveness of the Patient Evaluation Measure as an Outcome Measure for Carpal Tunnel Syndrome
Hobby JL, Watts C, Elliot D (North Hampshire Hosp, Basingstoke, England; Broomfield Hosp, Chelmsford, England)
J Hand Surg [Br] 30-B:350-354, 2005   15–6

The aim of this study was to assess the validity of the Patient Evaluation Measure questionnaire (PEM) as an outcome measure in carpal tunnel syndrome. The PEM was compared to the DASH questionnaire and to objective measurements of hand function. We also compared its responsiveness to changes following carpal tunnel release with that of the DASH score. Twenty-four patients completed the PEM and DASH questionnaires before and 3 months after open carpal tunnel release. Grip strength, static two-point discrimination and the nine-hole peg test were measured. There was a significant correlation between individual items of the PEM and the objective measures. There was also strong correlation between PEM and DASH scores. The PEM showed a greater responsiveness to change (effect size 0.97) than the DASH score (effect size 0.49). The PEM correlates well with objective measures of hand function and the DASH score when used in carpal tunnel syndrome. It is more responsive to change than the DASH score. It is very simple to complete and score and is an appropriate and practical outcome measure in carpal tunnel syndrome.

▶ One of the maddening things about articles on validated outcome instruments is that they typically do not include the questionnaires in the body of the article. It's like reading about the beauty of iambic pentameter in *Cliff's Notes* without ever reading a line of Shakespeare. Hobby and colleagues compare the PEM, commonly used in the United Kingdom, to the DASH.

The PEM is a simple, 18-question psychometric test which probes the patient's perception of the doctor, treatment, and the state of the medical condition. The DASH is known to lack sensitivity to specific conditions since it asks about total limb, rather than joint-specific disability. It also shows great variability between chronic conditions, such as rheumatoid arthritis, compared to acute trauma. The Patient Rated Wrist Evaluation[1] probably shows the most promise in comparing patient scores to objective scores. Nonetheless, continued efforts to understand the morass of outcome measurements is welcome.

A. L. Ladd, MD

Reference

1. MacDermid JC, Turgeon T, Richards RS, et al: Patient rating of wrist pain and disability: A reliable and valid measurement tool. *J Orthop Trauma* 12:577-586, 1998.

Potential MR Signs of Recurrent Carpal Tunnel Syndrome: Initial Experience
Wu H-TH, Schweitzer ME, Culp RW (Natl Yang Ming Univ, Taipei, Taiwan; New York Univ; Philadelphia Hand Ctr, King of Prussia, Pa)
J Comput Assist Tomogr 28:860-864, 2004   15–7

Objective.—In nonoperated patients, the MR diagnosis of carpal tunnel syndrome (CTS) is difficult. In the postoperative patient this difficulty is compounded. Consequently, we sought to evaluate for potential MR signs of postoperative CTS.

Methods.—At 1.5 T, 41 wrists in 37 patients with previous CTS release were evaluated by two observers for 1) flexor retinacular regrowth; 2) median nerve: a) high T2 signal, b) proximal enlargement, c) fibrous fixation, d) neuroma, and e) entrapment; 3) flexor tenosynovitis; 4) mass, bursitis, accessory muscle, distal belly progression, or excessive deep fat; 5) hamate fracture; and 6) volar nerve migration. Electromyography (EMG), operative findings, and clinical follow-up were used to determine the presence of recurrent CTS.

Results.—Fifteen of 41 wrists had recurrent CTS. Retinacular regrowth was seen in 4/15 (27%) with and 7/26 (27%) without recurrent CTS ($P = 0.7$). Excessive fat was seen in 1/15 (7%) with and 2/26 (8%) without CTS ($P = 0.19$). No patient had incomplete resection of flexor retinaculum, scarring, neuroma of nerve, or tendon laceration; bursitis, accessory or distal muscle progression of muscle belly, or hamate fracture. Nerve edema with high T2 signal was seen in 4/15 (27%) with and 3/26 (12%) without CTS ($P = 0.16$); proximal enlargement was seen in 6/15 (40%) with CTS and 2/26 (8%) without CTS ($P = 0.007$). Also, 1 patient with recurrent disease demonstrated a mass and 1 other patient without CTS had nerve entrapment. Tenosynovitis was seen in 9/15 (60%) with and 9/26 (35%) without recurrent CTS ($P = 0.02$). Counterintuitively, the nerve was more palmar with recurrent CTS than without (mean 6.9/8.9 mm).

Conclusion.—Only proximal enlargement, tenosynovitis, and the rare mass may help to diagnose recurrent CTS by MR. However, there appears to be a subgroup of patients with recurrent neuropathy related to an excessively superficial median nerve.

▶ The use of MRI for the diagnosis of CTS has been complicated by the inconsistency of findings for both primary and recurrent CTS. Most clinicians and radiologists would agree that MRI is most valuable for recurrent CTS after release in assessing complications, incomplete resection of the transverse carpal ligament, and other variables, and this group has rightfully focused on the specific problem of recurrent CTS. That authors looked at retinacular "regrowth," excessive fat, increased T2 signal, proximal enlargement of the median nerve, presence of mass lesions, and tenosynovitis. Only the presence of flexor tenosynovitis and enlargement of the median nerve proximal to the carpal tunnel were statistically significant. The authors did not assess thenar musculature for denervation changes and did not separately address the issue of entrapment of the nerve in scarring, even though they show an example (Fig 1 in the original article).

This is a small study, and the authors acknowledge significant limitations. They state that MRI may be more valuable when preoperative imaging is available, which is an unlikely scenario when the diagnosis of CTS is commonly made clinically with the support of EMG. MRI continues to have value in assessing complications of CTS surgery or incomplete resection of the transverse carpal ligament; nonetheless, it is still a supportive test, secondary to clinical and EMG findings, rather than a primary test for the diagnosis of either primary or recurrent CTS.

K. K. Amrami, MD

16 Hand: Peripheral Nerve

Comparison of Transthecal Digital Block and Traditional Digital Block for Anesthesia of the Finger
Keramidas EG, Rodopoulou SG, Tsoutsos D, et al (Gen State Hosp of Athens "G Gennimatas," Greece; Northern Gen Hosp, Sheffield, England)
Plast Reconstr Surg 114:1131-1134, 2004   16–1

A randomized, double-blind study was performed in 50 patients to compare the transthecal and traditional subcutaneous infiltration techniques of digital block anesthesia regarding the onset of time to achieve anesthesia and pain during the infiltration. All the patients had sustained injury involving two or four fingers of the hand. Each patient served as his or her own control, having one finger infiltrated with the transthecal technique and the other with the subcutaneous infiltration technique. Time to loss of pinprick sensation and pain (at the time of the infiltration and 24 hours postoperatively) were assessed using a visual analogue scale and verbal response score. A total of 104 blocks (52 transthecal and 52 subcutaneous infiltration) were performed. All of these blocks were successful. Mean time to achieve anesthesia with the transthecal block was 165 seconds, compared with 100 seconds for the subcutaneous infiltration block. The mean analogue pain score was higher for transthecal blocks than for subcutaneous infiltration blocks (3.2 ± 0.19 versus 1.6 ± 0.14). Twenty-four hours postoperatively, 24 patients who had the transthecal block experienced pain at the injection site of the digit. However, none of the patients who received the subcutaneous infiltration block complained of pain at the digit. The technique of anesthesia preferred by patients for their finger was the subcutaneous infiltration block, because it causes less pain. Our results confirm the efficacy of the transthecal block for achieving anesthesia of the finger; however, because it is a more painful procedure, it is not recommended.

▶ The authors present a very well-done prospective randomized study comparing 2 types of digital anesthesia. The findings demonstrate that the subcutaneous (2-injection) dorsal technique provided faster anesthesia and caused less pain from the injection than did a single transthecal injection. Furthermore, at 24 hours after the injection, a significant number of patients who had the transthecal injection had pain at the injection site. I found it interesting that the same amount (2 mL) of total lidocaine was used to anesthetize with either technique. The vast majority of patients preferred the subcutaneous blocks. As someone who does both techniques, I find that the results of this study make a strong argument for the subcutaneous method.

M. Rizzo, MD

The Effect of Long-Distance Bicycling on Ulnar and Median Nerves: An Electrophysiologic Evaluation of Cyclist Palsy

Akuthota V, Plastaras C, Lindberg K, et al (Univ of Colorado, Denver; Rehabilitation Inst of Chicago; Univ of Chicago; et al)

Am J Sports Med 33:1224-1230, 2005   16–2

Background.—Distal ulnar neuropathies have been identified in cyclists because of prolonged grip pressures on handlebars. The so-called cyclist palsy has been postulated to be an entrapment neuropathy of the ulnar nerve

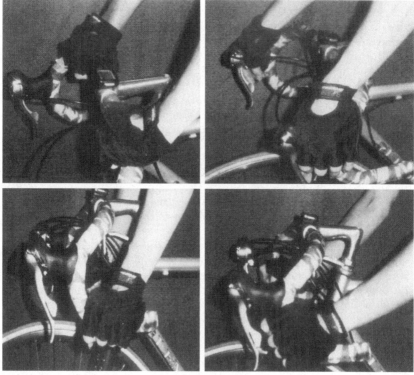

FIGURE 4.—A variety of hand positions available for road cycling. (Courtesy of Akuthota V, Plastaras C, Lindberg K, et al: The effect of long-distance bicycling on ulnar and median nerves: An electrophysiologic evaluation of cyclist palsy. *Am J Sports Med* 33:1224-1230, 2005.)

in the Guyon canal of the wrist. Previous studies utilizing nerve conduction studies have typically been either case reports or small case series.

Hypothesis.—Electrophysiologic changes will be present in the ulnar and median nerves after a long-distance multiday cycling event.

Study Design.—Cohort study; Level of evidence, 2.

Methods.—A total of 28 adult hands from 14 subjects underwent median and ulnar motor and sensory nerve conductions, which were performed on both hands before and after a 6-day, 420-mile bike tour. A ride questionnaire was also administered after the ride, evaluating the experience level of the cyclist, equipment issues, hand position, and symptoms during the ride.

Results.—Distal motor latencies of the deep branch of the ulnar nerve to the first dorsal interosseous were significantly prolonged after the long-distance cycling event. The median motor and sensory studies as well as the ulnar sensory and motor studies of the abductor digiti minimi did not change significantly. Electrophysiologic and symptomatic worsening of carpal tunnel syndrome was observed in 3 hands, with the onset of carpal tunnel syndrome in 1 hand after the ride.

Conclusion.—Long-distance cycling may promote physiologic changes in the deep branch of the ulnar nerve and exacerbate symptoms of carpal tunnel syndrome (Fig 4).

▶ The authors have taken the effort to document what many of us have seen clinically: Long-distance cyclists put chronic compressive loads on Guyon's canal, and, by proximity, on the carpal tunnel. The authors note the cyclists wore gloves, and, in all but 1 case, used padded handlebars.

The authors do not comment on whether all cyclists had drop handlebars, nor do they comment on the different hand positions that may provoke the compression, as seen in Figure 4. Furthermore, they do not discuss modifications of handlebars such as aerodynamic handlebars (Aerobars) and whether modifications improve ergonomics and nerve compression. Most importantly, they do not discuss prevention or treatment of the problem, not even the assumed recommendation: "Stop cycling!"

A. L. Ladd, MD

Resistance to Disruption and Gapping of Peripheral Nerve Repairs: An In Vitro Biomechanical Assessment of Techniques
Temple CLF, Ross DC, Dunning CE, et al (Univ of Western Ontario, London, Canada)
J Reconstr Microsurg 20:645-650, 2004   16–3

One potential cause of suboptimal results after nerve repair is disruption or gapping of the neurorrhaphy in the postoperative period. This study assesses the biomechanical strength of five nerve repair techniques: fibrin glue, simple epineurial sutures, and three other novel neurorrhaphy methods. Fifty rabbit sciatic nerve segments were divided and repaired utilizing one of five different methods, producing five groups of ten specimens. Fibrin glue and four epineurial suture techniques (simple, horizontal mattress, "Tajima," "Bunnell") were employed. Repaired nerve segments were ramp-loaded to failure on an Instron 8300 materials-testing machine at a displacement rate of 5 mm/min. Gapping at the repair site was captured using high-resolution video. Differences among the five groups were assessed for significance using ANOVA and Fisher's protected least squares differences post-hoc testing. The mean force to produce disruption was higher for mattress suture repairs relative to simple repairs, but not significantly so ($p = 0.31$). Both were significantly stronger than fibrin glue repairs ($p < 0.0001$). "Tajima" and "Bunnell" repairs were both statistically stronger than glue ($p < 0.0001$), simple ($p < 0.0001$), or mattress ($p = 0.0004$) repairs, but not significantly different from one another ($p = 0.48$). Data for gapping at the repair site were similar with all suture techniques outperforming fibrin glue ($p = 0.003$). "Bunnell" repairs demonstrated the most resistance to gapping, compared to glue ($p < 0.0001$), simple ($p = 0.0001$), mattress ($p = 0.007$) and "Tajima" repairs ($p = 0.01$). These data demonstrate that repairs done utilizing fibrin glue are significantly weaker than all types of suture repairs. Two novel techniques for nerve repair (epineurial "Tajima" and "Bunnell") are significantly more resistant to disruption and gapping. Further evaluation to assess the effect of these repair techniques on function is required.

▶ Despite advances in microsurgery, peripheral nerve repairs continue to often have suboptimal results. The authors have attempted to determine the optimal suture technique to help reduce the amount of gapping by evaluating repair strength with a time-zero biomechanical study in a manner that is analogous to most flexor tendon repairs. They demonstrated that locking epineurial sutures, such as the Tajima and Bunnell techniques, provided the greatest resistance to gapping and mechanical disruption of nerve repairs.

Although the investigators used an animal model (rabbit sciatic nerve), they failed to use the full potential of an animal study to evaluate healing and outcomes after nerve coaptation. While the strongest techniques may certainly have the greatest time-zero strength, the locking epineurial sutures may also produce the greatest fibrosis and induce formation of an intraneural neuroma.

It is important to recognize that although fibrin glue had the poorest mechanical strength, this may not be of importance with proximal injuries such as brachial plexus injuries where there is limited movement. While initial resistance to gapping is certainly important when performing nerve coaptation, outcomes evaluation with histology and electrophysiology are of paramount importance prior to determining if either of the locking epineurial suturing techniques has clinical applicability.

R. Gupta, MD

Nerve Repair Using a Vein Graft Filled With Collagen Gel
Choi B-H, Zhu S-J, Kim S-H, et al (Yonsei Univ, Seoul, Korea; Yonsei Univ, Wonju, Korea; Univ of Ulsan, Gangneung, Korea; et al)
J Reconstr Microsurg 21:267-272, 2005   16–4

Abstract.—It has been shown that a vein graft provides a good environment for axon regeneration in short nerve gaps. But the use of a vein graft for long nerve gaps is controversial because veins may collapse, due to their thin walls, and the surrounding scar tissue can cause constriction. In an attempt to improve results using the vein graft, the authors conducted the reported experiment by filling the lumen of the vein with collagen gel. A 15-mm rabbit peroneal nerve defect was bridged with a collagen-filled vein graft. On the contralateral side, the defect was bridged with the vein alone. When the regenerated tissue was examined 4 weeks, 8 weeks, and 12 weeks after grafting, the number and diameter of myelinated fibers were significantly increased, compared with the control group without collagen gel. This study found that in order to increase the efficacy of a vein graft for axonal regeneration, collagen gel might be an appropriate matrix material with which to fill the vein graft.

▶ Vein graft conduit is commonly used for small-segment nerve grafting in the hand. While its use is generally accepted for short defects less than 3 cm, it is acknowledged that longer defects are associated with poorer outcomes. The main advantage of the use of a vein conduit is its easy availability within the operative site and the lack of cost compared with a synthetic nerve conduit. This work suggests that collagen I–filled veins may be a method to improve the outcome with the use of such conduits. The authors' findings are consistent with others who have shown the importance of various extracellular elements in peripheral nerve regeneration. However, the presence of more and larger axons does not provide definitive evidence that there will be improved end-organ reinnervation and functional recovery. Further work is necessary to truly establish the effect of a collagen gel matrix with respect to peripheral nerve regeneration outcomes. At present, various strategies are being explored to improve the result of peripheral nerve regeneration, including the use of growth factors, stem cells, and extracellular matrix proteins.

A. Chong, MD

End-to-Side Neurorrhaphy for Defects of Palmar Sensory Digital Nerves
Voche P, Ouattara D (Clinique La Francilienne, Pontault-Combault, France)
Br J Plast Surg 58:239-244, 2005   16–5

Background.—A number of techniques are available for use when a nerve defect cannot be repaired by end-to-end neurorrhaphy. Nerve graft is the standard, but nerve conduits can be used as an alternative for defects of less than 3 to 5 cm. In recent years, end-to-side (ETS) neurorrhaphy has been added to the surgical options, although this technique was first described in

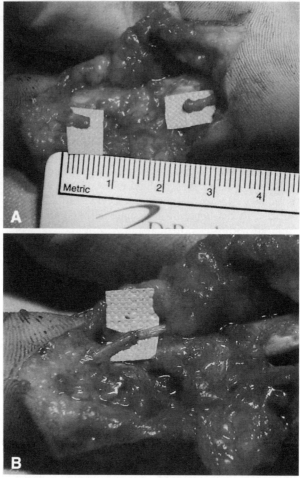

FIGURE 1.—A, Two-centimeter defect of the ulnar collateral nerve of a little finger at P1 level). B, End-to-side neurorrhaphy to the radial collateral nerve of the same finger. (Reprinted by permission of the publisher from Voche P, Ouattara D: End-to-side neurorrhaphy for defects of palmar sensory digital nerves. *Br J Plast Surg* 58:239-244. Copyright 2005 by Elsevier.)

the early 1900s. The use of ETS neurorrhaphy in a series of patients at one French center was reported.

Methods.—Ten traumatic nerve defects at the palm or digital level were treated with ETS neurorrhaphy by one surgeon from October 1999 to June 2003. The patients included 7 men and 3 women with an average age of 30 years (range, 9 to 55 years). The mean follow-up was 16 months (range, 9 to 29 months). The injuries were the result of dog bite in 3 patients, crushing in 2 patients, ballistic trauma in 1 patient, a barb-wire wound and a car accident in 1 patient each, and multilevel clean-cut lacerations in 2 patients. Three of the injuries were work related.

Under microscopic magnification, the proximal end of the injured nerve was left free, avoiding direct placement under the skin incision. The distal end was freed distally to provide sufficient mobility to reach the donor nerve without tension (Fig 1). After a donor nerve was selected and exposed, a small epineurial window was removed, with the intended area selected so as to avoid any tension on the suture site. Care was taken to avoid damaging the perineurium and the underlying fascicules. ETS neurorrhaphy was then performed without tension. An average of 6 to 8 epineurial 10-0 stitches were placed, and the wound was closed in a standard manner with polypropylene 3-0 interrupted sutures.

Results.—Static and 2-point discrimination tests (2-pd) were scored on pulps depending on the repaired nerve and donor nerve. Cold intolerance was rated subjectively by the patient. Static 2-pd scores averaged 9.1 mm on the repaired nerve, compared with an average of 4.6 mm on the control side. Moving 2 pd scores averaged 7 mm on the repaired nerve, compared with an average of 2.6 mm on the control side. One patient experienced impairment of the donor nerve. Seven patients were able to return to their previous jobs; 2 were required to modify their functions.

There was no occurrence of neuroma on the proximal end of the injured nerve, but 1 patient complained of tingling that was relieved by local massage. Three patients reported cold intolerance.

Conclusion.—ETS neurorrhaphies are effective and can provide results comparable with those of nerve grafts or vein conduits.

▶ Mutilating hand injuries often result in nerve transections that are not amenable to primary repair or require excessive tension to achieve nerve repair. Nerve grafts, vein conduits, and synthetic nerve conduits have been used with success in these lesions. The authors report their series of 10 patients with nerve defects ranging from 1.5 to 4 cm.

In these patients, they used ETS nerve repairs by coapting the distal affected nerve to the closest adjacent noninjured nerve—proper digital or common digital. They used an epineurial window and 10-0 nylon microsurgical repair. They noted nerve recovery from 6 to 11 mm of static 2-point discrimination and 4 to 10 mm of moving 2-point discrimination. All patients recovered protective sensation.

Although the results are acceptable, surgeons should consider that a proximal digital neuroma will develop in the unrepaired proximal stump and may be bothersome to the patient. For this reason, repair with grafting or nerve conduit is preferable in most cases. Additionally, if this technique is used and flexor tenolysis must later be performed, extra caution must be applied for ETS neurorraphies that cross over a tendon.

R. Buntic, MD

Limited, Protected Postsurgical Motion Does Not Affect the Results of Digital Nerve Repair

Yu RS, Catalano LW III, Barron OA, et al (St Lukes'-Roosevelt Hosp Ctr, New York)

J Hand Surg [Am] 29A:302-306, 2004   16–6

Background.—Since 1921, the rehabilitation after repair of digital nerve laceration has included cast immobilization for 3 weeks, but fingers with flexor tendon injuries have had improved outcomes when finger motion is allowed soon after surgery. When flexor tendon injuries coexist with digital nerve injuries, early, limited motion is used to rehabilitate the tendon repair but subjects the nerve repair to the same motions. The outcomes of primary nerve repairs followed by immobilization or early mobilization were compared in a retrospective review.

Methods.—The patients were older than 25 years and had primary surgical repair of isolated digital nerve lacerations (25 patients) or combined digital nerve and flexor tendon lacerations (20 patients). Immediately after surgery, patients with combined injuries began a protocol of active extension and passive flexion in an extension-block splint assisted by a rubber band attached to the fingernail and incorporated into the splint. The groups were compared on the basis of range of motion at the metacarpophalangeal, proximal interphalangeal, distal interphalangeal, and wrist joints; static 2-point discrimination; and Semmes-Weinstein monofilament testing.

Results.—The arcs of motion of the 2 groups were similar when compared with contralateral fingers. The final 2-point discrimination and Semmes-Weinstein monofilament testing showed statistically significant differences between the injured and contralateral uninjured digits but did not differ significantly between the groups.

Conclusions.—The loss of sensibility of the injured digits did not differ significantly between patients treated with immobilization and those treated with early mobilization. Digital nerve repairs appear to require less than the 3 weeks of immobilization traditionally allotted for them. By initiating digital motion shortly after surgery, the short-term stiffness of the fingers that accompanies cast immobilization may be avoided or reduced. Further study using a prospective, randomized format is warranted.

▶ This is a retrospective review of patients who had either an isolated digital nerve laceration or combined digital nerve and flexor tendon lacerations. The authors sought to compare these 2 groups with respect to the effect of mobilization or immobilization on the outcome of nerve recovery. The dogma is that patients who undergo an early range-of-motion protocol may have diminished sensory recovery because of early motion to the injured nerve. The authors, in a retrospective review, identified 14 patients (16 digits) who had isolated nerve repairs, and 12 patients (14 digits) with combined nerve and tendon repairs who underwent an early, passive, range-of-motion protocol. This protocol essentially was active extension and passive flexion in an extension block splint assisted by a rubber band attached to the fingernails and incorporated into the splint. Overall, the 2 groups were statistically similar. With respect to outcome, the range of motion and arcs of motion were similar in all patients. The ultimate outcome demonstrated no statistical significance between both groups as determined by 2-point discrimination ($P = .814$) and Semmes-Weinstein testing ($P = .974$). The authors conclude that the sensibility of the injured digits, as measured by 2-point discrimination and Semmes-Weinstein monofilament testing, was not different between the 2 study groups. They also challenge the dogma that digital nerve repairs require 3 weeks of immobilization as long as there is a tension-free repair. The authors suggest that a prospective, randomized study is required to truly evaluate this group.

Although this is an interesting study, it lacks several basic tenets of retrospective reviews and statistical analysis, including a power analysis. In order to state that there was no clinically relevant statistical difference, the authors should have performed a power analysis based on a previous literature review. In addition, I am in agreement with the authors that a prospective, randomized study comparing the results of isolated digital nerves treated with early versus no immobilization is necessary, and we wait for the authors to provide us with this information.

A. Y. Shin, MD

Coverage of Painful Peripheral Nerve Neuromas With Vascularized Soft Tissue: Method and Results

Krishnan KG, Pinzer T, Schackert G (Technical Univ of Dresden, Germany)
Neurosurgery 56:ONS-369–ONS-378, 2005   16–7

Objective.—Our goals are to describe a method of treating painful peripheral nerve neuromas by means of vascularized tissue coverage, report the results in seven patients, and discuss the indications for this treatment modality. An analysis of pain, functionality of the affected body part, professional activities of the patients, and medications before and after surgery is presented.

Methods.—Seven male patients (mean age, 45.1 yr) with posttraumatic nerve injuries, who had developed painful stump neuromas or neuromas-in-continuity, and who had unsuccessfully undergone several treatment procedures, were selected for the surgery described here. The operation included resection of the stump neuroma (four patients) or neurolysis of the neuroma-in-continuity (three patients) and coverage of the nerve with a vascularized fascial, fasciocutaneous, or perforator flap (three pedicled regional flaps and four free flaps). A modified quadruple visual analog scale was used to quantify pain before and after surgical treatment. The mean follow-up was 16.6 months.

Results.—The mean values of the quadruple visual analog scale (pain now/typically/at its best/at its worst) before surgery were 6.5/6.5/4.7/7.9. These values changed to 0.3/0.4/0/0.9 at a mean follow-up of 16.6 months after surgery. Five patients returned to their original profession, one receives a pension, and one began a less demanding job after undergoing surgery. Six of the seven patients received opioids before surgery (one had a spinal cord stimulator). After surgery, all patients stopped taking regular pain killers and the spinal cord stimulator was deactivated in one; two patients still take nonsteroidal anti-inflammatory drugs occasionally, but not on a regular basis.

Conclusion.—Vascularized soft tissue coverage of painful peripheral nerve neuromas seems to be an effective and attractive, but also complex, method of treatment. This option may be considered and reserved for patients who have already undergone several pain treatment modalities without success.

▶ Recalcitrant neuromas remain extremely difficult problems to treat. Multiple treatment options have been described. The basic principles remain the same: adequate soft tissue coverage and prevention of neuroma recurrence.

The authors describe their experience in treating this problem with vascularized soft tissue flaps, free or pedicled. Their experience is unique in that neuromas were treated in every part of the body—hand, lower extremity, face, and trunk. Results are very good after neurolysis and soft tissue coverage in their small series. It is likely that this combination plays a strong role in neuroma prevention. Long-term follow-up will be of great interest.

C. Lee, MD

Nerve Decompression for Complex Regional Pain Syndrome Type II Following Upper Extremity Surgery
Placzek JD, Boyer MI, Gelberman RH, et al (Washington Univ, St Louis; Oakland Univ, Rochester, Mich; Milliken Hand Rehabilitation Ctr, St Louis)
J Hand Surg [Am] 30A:69-74, 2005   16–8

Purpose.—To evaluate the results of nerve decompression for the symptoms of complex regional pain syndrome that developed after upper-extremity surgery.

Methods.—Eight patients (5 men, 3 women) developed worsening severe pain, swelling, and loss of range of motion after an upper-extremity surgery. The diagnosis of complex regional pain syndrome was made at an average of 6 weeks (range, 1-10 weeks) after the surgical procedure. A clinical diagnosis of either median or combined median and ulnar nerve compression at the wrist was confirmed in all patients with electrophysiologic testing. Nerve decompression was performed at a mean of 13 weeks after the procedure. Subjective (Disabilities of the Arm, Shoulder, and Hand questionnaire; visual analog pain scale) and objective (forearm, wrist, and finger range of motion; grip strength) data from before and after nerve decompression were reviewed.

Results.—The average score on the Disabilities of the Arm, Shoulder, and Hand questionnaire decreased from 71 to 30 (p < .05). The mean visual analog pain score decreased from 7.5 to 1.8. (p < .05) There was immediate and near-complete resolution of all somatic complaints including hypersensitivity to touch, hyperhydrosis, swelling, and cold sensitivity. Range of motion and grip strength improved.

Conclusions.—Traditionally surgical treatment has been avoided in patients with complex regional pain syndrome; however, in the setting of clinical and electrophysiologic evidence of nerve compression surgical intervention may hasten recovery in these patients.

▶ Diagnosis of complex regional pain syndrome (CRPS) after an upper extremity operation requires careful analysis to consider secondary causes such as an identifiable nerve lesion, as in CRPS type II, which may respond to operative nerve decompression. This study addresses this problem by identifying a group of patients diagnosed with CRPS after an upper extremity operation. These patients were stratified into type II who underwent diagnostic testing to confirm nerve compression. Eight of 14 patients underwent median nerve decompression, ulnar nerve decompression, or both at the wrist, with a significant decrease in pain. This represents a greater than 50% response rate for surgical decompression.

Preoperative nerve examinations before the first surgery are not documented (ie, preexisting nerve compression), and the intraoperative findings that could have led to avoidance of secondary nerve decompression are not addressed. Nevertheless, this small but significant study emphasizes the importance of potential secondary causes of chronic hand pain after upper extremity surgery.

C. Lee, MD

Idiopathic Arm Pain
Ring D, Guss D, Malhotra L, et al (Massachusetts Gen Hosp, Boston)
J Bone Joint Surg Am 86-A:1387-1391, 2004   16–9

Background.—Arm pain with little or no objective abnormality (referred to herein as idiopathic arm pain) is a common and frustrating problem for both patients and physicians. We investigated the relative effect of idiopathic arm pain and arm pain due to a discrete diagnosis on upper-extremity-specific health status.

Methods.—The Disabilities of the Arm, Shoulder and Hand (DASH) questionnaire was completed by 3888 patients seen over a twelve-month period. Scores for the entire sample, for 496 patients diagnosed with idiopathic arm pain, and for 1379 patients diagnosed with one of twenty-one discrete conditions were compared.

Results.—Patients with idiopathic pain reported substantial and highly variable upper-limb-specific dysfunction (average DASH score [and standard deviation], 36 ± 24 points). Patients with discrete diagnoses also exhibited substantial variation (average standard deviation, 25; range, 6 to 27) as well as long right tails indicating floor effects, particularly for less severe conditions (Pearson correlation of $r = -0.87$ between the mean DASH score and skewness). Analysis of variance confirmed the ability of the DASH instrument to discriminate among groups of diagnoses of varying severity, but post hoc Tukey analysis identified ten subgroups with substantial overlap of the DASH scores.

Conclusions.—Patients with idiopathic arm pain report substantial and highly variable upper-extremity dysfunction. The wide variations observed in the DASH scores of the patients with idiopathic pain and those with discrete diagnoses are greater than would be expected on the basis of the variations in the objective pathological conditions and may reflect the strong influence of psychological and sociological factors on health status measures.

▶ The wide variation in DASH scores is far greater than one would expect for several of these conditions. For example, the DASH score for patients with a single isolated condition such as trigger finger should be more uniform than in complex and varied problems such as distal radius fractures. However, this study demonstrates that DASH scores are actually not very useful in determining the severity of hand and upper extremity conditions. Serial observation and time are often more useful diagnostic measures. The wide variation in the DASH scores for the specific diagnoses and the substantial dysfunction in the absence of objective findings noted in this report reflect the strong influence of psychologic and sociologic factors. Supportive treatment may be needed to address psychosocial factors that may be contributing to these higher DASH scores.

B. Wilhelmi, MD

17 Hand: Tendon

The Terminal Tendon of the Digital Extensor Mechanism: Part I, Anatomic Study
Schweitzer TP, Rayan GM (Univ of Oklahoma, Oklahoma City; Integris Baptist Med Ctr, Oklahoma City)
J Hand Surg [Am] 29A:898-902, 2004   17–1

Background.—The term *terminal tendon* (TT) is applied to the most distal part of the extensor mechanism near the distal interphalangeal joint that inserts into the dorsal base of the distal phalanx. Normal function of the TT requires competent extrinsic and intrinsic muscles. The anatomy of the TT and its relationships to surrounding structures were examined.

Methods.—Eight female and 6 male cadaver specimens were used to obtain 15 human hands (56 digits). Anatomic dissection was carried out, and the TT and lateral bands of these digits were evaluated, noting the retinacular structures near the TT and the oblique retinacular ligament when possible.

Results.—The specific site of the TT is defined as that segment found between the convergence of the lateral bands proximally and the bony insertion in the phalanx distally. It is a flat and thin but relatively strong structure. Its radial bands are not as thick as its ulnar lateral bands (average, 3.6 mm vs 4.0 mm). The TT insertion is about 1.4 mm from the germinal matrix of the nail bed. The average TT length (from visible convergence of lateral bands over middle phalanx to most distal aspect of its insertion) is 10.1 mm, and the average TT width (directly over distal interphalangeal joint) is 5.6 mm. These values vary from digit to digit. The thin layer of transverse fibers between the lateral bands proximal to the TT is termed the triangular ligament (TL). It has a poorly defined proximal border. The average TL length is 13.7 mm, and the average TL width at its base is 5.4 mm. The sizes of the TT and TL vary with respect to the size of the digit. The largest dimension is often found in the middle finger, with progressively smaller dimensions found in the ring, index, and small fingers. Dorsally, the transverse retinacular ligament (TRL) is attached to the lateral bands. It is not directly attached to the TT. The TRL is more defined and distinct than the oblique retinacular ligament. Ulnar TRLs are often thicker than radial TRLs.

Conclusions.—The TT appears to be the primary structure responsible for extending the distal interphalangeal joint, aided by intrinsic muscles. Adjacent retinacular structures appear to provide stability for the TT. During surgery, the characteristics of the TT to remember are its thinness and proximity to the nail matrix.

▶ This is an important contribution to further our understanding of the precise anatomy and range of variations of the TT in the extensor mechanism in normal adult fingers. For all who perform surgery in and around this area and treat injuries and pathologic conditions, this is an excellent reference article that highlights the critical relationship of the TT to the germinal matrix and draws some functional conclusions and even raises some questions about the importance of other structures such as the oblique retinacular ligament. As an anatomist, I certainly encourage all hand surgeons to become familiar with this work.

R. A. Berger, MD, PhD

The Terminal Tendon of the Digital Extensor Mechanism: Part II. Kinematic Study
Schweitzer TP, Rayan GM (Univ of Oklahoma, Oklahoma City)
J Hand Surg [Am] 29A:903-908, 2004   17–2

Purpose.—To conduct kinematic analyses of both intact and sectioned terminal tendon (TT) of multiple fingers in the hand.

Methods.—The TTs of 36 fresh-frozen cadaveric digits were used in this study. TT excursion was assessed along with the influence on proximal joint motion. The influence of TT lengthening and shortening on distal interphalangeal (DIP) joint motion were investigated.

Results.—TT excursion averaged 1 mm at the DIP joint and was influenced by the proximal interphalangeal (PIP) joint but not the position of other joints in the hand and wrist. The greatest degree of DIP joint motion averaged 86° when the PIP joint was in full flexion, whereas the least motion averaged 45° when this joint was in neutral position. Lengthening of the TT resulted in angular deformity at the DIP joint. Average flexion deformities reached 25° at 1 mm, 36° at 2 mm, 49° at 3 mm, and 63° at 4 mm of lengthening. The middle finger showed the greatest flexion deformity, followed by the ring, small, and index fingers. Shortening the TT by as little as 1 mm resulted in difficult tendon repair because of excessive tension and minimal or no DIP joint flexion was obtained.

Conclusion.—Only DIP and PIP joints affect TT excursion; hence these are the main joints to be immobilized to protect TT repair. The middle finger TT showed the least tolerance to lengthening with potential for mallet deformity. Joint flexion deformity is proportional to tendon lengthening. Only 1 mm of TT lengthening results in ~25° of DIP joint extension lag, and 4 mm of TT lengthening results in DIP joint flexion deformity greater than 60°. Even 1 mm of TT shortening will seriously restrict DIP joint flexion.

▶ This careful anatomical study emphasizes the importance of anatomical perfection in digit function. Even 1 mm of lengthening of the terminal tendon after mallet injury will result in a 25° extensor lag; overtightening a similar amount will result in a similar loss of flexion (assuming that the much stronger profundus cannot stretch out the tight extensor).

P. C. Amadio, MD

The Effect of Partial A2 Pulley Excision on Gliding Resistance and Pulley Strength *In Vitro*
Tanaka T, Amadio PC, Zhao C, et al (Mayo Clinic Rochester, Minn)
J Hand Surg [Am] 29A:877-883, 2004   17–3

Background.—Injuries to the digital pulleys can be associated with flexor tendon injury, the repair of which is complex and challenging. Finger motion can be notably affected by total or partial loss of the digital pulleys. Mechanically, the A2 and A4 pulleys are stronger, less compliant, and less deformable than the A1, A3, and A5 pulleys. When both the A2 and A4 pulleys are injured, joint motion can decline by 10%. During flexor tendon repair, not only must surgeons avoid traumatic injury to the pulley, but in the course of the process they may need to excise part of a pulley to obtain exposure and facilitate the surgical process. Whether the pulley, especially the A2 and A4, would then need complete repair has been questioned. The gliding resistance of the interface between the tendon and a partially excised pulley and the strength of the remaining pulleys were investigated.

Methods.—Eleven human cadavers were used to harvest 32 fingers. The A2 pulley was then excised 25%, 50%, and 75% progressively, with cuts made either from distal to proximal or from proximal to distal. Peak gliding

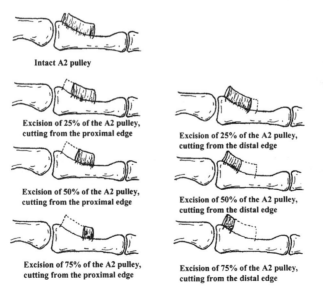

Intact A2 pulley

Excision of 25% of the A2 pulley, cutting from the proximal edge

Excision of 25% of the A2 pulley, cutting from the distal edge

Excision of 50% of the A2 pulley, cutting from the proximal edge

Excision of 50% of the A2 pulley, cutting from the distal edge

Excision of 75% of the A2 pulley, cutting from the proximal edge

Excision of 75% of the A2 pulley, cutting from the distal edge

FIGURE 2.—Testing groups. (Reprinted from Tanaka T, Amadio PC, Zhao C, et al: The effect of partial A2 pulley excision on gliding resistance and pulley strength *in vitro. J Hand Surg [Am]* 29A:877-883. Copyright 2004, with permission from The American Society for Surgery of the Hand.)

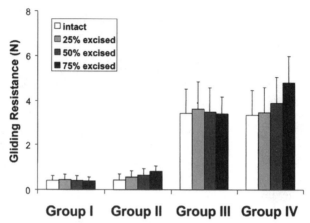

FIGURE 4.—Peak gliding resistance. *Open box,* Intact; *lightly shaded box,* 25% excised; *medium-shaded box,* 50% excised; *solid black box,* 75% excised. (Reprinted from Tanaka T, Amadio PC, Zhao C, et al: The effect of partial A2 pulley excision on gliding resistance and pulley strength *in vitro. J Hand Surg [Am]* 29A:877-883. Copyright 2004, with permission from The American Society for Surgery of the Hand.)

resistance was measured under 4 conditions (Fig 2). Measurement of the pulley breaking strength and stiffness was also obtained.

Results.—The intact and repaired tendon groups had similar trends in peak gliding resistance (Fig 4). Moving the cut from distal toward proximal had no significant effect on peak gliding resistance. Cutting from proximal toward distal produced a significant increase in peak gliding resistance when 25% of the pulley remained distally compared with intact, 75%, and 50% of the pulley remaining proximally. The breaking strength of the 25% distal portion of the A2 pulley was significantly greater than that of the 25% proximal portion (160 N vs 96.7 N). Stiffness showed a similar pattern, with the distal portion having a value of 120 N/mm and the proximal portion 70.5 N/mm.

Conclusions.—A2 and A4 pulleys are crucial to the optimal function of the digital flexor tendon. The A2 pulley is thickest in its distal aspect. The strength of the distal 25% of this pulley is about 65% greater than that of the proximal 25%. The stiffness is similarly greater. When the distal short segment is the only portion left, gliding resistance is increased. If 50% of the A2 pulley remains, either proximally or distally, the gliding resistance does not increase dramatically, and the pulley's retained strength is substantial. Thus, the better clinical practice when excision of the A2 pulley is needed is to limit it to 50%.

▶ It is well recognized that retention of the A2 pulley is critical in the return of digital motion after zone 2 flexor tendon injury and subsequent repair. From a practical standpoint, exposure is very important in obtaining a quality flexor tendon repair in zone 2. In some instances, the A2 pulley may be lacerated or partially excised at the time of repair in order to fully expose either the flexor digitorum superficialis laceration or lacerations of both flexor digitorum superficialis and flexor digitorum profundus tendons.

This is a very well-designed cadaveric biomechanical study evaluating the strength and resistance to gliding of various portions of the A2 pulley. The authors have found that with the A2 pulley cut from proximal to distal, there was a significant increase in peak gliding resistance and a significantly higher breaking strength with the distal 25% of the A2 pulley left intact compared with the proximal 25%. The authors also found that if the A2 pulley is limited to a 50% excision of any portion, there is little increase in gliding resistance and little decrease in breaking strength. This enables the authors to conclude that partial excision of any 50% of the A2 pulley to facilitate exposure for tendon repair is clinically feasible. A relevant additional question of interest not examined in this study is, what effect does additional complete or partial incision of the A1, C1, A3, and C2 pulleys have in the clinical setting of partial A2 pulley excision? This is often a dilemma facing surgeons embarking on repair of zone 2 flexor tendon injuries. It would seem that removal of portions of A1, C1, A3, and C2 pulleys would enhance the importance of retaining more of the A2 pulley.

P. M. Murray, MD

A1 Pulley Release of Locked Trigger Digit by Percutaneous Technique

Park MJ, Oh I, Ha KI (Sungkyunkman Univ, Seoul, Korea; Eulji Univ, Daejeon, South Korea)
J Hand Surg [Br] 29B:502-505, 2004   17–4

Abstract.—We performed 118 percutaneous releases of the locked trigger digits in an office setting using a specially designed knife (Fig 2, b). Thirty-five digits were locked in flexion, 79 digits in extension and the remaining four were fixed in a semiflexed position. Successful percutaneous release was

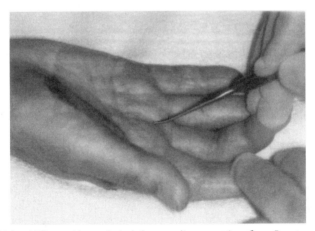

FIGURE 2, b.—A 73-year-old man who had a long-standing severe trigger finger. Percutaneous A1 pulley release was performed using the specially designed knife. (Reprinted from Park MJ, Oh I, Ha KI: A1 pulley release of locked trigger digit by percutaneous technique. *J Hand Surg [Br]* 29B:502-505. Copyright 2004, with permission from The British Society for Surgery of the Hand.)

achieved for 107 digits (91%), with the remaining 11 digits requiring an open surgical procedure. Although there were no persistent triggering in 98 digits with a follow-up of at least 6 months, painful stiffness at the interphalangeal joints remained in ten digits despite of physical therapy. No neurovascular injury occurred. We suggest that a locked trigger digit can be successfully released with the percutaneous technique.

▶ One hundred seven of 118 digits that underwent percutaneous trigger release for locked fingers had successful release with a custom-designed knife. Of the 11 incomplete releases, 6 A1 pulleys were incompletely released proximally and 5 distally. Use of our previously published transverse landmarks for percutaneous trigger release could have potentially reduced these failures.[1] Several studies have reported success with percutaneous release of trigger fingers, using a needle. In these other reports, there have been complications of neurovascular injuries for the thumb, small, and index fingers. We described longitudinal anatomic landmarks based on cadaver studies to minimize this risk for neurovascular injuries.[2] In their report, these authors had no such injuries. Their new instrument may decrease the risk for these injuries. Another concern with their technique is their use of a distal to proximal maneuver, which poses a theoretic risk of injuring transversely oriented anatomic structures in the palm with overrelease.

B. J. Wilhelmi, MD

References

1. Wilhelmi BJ, Snyder N, Verbesey JE, et al: Trigger finger release with hand surface landmark ratios: An anatomic and clinical study. *Plast Reconstr Surg* 108:908-915, 2001.
2. Wilhelmi BJ, Neumeister MW, Mowlavi A, et al: The safe treatment of trigger finger with longitudinal and transverse landmarks: An anatomic study of the border fingers for percutaneous release. *Plast Reconstr Surg* 112:993-999, 2003.

Dental Rolls: A Suitable Model for Practising Tendon Repair Techniques
Tare M (Broomfield Hosp, Chelmsford, Essex, England)
J Hand Surg [Br] 29B:506-507, 2004   17–5

Background.—Surgical training in the United Kingdom (UK) has always been based on the apprenticeship and the "see one and then do one" concept. However, there have been many changes in surgical training in the past decade. The Calman system of training and the European working time directives have altered the tradition of long working hours and a lengthy career path. Although these changes are important for ensuring adequate health and safety, they have slowed the process of acquiring surgical skills and dexterity. With working time reduced, trainees will face the choice of increasing the length of training (which has already been stretched to 6 years) or to utilizing their free time to acquire knowledge and skills. It is likely that training with simulators and practice models will play an increasingly important role

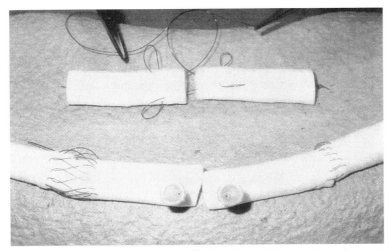

FIGURE 1.—(Reprinted from Tare M: Dental rolls: A suitable model for practicing tendon repair techniques. *J Hand Surg [Br]* 29B:506-507. Copyright 2004, with permission from The British Society for Surgery of the Hand.)

in surgical training in the UK. An easily assembled and economical simulator for practicing various flexor tendon repairing knots was presented.

Methods.—The most commonly used techniques for suturing of the flexor tendon are the Bunnell, Kessler, modified Kessler, Silfverskiöld, Tsuge, and Strickland repairs. Some of these knots are complex and difficult to comprehend from illustrations. This simulator is constructed of a disposable cardboard kidney tray, which acts as the platform. Two dental rolls made of compact cotton wool are used to represent the cut ends of a tendon (Fig 1). The diameter of the dental roll is roughly equivalent to that of a round tendon of flexor carpi radialis, and the resistance offered by the compact cotton wool to the suture needle is comparable with that of a tendon. The dental rolls are fixed to the kidney tray either by two disposable needles or with sutures. Almost any suture technique can be demonstrated and practiced with this model.

Conclusions.—The simulator described here is easily built and can aid trainees in understanding the basic principles of various knots and improving their understanding of the distance and depth of each "bite" taken while repairing the tendon.

▶ This short article makes a useful point. It is possible to practice tendon repairs before doing them clinically. The simple expedient of a dental roll makes it possible for students, fellows, and residents to practice the throws literally hundreds of times, as they do with knot tying over hooks, chair legs, etc. The authors do not mention, but I would recommend, a second step: practice in animal tendons, which then can be tested for gapping and breaking strength, using only a simple fish scale. Clinical tendon repairs are not all that commonly performed, but these methods make it possible for even the occasional tendon surgeon to perfect the necessary skills.

P. C. Amadio, MD

A Comparative Analysis of the Biomechanical Behaviour of Five Flexor Tendon Core Sutures

Viinikainen A, Göransson H, Huovinen K, et al (Univ of Helsinki; Helsinki Univ Central Hosp; Tampere Univ of Technology, Finland)
J Hand Surg [Br] 29B:536-543, 2004   17–6

Abstract.—Five core suture techniques were compared by static tensile testing in vitro. Fifty porcine tendons were used. The core sutures were performed with 3-0 or 4-0 braided polyester suture (Ticron®) and the over-and-over running peripheral sutures with 6-0 monofilament polypropylene (Prolene®). The core sutures were: (1) Pennington modified Kessler (3-0), (2) Double Pennington modified Kessler (3-0), (3) 4-strand Savage (3-0), (4) 4-strand Savage (4-0), and (5) 6-strand Savage (4-0). Repairs were compared as paired in regard to one variable: the number of core suture strands, the suture calibre, or the suture configuration. Biomechanical differences between the repair groups started during the linear region, with the yield force and stiffness increasing along with the number of core suture strands. All three variables influenced the strain at the yield point. Thus, the strength of the intact repair can be improved by modifying the core suture. In all repairs gap formation started near the yield point after failure of the peripheral suture. The yield force represents the strength of the intact repair composite and should be considered the strength of the tendon repair.

▶ This study examined the variables of different core suture configurations, suture caliber, and number of strands on the biomechanical behavior of the intact repair in relation to static tensile testing. This study supported previous reports that increasing the number of strands across the repair site enhances the yield force and ultimate force. The suture caliber and the suture configuration had no significant influence on the yield force. However, the authors did not compare different suture calibers with the Kessler group. The weakness of this study is that the gap forces measured from the static tensile tests are not directly comparable to the biomechanical behavior of flexor repairs during postoperative mobilization in which the tendon is subjected to cyclical loading. This cyclical loading has been shown to cause gap formation at significantly lower loads than static testing. Previous reports have considered the force as the strength of a repair, despite the gap that develops before the force causes the rupture. Since gapping attenuates the repair strength and increases the risk of rupture during rehabilitation, this study demonstrates that the yield force, which represents the force that produces gapping of the repair, should be considered the strength of the repair.

B. Wilhelmi, MD

Prevention of Peritendinous Adhesions Following Flexor Tendon Injury With Seprafilm

Menderes A, Mola F, Tayfur V, et al (Dokuz Eylul Univ, Izmir, Turkey)
Ann Plast Surg 53:560-564, 2004   17–7

Abstract.—Peritendinous adhesions are the most important complication of flexor tendon injury. In this study, Seprafilm was used for the prevention of peritendinous adhesions following flexor tendon repair. Seprafilm Bioresorbable Membrane (Genzyme Corporation, Cambridge, MA) contains sodium hyaluronate and carboxymethyl cellulose. Thirty New Zealand white male rabbits were divided equally into 3 groups. In all groups, the deep flexor tendon of the third finger of the left back foot was cut and repaired by Kessler-Tajima suture technique. In the first study group following tendon repair, Seprafilm was wrapped around the repaired tendon. In the second study group, sodium hyaluronate gel was injected to the operation field after tendon repair. In the control group, no external material was applied to the field. The study groups had better range of motion. Histopathologically, study groups had less adhesions compared with the control groups. As a result, it was concluded that in rabbit the peritendinous adhesions following flexor tendon repairs could be lowered with Seprafilm and hyaluronic acid.

▶ This article describes experimental work on one of the most elusive and difficult problems in hand surgery: how to modulate wound healing such that part of the wound (surrounding the tendon) does not form scar, while another part of the wound (within the tendon substance) heals normally. Many previous investigators have examined topical agents (corticosteroids, anti-neoplastic agents, other modulators of metabolism) as well as different physical barriers (autologous vein, artificial skin) as possible means to this end.

Menderes et al have proposed using Seprafilm, a commercially available product currently used to minimize intestinal adhesions after laparotomy. A unique feature of this physical barrier is that this product swells after placement; this may be problematic with regard to early mobilization (in this study, immediate mobilization). It would have been interesting to examine repaired tendons within 24 to 48 hours after repair. In the tightly constrained anatomy of the distal rabbit foot, it would seem probable that this Seprafilm would be displaced with early motion.

Similar displacement may occur in human zone II tendon repairs. Regardless, I am eagerly awaiting the development of products such as this that may modulate healing at different portions of the same wound.

M. Concannon, MD

Early Active Mobilization of Primary Repairs of the Flexor Pollicis Longus Tendon With Two Kessler Two-Strand Core Sutures and a Strengthened Circumferential Suture

Sirotakova M, Elliot D (Broomfield Hosp, Chelmsford, England)
J Hand Surg [Br] 29B:531-535, 2004   17–8

This study reports our treatment of divided flexor pollicis longus (FPL) tendons by primary repair from 1999 to 2002. Forty-eight FPL repairs were performed using two Kessler two-strand repairs with a cross-linked Silfverskiold circumferential suture. All were rehabilitated by early active mobilization. Excellent or good results were observed in 73/77% of cases (White/Buck-Gramcko assessments, respectively). No patients (0%) ruptured their repair as a result of early active mobilization. Two patients (4%) developed post-operative infections with wound and tendon dehiscence. This combination of repairs addresses the problem of rupture of FPL during early mobilization which we experienced in previous studies. Its problems and alternatives are discussed.

▶ This article serves as an excellent review of various approaches to flexor tendon repairs. It also confirms the phenomenon that additional strands across the tendon repair result in a stronger repair.

In this work, the authors focus on the FPL tendon with its unique characteristics. The FPL typically retracts more than other flexor tendons, and thus it has more tension on the repair, making it more likely to rupture with a conventional 2-strand repair technique. The greater retraction of the FPL is due partially to the fact that it does not share a common muscle belly or other interconnection with adjacent flexor tendons. Of even greater importance, (not noted in this article) is that it does not have a lumbrical insertion, which typically limits the degree of flexor digitorum profundus retraction at exploration.

The authors make note of recommendations to either step cut or "Z-lengthen" the tendon at the musculotendinous junction when the FPL is noted to be retracted. This is rarely, if ever, indicated in a primary tendon laceration without tendon loss, and its use should be strongly discouraged.

The main message of this article is that multiple strands across the tendon repair, combined with an epitendinous repair, are strong enough to allow for early active mobilization. This confirms earlier work done by other investigators. The authors also point out that while these multistrand repairs are strong, they are also bulky and therefore may be more problematic in the precise areas where they would be of most use: zone II.

M. Concannon, MD

Expression of Growth Factors in Canine Flexor Tendon After Laceration In Vivo

Tsubone T, Moran SL, Amadio PC, et al (Mayo Clinic, Rochester, Minn)
Ann Plast Surg 53:393-397, 2004   17–9

Abstract.—Growth factors, transforming growth factor β (TGF-β), epidermal growth factor (EGF), platelet-derived growth factor (PDGF), insulin-like growth factor (IGF), basic fibroblast growth factor (bFGF), and vascular endothelial growth factor (VEGF), are critical components of the cutaneous wound healing process. Little is known, however, about the expression of these growth factors in normal flexor tendon healing. In this study, we wished to examine which of these growth factors are present at 10 days following tendon injury in a canine flexor tendon repair model.

Using immunohistochemical analysis, we found positive staining for all growth factors in both timing groups. TGF-β was detected around the repair site and proximal to it. PDGF-AA, PDGF-BB and VEGF appeared in the whole tendon section following repair. EGF, IGF and bFGF were not seen in tenocytes but were present in inflammatory cells surrounding the repair site. These findings provide evidence that TGF-β, EGF, PDGF-AA, PDGF-BB, IGF, bFGF and VEGF are all expressed at 10 days after tendon injury but by different cell types and in different locations. The time course of growth factor expression is an important element in wound healing, and a better understanding of where and when such factors are expressed may help in the development of methods to manipulate this expression, accelerate healing, and reduce adhesions.

▶ The authors performed immunohistochemical analysis of repaired canine flexor tendons 10 days after zone II equivalent injury and suture repair. The dogs were randomly assigned to either passive digital motion starting postoperative day 1 or postoperative day 5. The authors found the presence of a variety of growth factors in both groups, varying in different locations and cell types. The findings in the article corroborate data from other models of tissue healing, and published research on tendon healing specifically. Other than a slightly increased TGF-β staining in the day-5 therapy group, no other differences were noted between the 2 groups. However, the small sample size and the lack of any quantitative analysis techniques restrict the authors' ability to make comparisons. The use of only one time period limits the usefulness of the study in elucidating growth factor expression during the temporal course of tendon healing. This report highlights once again that tissue healing is a complex dynamic process involving the interplay of multiple growth factors and cytokines. It provides a starting point for further work on the molecular biology underlying tendon healing and adhesion formation.

A. Chong, MD

Tendon Healing *In Vitro*: Genetic Modification of Tenocytes With Exogenous PDGF Gene and Promotion of Collagen Gene Expression

Wang XT, Liu PY, Tang JB (Boston Univ, Providence, RI; Nantong Med College, Jiangsu, China)

J Hand Surg [Am] 29A:884-890, 2004

17–10

Purpose.—Promotion of collagen production can increase tendon healing strength and reduce repair ruptures. Transfer of an exogenous growth factor gene to tenocytes of intrasynovial tendons may enhance the capacity of cells to produce collagen. We transferred the platelet-derived growth factor B (PDGF-B) gene to tenocytes and investigated its effects on the expression of the PDGF gene and the type I collagen gene in an in vitro tenocyte culture model.

Methods.—Tenocytes obtained from explant cultures of rat intrasynovial tendons were treated for 12 hours with the plasmid containing the PDGF complementary deoxyribonucleic acid (cDNA) with liposome and were then cultured for 6 additional days. The control tenocytes did not receive the exogenous gene and liposome. Efficiency of the gene transfer was evaluated by using reverse transcription polymerase chain reactions (RT-PCR) to detect the presence of the transferred gene in the tenocytes. Enhancement of the expression of the target gene was assessed by RT-PCR with primers effective to amplify both internal and transferred genes. Expression of the type I collagen gene was determined by quantitative analysis of the products of RT-PCR.

Results.—Levels of expression of the type I collagen gene by tenocytes were increased significantly by transfer of the exogenous PDGF gene to the tenocytes. Efficiency of the gene transfer was confirmed by the presence of exogenous PDGF cDNA in the tenocytes receiving the transferred gene. Expression of the PDGF gene increased significantly in the cells treated with exogenous PDGF cDNA.

Conclusions.—Exogenous PDGF genes can be transferred effectively into intrasynovial tenocytes and the transfer increases significantly the expression of genes for PDGF and type I collagen. Transfer of the PDGF gene may offer a novel way of effectively promoting healing of intrasynovial flexor tendons. The findings warrant future in vivo study to test the effectiveness of gene therapy to promote flexor tendon healing.

▶ This is a proof of concept article, showing that it is possible to use gene therapy to affect what tendon cells make. The mode, however, is highly artificial; the cells are in culture, not in a tissue. The plasmid vector used to insert the new genetic material is not effective clinically, and this method of gene therapy has only transient effects. The effects of PDGF on other genes was not assessed, yet a growth factor is likely to affect the synthesis of many genes both helpful and harmful to tendon healing. Despite all the hype in the lay press, we have a long way to go before gene therapy plays a role in tendon repair.

P. C. Amadio, MD

18 Hand: Bone & Ligament

Three Cast Techniques for the Treatment of Extra-articular Metacarpal Fractures: Comparison of Short-term Outcomes and Final Fracture Alignments
Tavassoli J, Ruland RT, Hogan CJ, et al (Bone and Joint/Sports Medicine Inst, Portsmouth, Va)
J Bone Joint Surg Am 87-A:2196-2201, 2005   18–1

Background.—Most extra-articular metacarpal fractures can be managed nonoperatively. While the conventional wisdom is that the metacarpophalangeal joint should be immobilized in a position of flexion, alternative methods for cast immobilization have been described. The purpose of this study was to retrospectively evaluate three methods of closed treatment; specifically, we investigated whether the position of immobilization of the metacarpophalangeal joint or the absence of a range of motion of the interphalangeal joints affected the short-term outcome or fracture alignment.

Methods.—Between November 2000 and April 2004, extra-articular metacarpal fractures were immobilized for five weeks in one of three ways: with the metacarpophalangeal joints in flexion and full interphalangeal joint motion permitted (Group 1); with the metacarpophalangeal joints in extension and full interphalangeal joint motion permitted (Group 2); and with the metacarpophalangeal joints in flexion, the interphalangeal joints in extension, and no interphalangeal joint motion permitted (Group 3). Radiographs and the range of motion were evaluated at five weeks after application of the cast, and the range of motion and grip strength were assessed at nine weeks.

Results.—Two hundred and sixty-three patients met the inclusion criteria. At five weeks, there was no difference among the treatment methods with regard to the range of motion or the maintenance of fracture reduction. At nine weeks, there was no significant difference with regard to the range of motion or grip strength.

Conclusions.—When immobilization was discontinued by five weeks, the position of the metacarpophalangeal joints and the absence or presence of interphalangeal joint motion during the immobilization had little effect on motion, grip strength, or fracture alignment. This finding contradicts the conventional teaching that the metacarpophalangeal joint must be immobilized in flexion to prevent long-term loss of joint extension. Patient comfort, ease of application, and the surgeon's familiarity with the technique should influence the choice of immobilization.

▶ The authors report that no significant difference was found in the range of motion at 5 and 9 weeks after 3 different cast treatments for extra-articular metacarpal fractures. The 3 casted positions included (1) metacarpophalangeal (MP) joint flexed, proximal interphalangeal (PIP) joint free, (2) MP joint extended and IP joint free, and (3) MP joint flexed with IP joint extended. The authors also report no significant change in fracture alignment between groups and acceptable alignment at union.

Specifically, this article is important because it illustrates that immobilization for the MP joint in the extended position with the PIP joints free does not lead to significant stiffness at the MP joint. King et al[1] have reported previously on this finding for 5th metacarpal neck fractures in 1999. This method has been used at our institution for quite some time with excellent motion and acceptable fracture alignment results.

The authors do not report on the exact timing of the reduction and casting. The technique as described by King et al incorporates a delayed traction reduction with cast application and 3-point molding with the MP joints extended and the PIP joints free. They described initial splint immobilization followed by elective traction reduction (with or without local anesthetic) at 3 to 7 days after the injury. In particular, the cast is applied with extra padding in the expected region of molding, and the cast is applied while the fracture is under traction. The importance of the cast is not only the 3-point bending mold but also molding the cast to the transverse arch of the palm, therefore fixing the position of the bending mold to the fracture site.

Reduction and application of the cast at this slightly delayed time allows better fitting of the cast and mold because less edema and soft tissue swelling occurs. This technique (traction reduction and cast application with MP joints extended and PIP joints free) is also very easy because the finger traps provide excellent positioning of the fracture and the hand for cast application. In addition, the fingers may be buddy (ie, taped for further protection).

D. G. Dennison, MD

Reference

1. King JC, Nettrour JF, Beckenbaugh RD: Traction reduction and cast immobilization for the treatment of boxer's fractures. *Tech Hand Upper Extremity Surg* 3:174-180, 1999.

Use of Bioabsorbable Osteofixation Devices in the Hand

Waris E, Ashammakhi N, Kaarela O, et al (Univ of Helsinki; Oulu Univ, Finland; Tampere Univ of Technology, Finland; et al)
J Hand Surg [Br] 29B:590-598, 2004   18–2

Bioabsorbable internal fixation by means of pins, tacks, screws and miniplates offers an alternative to metallic osteofixation for the stabilization of small bone fractures, osteotomies, ligament injuries and fusions in the hand. The advantages of using them include avoidance of metallic-implant-related long-term complications and a secondary removal operation. Currently the most commonly used devices are made of poly L-lactide (PLLA) and copolymers of polylactides (P(L/DL)LA) and polyglycolide (PLGA). In areas of mechanical stress, the use of ultra-high-strength self-reinforced devices is recommended. Biomechanical studies on fresh frozen bones have shown that the fixation rigidity achieved with self-reinforced devices approaches that of metallic osteofixation methods. The reliability of modern implants has been confirmed in several experimental and clinical studies (Fig 1).

▶ The authors present a very useful and timely review of important concepts related to the use of bioabsorbable implants in general and as they relate to hand surgery in particular. Historically, PLGA and PLLA have been used most commonly as polymers in bioabsorbable implants. Previous problems with foreign body reactions, osteolysis, and sinus formation may have been related to color dyes used and/or crystal deposits resulting from the formulation of implants.

Newer methodologies for implant manufacture seem to avoid those problems while producing devices with bending and torsion strengths similar to

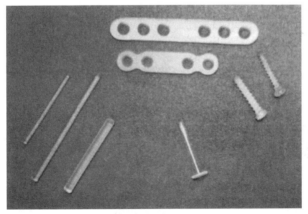

FIGURE 1.—Self-reinforced poly-L-lactide (SR-PLLA) and poly-L/DL-lactide (SR-P(L/DL)LA) miniplates, pins (diameter 1.5, 2.0 and 3.2 mm), tacks and screws (diameter 2.0 and 1.5 mm) for bone fixation in the hand. (Reprinted from Waris E, Ashammakhi N, Kaarela O, et al: Use of bioabsorbable osteofixation devices in the hand. *J Hand Surg [Br]* 29B:590-598. Copyright 2004, with permission from The British Society for Surgery of the Hand.)

small titanium plates and screws. The bending modulus of self-reinforced polymers is close to that of cortical bone, which helps avoid stress risers unlike the case for high-modulus stainless steel.

The authors suggest advantages to using bioabsorbable implants, including no need of metal plates in children with growing skeletons; no hardware removal required; no stress shielding, with gradual resorption as adjacent bone strength increases; and avoidance of bulky metal devices or titanium debris interfering with tendon and soft tissue gliding in the hand. Disadvantages include the fact that currently available bioabsorbable implants cannot be self-drilling or self-tapping, are unforgiving and require precise placement the first time, and cannot be seen on radiographs or with fluoroscopy. The authors have previously published the results of experimental studies using bioabsorbable implants and hint at future work that may be forthcoming from their group, including investigating ways to combine the implants with antibiotics or growth factors that could leach from the devices as the bioabsorption occurs.

R. R. Slater, Jr, MD

Base of Distal Phalanx Fracture in Children: A Mallet Finger Mimic
Ganayem M, Edelson G (Poriya Government Hosp, Tiberias, Israel)
J Pediatr Orthop 25:487-489, 2005   18–3

Background.—Prior to closure of the epiphyses, fractures usually occur through the growth plate, Salter-Harris type I or II, or through the juxtaepiphyseal region 1 to 2 mm distal to the growth plate. Because of the asymmetry of the insertions of the extensor and the flexor digitorum profundus tendons, the clinical manifestation of this injury in young children mimics a finger mallet deformity. However, unlike mallet finger, the juxtaepiphyseal fracture does not involve a tear or avulsion of the extensor tendon itself. The fracture is usually an open injury and may be mistaken for a distal interphalangeal joint dislocation. A series of juxtaepiphyseal fractures at the base of the distal phalanx of the finger was presented.

Methods.—Seven fractures at the base of the distal phalanx were identified in seven children ranging in age from 4 to 10 years. The mechanism of injury was hyperflexion of the distal phalanx by a heavy object hitting the digit or entrapment of the digit in a closing door. Six of the injuries were open and consistently displayed a transverse laceration of the nail matrix, with the nail degloved from under the nail fold. One injury was closed. The six open injuries were treated according to a standard protocol involving thorough debridement under regional anesthesia with IV antibiotic coverage. The nail was replaced under the proximal nail fold, and the fracture reduced by applying hyperextension force to the terminal phalanx. In two cases the nail fold presented an obstacle to reduction, and reduction was accomplished by elevating a flap via two incisions perpendicular to the eponychium. A Kirschner wire was used to reattach the shaft to the epiphyses and concomitantly to immobilize the distal interphalangeal joint. Intravenous antibiotics were continued for 3 days after surgery. The one case of close injury was treated with closed reduction and splinting.

Results.—The Kirshner wires and the splint were removed at 3 weeks. There were no infections present, and the fractures healed with no significant deformity at an average follow up of 18 months (range, 1-2.5 years).

Conclusions.—Fractures of the base of the distal phalanx in children may at first appear to be classic mallet finger deformities, but they are anatomically different and potentially more problematic. The fractures are usually unstable, and reduction should be maintained by fixation with Kirschner wires with fluoroscopic guidance.

▶ The authors report 7 juxta-epiphyseal distal phalanx injuries with subluxed nail plates in children between 4 and 10 years of age. They have reminded us of the extremely important differences between adult mallet injuries and open fractures of the distal phalanx in children. They report successful treatment of all fractures with debridement, reduction, nail bed repair, and antibiotics. Any history of trauma with a "mallet type" deformity and subluxed nail plate (or subungual hematoma) in a child, should raise the suspicion of an underlying Seymour fracture.

Proper identification of this injury, by physical exam and radiographs, followed by debridement and reduction of the fracture, along with repair of the nailbed, are the key points in treatment. The authors used IV antibiotics for 3 days postoperatively. Although I am not certain that there is any significant benefit of antibiotics beyond 24 hours, I would expect that after initial debridement, irrigation, and IV antibiotics that either no further antibiotics or oral antibiotics for the next 48 hours would be reasonable (in acute, non-contaminated wounds). Pin immobilization may be necessary, but re-insertion of the nail plate with absorbable sutures may often provide acceptable splinting of the fracture.

D. G. Dennison, MD

Principles of Metacarpal and Phalangeal Fracture Management: A Review of Rehabilitation Concepts
Hardy MA (Univ of Mississippi, Jackson)
J Orthop Sports Phys Ther 34:781-799, 2004   18–4

Patients with common hand fractures are likely to present in a wide variety of outpatient orthopedic practices. Successful rehabilitation of hand fractures addresses the need to (1) maintain fracture stability for bone healing, (2) introduce soft tissue mobilization for soft tissue integrity, and (3) remodel any restrictive scar from injury or surgery. It is important to recognize the intimate relationship of these 3 tissues (bone, soft tissue, and scar) when treating hand fractures. Fracture terminology precisely defines fracture type, location, and management strategy for hand fractures. These terms are reviewed, with emphasis on their operational definitions, as they relate to the course of therapy. The progression of motion protocols is dependent on the

TABLE 1.—Potential Problems With Metacarpal Fractures and Strategies for Therapeutic Intervention

Potential Problems	Prevention and Treatment
Dorsal hand edema	Coban wrap compression, ice, elevation, high-voltage stimulation
Dorsal skin scar contracture that prevents full fist	Silicone TopiGel, simultaneous heat and stretch with hand wrapped in a fisted position; friction massage
MP joint contracted in extension	Initially: position MP joint at 70° flexion in protective splint Late: dynamic or static progressive MP joint flexion splint
Adherence of EDC tendon to fracture with limited MP joint flexion	Initially: teach EDC glide exercises to prevent adherence; splint IP joint in extension during exercise to concentrate flexion power at MP joint Late: dynamic MP flexion splint; NMES of EDC with on > off cycle
Intrinsic muscle contracture secondary to swelling and immobilization	Initially: teach intrinsic stretch (intrinsic minus position) Late: static progressive splint in intrinsic minus position
Dorsal sensory radial/ulnar nerve irritation	Desensitization program; iontophoresis with lidocaine
Attrition and potential rupture of extensor tendon over prominent dorsal boss or large plate	Rest involved tendon; contact physician if painful symptoms with AROM persist
Scissoring/overlapping of digits with flexion	Slight: buddy tape to adjacent digit Severe: malrotation deformity requiring ORIF
Absence of MP head	Shortening of metacarpal; may not be functional problem
Absence of MP head and MP joint extension lag	Shortening of metacarpal with redundancy in extensor length; splint in extension at night; strengthen intrinsics abduction/adduction; NMES of intrinsics with off > on cycle
Absence of MP head with volar prominence and pain with grip	Neck fracture angulated volarly; minor; padded work glove; major: reduction of angulation required

Abbreviations: AROM, Active range of motion; *EDC,* extensor digitorum communis; *MP,* metacarpophalangeal; *IP,* interphalangeal; *NMES,* neuromuscular electrical stimulation.
(Reprinted from Hardy MA: Principles of metacarpal and phalangeal fracture management: A review of rehabilitation concepts. *J Orthop Sports Phys Ther* 34:781-799, 2004, with permission of the Orthopaedic and Sports Sections of the American Physical Therapy Association.)

type of fracture healing, either primary or secondary, which in turn is determined by the method of fracture fixation. Current closed- and open-fixation methods for metacarpal and phalangeal fractures are addressed for each fracture location. The potential soft tissue problems that are often associated with each type of fracture are explained, with preventative methods of splinting and treatment. A comprehensive literature review is provided to compare evidence for practice in managing the variety of fracture patterns associated with metacarpal and phalangeal fractures, following closed- and open-fixation techniques. Emphasis is placed on initial hand positioning to protect the fracture reduction, exercise to maintain or regain joint range of motion, and specific tendon-gliding exercises to prevent restrictive adhe-

TABLE 2.—Potential Problems With Phalangeal Fractures and Strategies for Therapeutic Intervention

Potential Problems	Prevention and Treatment
Loss of MP flexion	Circumferential PIP and DIP extension splint to concentrate flexor power at MP joint; NMES to interossei
Loss of PIP extension	Central slip blocking exercises; during the day MP extension block splint to concentrate extensor power at PIP joint; at night PIP extension gutter splint; NMES to EDC and interossei with dual channel setup
Loss of PIP flexion	Isolated FDP tendon glide exercises; during the day MP flexion blocking splint to concentrate flexor power at PIP joint; at night flexion glove; NMES to FDS
Loss of DIP extension	Resume night extension splinting; NMES to interossei
Loss of DIP flexion	Isolated FDP tendon glide exercises; PIP flexion blocking splint to concentrate flexor power at DIP joint; stretch ORL tightness; NMES to FDP
Lateral instability any joint	Buddy strap or finger hinged splint that prevents lateral stress
Impending Boutonniere deformity	Early DIP active flexion to maintain length of lateral bands
Impending swan neck deformity	FDS tendon glide at PIP joint and terminal extensor tendon glide at the DIP joint
Pseudo claw deformity	Splint to hold MP joint in flexion with PIP joint full extensor glide
Pain	Resume protective splinting until healing is ascertained; address edema, desensitization program

Abbreviations: DIP, Distal interphalangeal; *EDC*, extensor digitorum communis; *FDP*, flexor digitorum profundus; *FDS*, flexor digitorum superficialis; *MP*, metacarpophalangeal; *NMES*, neuromuscular electrical stimulation; *ORL*, oblique retinacular ligament; *PIP*, proximal interphalangeal.
(Reprinted from Hardy MA: Principles of metacarpal and phalangeal fracture management: A review of rehabilitation concepts. *J Orthop Sports Phys Ther* 34:781-799, 2004, with permission of the Orthopaedic and Sports Sections of the American Physical Therapy Association.)

sions, all of which are necessary to assure return of function post fracture (Tables 1 and 2).

▶ This was an excellent review of the literature outlining hand fracture management, splinting for early protected motion, and rehabilitation. Successful hand fracture outcomes resulting in full unrestricted motion, especially for phalangeal fractures, can be a challenging process, and there are limited quick access reference tools available for therapists when they encounter problems.

I found the charts, Tables 1 and 2, outlining potential problems with metacarpal and phalangeal fractures (including strategies for therapeutic intervention) very helpful tools that will be incorporated into my clinical practice. Additionally, the diagrams of the various splints used to achieve goals are helpful. I recommend keeping a copy of this article in the clinic for reference for any therapist working in a high-volume hand practice. It is my hope that a greater number of early, controlled motion studies for hand fractures will be completed in the near future.

M. Outzen, MS, OTR/L

A Biomechanical Modeling of Injury, Repair, and Rehabilitation of Ulnar Collateral Ligament Injuries of the Thumb
Harley BJ, Werner FW, Green JK (State Univ of New York Upstate Med Univ, Syracuse)
J Hand Surg [Am] 29A:915-920, 2004   18–5

Purpose.—The use of early active motion protocols after repair of the thumb ulnar collateral ligament (UCL) theoretically could avoid the complications of postoperative immobilization and improve ligament healing. The goals of this study were as follows: (1) to develop an accurate model of acute UCL rupture, (2) to determine the strain pattern in the UCL during constrained active thumb motion in intact and repaired thumbs, and (3) to determine the load to failure and strain of the UCL during rupture in forced abduction.

Methods.—Sixteen fresh-frozen adult cadaver thumbs were mounted in a testing apparatus designed for testing the strain in the UCL during constrained active motion and abduction load to failure. Strain data for the UCL during motion were measured. Specimens were tested to failure using an MTS machine. Dynamic strain data were acquired throughout the loading cycle. Repair of the torn ligament was performed with a suture anchor technique. Strain and load-to-failure measurements then were repeated in the repaired specimens. Differences in the strain values and failure forces between the intact and repaired specimens then were compared.

Results.—A reliable model of a UCL rupture was created. Strains in the UCL were similar during active motion in both intact and repaired specimens. A significant decrease in maximum load to failure was noted in repaired specimens but failure reliably occurred at strains 3 times greater than expected with active motion.

Conclusions.—A controlled active motion therapy protocol after suture anchor repair of a ruptured UCL of the thumb is safe from a biomechanical point of view.

▶ The authors selected a relevant clinical problem and designed a biomechanical model to study it. Sixteen fresh frozen cadavers were used for biomechanical testing of both the creation of the injury and testing the repair. Two thirds of their specimens failed at the distal insertion, so the authors believe the study did simulate the clinical situation. After repair using a suture anchor, the strength of the repair was deemed sufficient to allow early protected range of motion. After repair, the ligament was found to be only 60% as strong as before injury, but the authors admit that this is because the model was in cadaver, with no healing of the ligament occurring. This study provides good information about the use of more aggressive therapy protocols for rehabilitation of a common injury.

J. A. Katarincic, MD

Effects of the Adductor Pollicis and Abductor Pollicis Brevis on Thumb Metacarpophalangeal Joint Laxity Before and After Ulnar Collateral Ligament Reconstruction

Draganich LF, Greenspahn S, Mass DP (Univ of Chicago)
J Hand Surg [Am] 29A:481-488, 2004   18–6

Background.—Patients with injuries to the stabilizing structures of the metacarpophalangeal (MCP) joints usually have altered kinematics, which can lead to constant subluxation of the joint, pain, and decreased strength during pinch and other important functions of the thumb. Joint laxity and instability of the injured MCP joint can be treated with surgical repair or reconstruction and arthrodesis of the joint.

The intrinsic muscles and ulnar capsuloligamentous structures (UCLS) which consist of the ulnar collateral ligament (UCL), accessory UCL, dorsal capsule, and volar plate of the MCP joint are important for controlling the motion and stability of the MCP joint during pinch. The purpose of this cadaveric study was to determine the effects of the adductor pollicis (AdP) and abductor pollicis brevis (APB) on 3-dimensional MCP joint laxity before transection of the UCLS and after reconstruction of the UCL and repair of the dorsal capsule.

Methods.—Loads were applied to the flexor pollicis longus (FPL) alone, to the AdP and FPL in combination, and to the ABP and FPL in combination in 11 cadavers. Loading was performed in the intact joint after the UCLS were transected and after the UCL was reconstructed for flexion angles of 0°, 15°, 30°, and 45°. The spatial positions of the proximal phalanx and the metacarpal of the MCP joint were measured with a 6-degrees-of-freedom digitizing system.

Results.—Combined loading of the AdP and FPL in the intact joint did not affect the position of the proximal phalanx. Combined loading of the APB and FPL altered the position of the phalanx from an ulnar to a radial shift and from an ulnar to a radial deviation and increased pronation. Combined loading of the FPL and AdP and transection of the UCLS increased supination of the MCP joint, and combined loading of the FPL and APB increased radial shift, radial deviation, and pronation of the joint.

Conclusion.—MCP joint motion was not affected by the AdP. The ABP produced a radial shift and radial deviation of the MCP joint and increased pronation of the thumb. Transection of the UCLS increased joint laxity for each of the combined loadings. Normal laxity to the MCP joint was restored by reconstruction of the UCL.

▶ This study evaluated the intrinsic muscle's effect on the thumb MCP joint following injury and subsequent reconstruction of the UCL. Although the primary effect on the MCP joint was noted during loading of the APB, the clinical consequence is of uncertain significance. Although the AdP did not have a significant effect on the MCP joint after ulnar collateral ligament sectioning, a more clinically appropriate question would be related to its potential secondary stabilization of the MCP joint.

Chronic UCL injuries of the thumb MCP joint have uncertain outcomes following reconstruction with tendon grafts. These cases may benefit from rehabilitation of secondary stabilizers of this joint. Future studies may be directed towards the intrinsic muscle's potential rehabilitative effect following injury.

R. Goitz, MD

Chronic Finger Joint Instability Reconstructed With Bone-Ligament-Bone Graft From the Iliac Crest

Wu WC, Wong TC, Yip TH (Pamela Youde Nethersole Eastern Hosp, Hong Kong)

J Hand Surg [Br] 29B:494-501, 2004   18–7

Background.—Nonrheumatoid chronic instability of digital joints is most commonly found at the metacarpophalangeal joint of the thumb and the proximal interphalangeal joint of the fingers. Significant functional disability can result and surgical treatment is often required. A new method using bone-ligament-bone (BLB) graft harvested from the iliac crest with overlying tendinous fibers to restore stability of the joint was presented.

Methods.—Five patients with chronic instability of joint of the thumb or fingers were treated between 1998 and 2001. The patients included 2 men and 3 women with a mean age of 41 years (range, 22-59 years). Three patients had thumb metacarpophalangeal joint involvement, 1 had instability of the proximal interphalangeal joint of the little finger, and 1 had instability of the thumb interphalangeal joint. The BLB graft is harvested from the iliac crest, usually on the side of the hand undergoing surgery. Once the graft is harvested, the size of the 2 bone pegs at either end is determined (Fig 1).

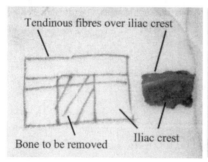 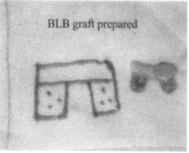

FIGURE 1.—Bone-ligament-bone graft harvested from the iliac crest. The tendinous part over the iliac crest is used to replace the collateral ligament. Two bone pegs were prepared from the iliac bone. (Reprinted from Wu WC, Wong TC, Yip TH: Chronic finger joint instability reconstructed with bone-ligament-bone graft from the iliac crest. *J Hand Surg [Br]* 29B:494-501. Copyright 2004, with permission from The British Society for Surgery of the Hand.)

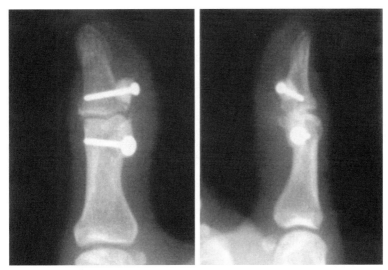

FIGURE 5.—A bone-ligament-bone graft has healed and restored stability of the joint. (Reprinted from Wu WC, Wong TC, Yip TH: Chronic finger joint instability reconstructed with bone-ligament-bone graft from the iliac crest. *J Hand Surg [Br]* 29B:494-501. Copyright 2004, with permission from The British Society for Surgery of the Hand.)

The prepared BLB is placed across the joint and its bone pegs are inserted into the proper troughs. After surgery, a boxing glove is worn for 1 or 2 days, and gentle mobilization exercises are started early. There is no need for plaster remobilization. Strengthening exercises are usually started about 1 month after the operation.

Results.—The mean duration of follow-up for these 5 patients was 3 years (range, 1 to 5 years). All patients achieved a pain-free joint with excellent stability after surgery, with no subsequent stretching of the reconstructed ligament (Fig 5). The range of motion, power grip, and pinch grip were the same or nearly the same as for the contralateral digit in 4 of the 5 cases. All patients returned to their original employment and sporting activities. One patient was advised to use a splint to protect the interphalangeal joint of the thumb during work.

Conclusion.—There are several advantages to the use of this new technique for correcting chronic finger joint instability, including no disruption of the finger tendons and minimal donor site morbidity.

▶ The authors present a technique for the treatment of nonrheumatoid chronic instability of the metacarpophalangeal and interphalangeal joints. A BLB construct harvested from the iliac crest was used to treat the digital joints of 5 patients. If in addition to the collateral ligament instability, there was significant dorsal or volar instability, the ligamentous portion of the BLB graft was attached to the dorsal capsule or volar plate. All 5 patients gained pain-free range of motion without instability. The range of motion was from full to 75% of the normal side, and the power grip and pinch strength were from 100% to 50% of the contralateral side.

Figure 5 shows a BLB graft used for repair of a thumb interphalangeal joint and highlights the requirement for accurate measurement and careful graft preparation. Despite a small series of 5 patients, this procedure provided good results, with early resumption of joint mobilization. One can add this operation to the list of possible procedures for the treatment of chronic finger joint instability.

K. Azari, MD

19 Hand: Arthritis & Arthroplasty

Modified Sauvé-Kapandji Procedure for Disorders of the Distal Radioulnar Joint in Patients With Rheumatoid Arthritis
Fujita S, Masada K, Takeuchi E, et al (Osaka Rosai Hosp, Japan)
J Bone Joint Surg Am 87:134-139, 2005   19–1

Background.—Operative problems may develop during treatment of disorders of the distal radioulnar joint in patients with rheumatoid arthritis of the wrist. Use of the Sauvé-Kapandji procedure has achieved good results in treating posttraumatic degeneration or rheumatoid arthritis. If the patient has poor distal ulnar bone stock, sufficient osseous support for the ulnar aspect of the carpus may be lacking. A modification of the procedure was developed to ensure sufficient support for the ulnar side of the carpus.

Technique.—The distal part of the ulna is resected, and a drill hole is made in the ulnar cortex of the distal part of the radius. The resected portion is then rotated 90° and inserted into the distal part of the radius. It is fixed at that site with a cancellous-bone screw (Fig 3, D).

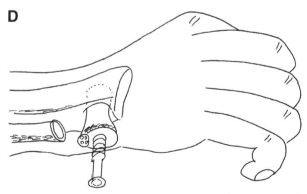

FIGURE 3.—D, The ulnar graft is inserted into the drill-hole and is fixed with a cancellous-bone screw. (Republished with permission of the Journal of Joint and Bone Surgery, Inc, from Fujita S, Masada K, Takeuchi E, et al: Modified Sauvé-Kapandji procedure for disorders of the distal radioulnar joint in patients with rheumatoid arthritis. *J Bone Joint Surg Am* 87-A:134-139, 2005. Reproduced by permission of the publisher via Copyright Clearance Center, Inc.)

Stability of the free end of the ulnar shaft is ensured by closing the periosteum and capsule over the bone end and along the length of the pseudarthrosis. This technique was used in 56 patients (66 wrists) with rheumatoid arthritis.

Results.—Patients' mean age was 59.3 years, and follow-up lasted a mean of 48 months. Postoperatively, all patients had osseous union and resolution of or a decrease in wrist pain. The mean total range of forearm rotation was 144° before surgery and increased to 167° at the latest follow-up evaluation. The surgery did not change the mean carpal translation index.

Conclusions.—Pain was reduced, forearm rotation was improved, and ulnar translation of the carpal bones was prevented with the modified Sauvé-Kapandji procedure. This procedure is designed to ensure that patients with poor distal ulnar bone stock because of rheumatoid degeneration can achieve adequate osseous support of the carpus.

▶ The authors have presented a novel modification of the classically described Sauvé-Kapandji procedure for patients who may have marginal bone stock under the hypothesis that rotating the resected head of the ulna 90° provides better fixation. What concerns me most about this procedure is that I remain unconvinced that the problem to be solved by this procedure actually exists. In their own description of the procedure and its indications, the authors state that the ulnar aspect of the distal ulna may have loss of structure because of the erosive changes of rheumatoid arthritis. While this is true, the examples that are cited in the radiographs show what appears to be a relatively robust ulnar cortex of the ulna, including the styloid process. By rotating the distal ulna 90°, any residual contact of the triangular fibrocartilage complex with the ulna is lost as well as the relationship of the extensor carpi ulnaris tendon subsheath to the ulna. While these can certainly be affected by the inflammatory process, rendering both essentially unreliable, the surgical procedure described by the authors would most certainly render both of these structures free floating. It just seems that the procedure is being modified in a manner that makes it more technically demanding without a substantially validated indication by their description. In my experience with the rheumatoid arthritis patient population, nonunion or loss of competency of the arthrodesed ulnar head has been a very infrequent occurrence. Great care must still be taken to try to stabilize the more proximal ulnar component as much as possible, which remains the greatest challenge in this population of patients with rheumatoid arthritis or other inflammatory arthropathies.

R. A. Berger, MD, PhD

A Crossover Trial of Custom-Made and Commercially Available Wrist Splints in Adults With Inflammatory Arthritis

Haskett S, Backman C, Porter B, et al (Vancouver Coastal Health Authority, BC, Canada; Univ of British Columbia, Vancouver, Canada)
Arthritis Rheum 51:792-799, 2004   19–2

Objective.—To compare the effect of 3 wrist splints (2 prefabricated commercial splints and 1 custom made) on perceived wrist pain, hand function, and perceived upper extremity function in adults with inflammatory arthritis.

Methods.—Subjects (n = 45, mean age 49 years, mean disease duration 8.6 years) were randomly assigned to treatment order in a 3-phase crossover trial. Splints were worn for 4 weeks, separated by 1-week washouts. Outcomes were assessed at baseline, after each splint phase and washout period, and at 6 months' followup using a pain visual analog scale (VAS), the Arthritis Hand Function Test, and McMaster-Toronto Arthritis Patient Function Preference questionnaire. Data were analyzed with multivariate analyses of variance (MANOVAs), t-tests, and chi-square tests.

Results.—There did not appear to be order or carryover effects. MANOVA indicated that wrist splints significantly reduced pain ($P = 0.007$). The custom leather splint was most effective in reducing pain, from 4.1 cm to 2.8 cm on the VAS ($P = 0.001$). All splints improved hand strength, and the commercial Rolyan splint provided significantly stronger grip than the Anatech commercial splint ($P = 0.04$). In contrast to previous studies, splints did not compromise dexterity. There were several significant differences among splints, depending on the outcome measure. Improvements were maintained at 6 months.

Conclusion.—After 4 weeks' use, wrist splints reduce pain, improve strength, and do not compromise dexterity. Similar improvements were achieved with the custom leather splint and Rolyan commercial splint, which were superior to the Anatech commercial splint.

▶ This was a very thought-provoking study in terms of custom versus prefabricated splinting options. As a practicing hand therapist, I find it is almost sacrilegious to consider that a custom and a prefabricated splint may provide an equal (or very similar) end result. Therefore, more studies comparing custom versus prefabricated splints are needed. It is helpful to know, however, that there are prefabricated splints being manufactured that are as good as custom splints and, furthermore, that splinting the inflamed, arthritic wrist for even 10 to 12 hours per week is effective in reducing pain and promoting some aspects of hand function.

This study may offer guidance to the hand therapist in his or her clinical decision-making process in today's cost-containing health care environment. For example, depending on constraints on time and costs, if a patient with inflammatory arthritis is referred for a wrist splint, a quality prefabricated splint that is comfortable to the patient can be issued in less time and overall cost to the patient and clinic versus construction of a splint, while still providing the same outcome. Conversely, this study may point to the fact that fitting a small, medium, or large prefabricated wrist splint to a patient takes minimal to no skill and is a task that may not necessarily need to be delegated to a hand or occupational therapist.

M. Outzen, MS, OTR/L

Early Failures With a Spheric Interposition Arthroplasty of the Thumb Basal Joint

Athwal GS, Chenkin J, King GJ, et al (Queen's Univ, Kingston, Canada; Univ of Western Ontario, London, Canada)

J Hand Surg [Am] 29A:1080-1084, 2004   19–3

Purpose.—The purpose of this study is to report the early results with the Orthosphere (Wright Medical Technology Inc, Arlington, TN) spheric interpositional arthroplasty.

Methods.—Six women and 1 man had Orthosphere arthroplasty between 2000 and 2001. The mean age at the time of surgery was 52 years (range, 24–73 years) and the mean duration of clinical and radiographic follow-up evaluation was 33 months (range, 29–44 months).

Results.—Six of 7 Orthosphere implants subsided into the trapezium resulting in pain, weakness, and stiffness (Fig 1). There was 1 implant dislocation. Five patients have had revision surgery to trapezial excision ligament reconstruction and tendon interposition arthroplasty. Of the remaining 2 patients 1 is contemplating presently revision surgery and the other is experiencing mild residual pain. No patients were satisfied completely with their Orthosphere results.

Conclusions.—In our experience the early outcome of the Orthosphere interpositional arthroplasty has been unacceptable. We no longer use the device at our institutions.

▶ The authors present their first 7 patients where a spheric interposition arthroplasty was performed. They concluded that the early outcomes from the use of the Orthosphere were unacceptable because of subsidence of the implant in the cancellous bone of the prepared trapezium. The resulting impingement of the base of the metacarpal on the trapezium caused pain and loss of function. One patient had a complete dislocation of the sphere. Based on this study, this editor questions the efficacy of this implant and would advise the surgeon who performs surgery for basilar joint arthritis to consider other proven techniques of reconstruction for this common problem.

C. Carroll IV, MD

FIGURE 1.—Varying degrees of subsidence of the Orthosphere spheric interpositional arthroplasty into the trapezium with resulting pain, weakness, and stiffness. (Reprinted from Athwal GS, Chenkin J, King GJ, et al: Early failures with a spheric interposition arthroplasty of the thumb basal joint. *J Hand Surg [Am]* 29A:1080-1084. Copyright 2004, with permission from The American Society for Surgery of the Hand.)

FIGURE 1.

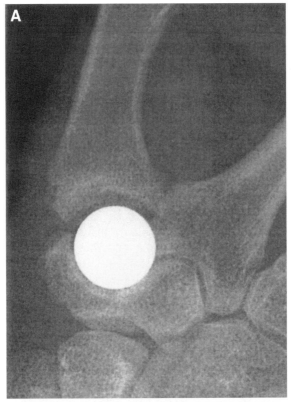

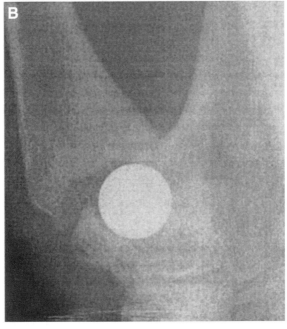

Use of the de la Caffinière Prosthesis in Rheumatoid Trapeziometacarpal Destruction

Skyttä ET, Belt EA, Kautiainen HJ, et al (Rheumatism Found, Heinola, Finland; Kanta-Häme Central Hosp, Hämeenlinna, Finland; Tampere Univ, Finland)
J Hand Surg [Br] 30B:395-400, 2005   19–4

This study evaluated the outcome of the de la Caffinière prosthesis in patients with an inflammatory arthropathy affecting the trapeziometacarpal joint. The procedure was performed in 57 thumbs for rheumatoid arthritis (41 cases), juvenile chronic arthritis (ten cases), psoriatic arthritis (four cases) and other inflammatory joint diseases (two cases). Survival analysis with a revision procedure or radiographic implant failure as end points was performed. Five loosened cups and two permanently dislocated prostheses underwent revision surgery. These were managed with a bone graft and tendon interposition technique. Radiographic follow-up yielded four additional implant failures (two loosened cups, one loosened metacarpal stem and one permanent dislocation). The implant survival rate based on revision operation was 87% (95% CI 73–94) at 10 years, and the total radiographic and implant failure rate based on radiographic findings was 15% (95% CI 7–29) at 10 years (Fig 5).

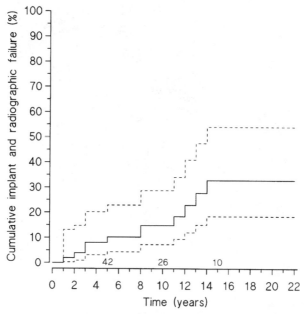

FIGURE 5.—The total implant failure rate of the de la Caffinière prostheses. Reoperated joints and radiographic implant failures are included in the survival analysis. (Reprinted from Skyttä ET, Belt EA, Kautiainen HJ, et al: Use of the de la Caffinière prosthesis in rheumatoid trapeziometacarpal destruction. *J Hand Surg [Br]* 30B:395-400. Copyright 2005, with permission from The British Society for Surgery of the Hand.)

▶ This long-term follow-up of the de la Caffinière prosthesis in patients with inflammatory arthritis provides useful information. The functional results are similar to resection arthroplasty, which is also the preferred method to use after an implant failure. The failure rate as marked by implant removal at 10 years is 13%, double that if gross loosening is used as the end point. It is clear that this implant can give reasonable results, but what is not clear to me is what, other than surgeon choice, would lead someone to use this device as an alternative to simple resection of the trapezium, ligament reconstruction and tendon interposition, or some other choice with a lower reoperation rate?

P. C. Amadio, MD

Excision of the Trapezium for Osteoarthritis of the Trapeziometacarpal Joint: A Study of the Benefit of Ligament Reconstruction or Tendon Interposition
David TRC, Brady O, Dias JJ (Queen's Med Centre, Nottingham, England; Pulvertaft Hand Centre, Derby, England; Glenfield Hosp, Leicester, England)
J Hand Surg [Am] 29A:1069-1077, 2004   19–5

Purpose.—To investigate whether palmaris longus interposition or flexor carpi radialis ligament reconstruction and tendon interposition improved the outcome of excision of the trapezium for the treatment of painful osteoarthritis of the trapeziometacarpal joint.

Methods.—183 thumbs with trapeziometacarpal osteoarthritis were randomized for treatment by either simple trapeziectomy, trapeziectomy with palmaris longus interposition, or trapeziectomy with ligament reconstruction and tendon interposition using 50% of the flexor carpi radialis tendon. A K-wire was passed across the trapezial void during each of the 183 surgeries to hold the base of the thumb metacarpal at the level of the index carpometacarpal joint and was retained for 4 weeks in every case. All patients wore a thumb splint for 6 weeks. Each patient had subjective and objective assessments of thumb pain, stiffness, and strength before surgery and at 3 months and 1 year after surgery.

Results.—The 3 treatment groups were well matched for age, dominance, and presence of associated conditions. Complications were distributed evenly among the 3 groups and no cases of subluxation/dislocation of the pseudarthrosis were observed. Of the 183 thumbs 82% achieved good pain relief and 68% regained sufficient strength to allow normal activities of daily living at the 1-year follow-up evaluation. Neither of these subjective outcomes nor the range of thumb movement was influenced by the type of surgery performed. Thumb key-pinch strength improved significantly from 3.5 kg before surgery to 4.6 kg at 1 year but the improvement in strength was not influenced by the type of surgery performed.

Conclusions.—The outcomes of these 3 variations of trapeziectomy were very similar at 1-year follow-up evaluation. In the short term at least there appears to be no benefit to tendon interposition or ligament reconstruction.

▶ The authors review the results of basilar joint arthroplasty and compare trapeziectomy, trapeziectomy with palmaris longus interposition, and trapeziectomy with ligament reconstruction and interposition with 50% of the flexor carpi radialis tendon. The study was prospective and randomized. The short-term results at 1-year follow-up were similar in all groups. The authors conclude that there are not any differences between the 3 techniques. Longer follow-up will be necessary to assess whether the interposition and ligament reconstruction will prevent proximal migration of the metacarpal base and allow for long-term maintenance of a satisfactory outcome when compared with trapeziectomy without any reconstruction. This is an excellent study and, when combined with the work of Roy Meals and others, it may change the way upper extremity surgeons treat basilar joint arthritis of the thumb.

C. Carroll IV, MD

Surgery of the Hand in Severe Systemic Sclerosis
Gilbart MK, Jolles BM, Lee P, et al (Univ of Toronto; Univ of Lausanne, Switzerland)
J Hand Surg [Br] 29B:599-603, 2004   19–6

Abstract.—Ten patients with scleroderma and severe hand problems required surgery, and seven were available for follow-up (two died from scleroderma-related complications and one was lost to follow-up). The mean duration of follow-up was 4 (range 1.5–9) years. Thirty-three procedures were carried out, including five metacarpophalangeal joint excisional arthroplasties, 13 proximal interphalangeal joint fusions, ten distal interphalangeal joint fusions, and one thumb interphalangeal joint fusion. The metacarpophalangeal joint excision arthroplasties and proximal interphalangeal joint fusions were performed for the correction of severe fixed "finger-in-palm" deformities. Lesions of cutaneous calcinosis were removed in four patients.

Fixation was satisfactory in all cases of interphalangeal joint fusion, with no cases of nonunion. Wound healing was satisfactory in six of seven patients. A second surgical procedure was required in three patients for the removal of tension band wires following interphalangeal fusion. Calcinosis was effectively removed using a high-speed dental burr. The results of hand surgery for systemic sclerosis are reliable, but goals must be limited and patient expectations should be modest.

▶ This study confirms some of the relative risks of operating on patients with scleroderma. With only 7 patients available for follow-up, there were complications in more than 50% of them. Three patients required hardware removal because of wire exposure from skin erosion, and 1 patient sustained digital ischemia and autoamputation of her index finger. However, there were no nonunions in 24 fusions, resulting in the authors' recommendation of the use of K-wires alone for fixation to minimize the risk of skin erosion and the need for wire removal. Although surgery on patients with scleroderma can have a high complication rate, proximal interphalangeal joint fusion can result in significant improvement in function because of a more optimal positioning of the digits. Preoperative discussion of these risks and benefits can improve patients' expectations and perceived outcome.

R. Goitz, MD

Value of C Reactive Protein in the Assessment of Erosive Osteoarthritis of the Hand
Punzi L, Ramonda R, Oliviero F, et al (Univ of Padova, Italy)
Ann Rheum Dis 64:955-957, 2005   19–7

Objective.—To investigate the value of serum C reactive protein (CRP) as a marker of erosive osteoarthritis (EOA) of the hand.

Methods.—Ninety eight patients, 67 with EOA and 31 with non-EOA of the hand, were included in the study and analysed for radiographic score (RS), number of erosions, and joint count (JC) at clinical observation and at bone scintigraphy. CRP was assayed in a serum sample by a highly sensitive immunonephelometric method.

Results.—The median (interquartile range) CRP level was 4.7 (2.4-6.9) mg/l in the EOA and 2.1 (0.5-4.9) mg/l in the non-EOA group (p=0.001). In all patients, CRP correlated with RS (r_s = 0.43, p<0.001), and mainly with JC at clinical observation (r_s = 0.72, p<0.001) and at bone scintigraphy (r_s = 0.47, p<0.001). The correlation of CRP with RS and JC was confirmed at clinical observation and at bone scintigraphy in the EOA subgroup, but only with JC at clinical observation in the non-EOA subgroup.

Conclusions.—CRP levels are higher in EOA than in non-EOA patients. These levels probably reflect the disease activity of EOA, as suggested by correlations between CRP and JC at clinical observation and at bone scintigraphy.

▶ EOA of the hand is an aggressive form of osteoarthritis (OA). It is unclear at present how EOA relates to the more common form of OA—whether it is a subset of OA or a phase in the evolution of normal OA. The authors show in this article, using a highly sensitive assay for CRP, that EOA patients have higher CRP levels compared with the non-EOA group. CRP levels correlated with RS and JC. As the authors point out, it is uncertain whether this higher level reflects greater inflammatory activity in the EOA group, or perhaps EOA patients have constitutionally higher CRP levels. Nevertheless, this report is an important step in the search for a useful serum marker for EOA.

A. Chong, MD

Grading of Radiographic Osteolytic Changes After Silastic Metacarpophalangeal Arthroplasty and a Prospective Trial of Osteolysis Following Use of Swanson and Sutter Prostheses

Parkkila TJ, Belt EA, Hakala M, et al (Rheumatism Found, Heinola, Finland; Oulu Univ, Finland)
J Hand Surg [Br] 30B:382-387, 2005   19–8

Background.—A symptomatic and destroyed metacarpophalangeal (MCP) joint is an indication for MCP joint arthroplasty. Silastic interposition arthroplasty has become the treatment of choice, and the Swanson silastic interposition arthroplasty is the gold standard against which other implants should be compared. The Swanson and Sutter implants both are made of Silastic, and the stems of these implants have the same shape. However, the hinge of the Swanson implant is U-shaped, whereas the hinge of the Sutter implant is rectangular and not as thin. The incidence of radiographic osteolysis after insertion of the Swanson and Sutter MCP implants in patients with rheumatoid arthritis was compared.

Methods.—A prospective study was conducted of patients with rheumatoid arthritis who underwent MCP joint replacement with the Swanson (89 implants in 25 hands) and Sutter (126 implants in 33 hands) MCP implants. The mean follow-up in the two groups was 57 (40 to 80) and 55 (36 to 79) months, respectively. All of the patients received intensive physiotherapy postoperatively.

Results.—A total of 45 (60%) metacarpal and 40 (53%) proximal phalangeal bones showed no osteolytic changes in the Swanson group. In the Sutter group, 23 (23%) of the metacarpal and 29 (29%) of the proximal phalangeal bones showed no osteolytic changes. Sclerotic changes occurred more frequently in the Swanson group than in the Sutter group. In the Swanson group, 29% had no sclerotic changes in the metacarpals, and 15% had no sclerotic changes in the proximal phalanges. In the Sutter group, 51% of the metacarpals and 43% of the proximal phalanges showed no evidence of sclerotic lines.

Conclusions.—A new method for classification of radiographic osteolysis is proposed. The significant number of osteolytic changes in the bones adjacent to MCP prostheses in this study is supportive of the view that silastic prostheses should only be used when other surgical alternatives cannot be used and that long-term control by radiography should be maintained after implantation of the silicone prostheses into the MCP joint. Osteolysis was more frequent in the Sutter than in the Swanson group at all of the classification grades in this study, which suggests that the use of the Sutter rather than the Swanson implant is questionable.

▶ The authors achieved their principal goal, that of determining and comparing the incidence of osteolysis, following insertion and function of silastic metacarpophalangeal implants (mean of 57 months for 89 Swanson silastic implants, 55 months for 126 Sutter silastic implants). To do so, they developed a new method of classifying radiological signs of osteolysis and this is the core value of this paper, particularly if sequencing from one grade to another can be established (only end-point findings were given here). They also present a method of evaluating sclerosis of bone as function time increases and suggest that this may be a useful biologic adaptation to the implant. This has been suggested before but never developed to the point of evaluation utility to my knowledge.

Though all surgery was done by one skilled surgeon, it is still remarkable that none of the common technical mistakes (implant malposition, unsuitable spacing, excessive cortex reaming, etc.) occurred nor was there any implant breakage or deformity reported. The type of silastic, which has been noted to affect the degree of particle shedding and reaction, was not discussed. Revision surgery was done for soft tissue problems, but it was recommended that reconstruction be considered for Grades III and IV osteolysis. Osteolysis (Grades II to IV) was more common in the Sutter patient group (67%) than the Swanson patient group (23%), but the incidence in both groups was considered high enough that the authors suggest that silastic implants be used only when other alternatives cannot be used.

The authors discuss briefly the alternative implant that they prefer, but give neither results nor references for this implant or any other of the non-silastic devices. This paper will best serve as an inducement for studies of the natural (perhaps unnatural) history of the biologic reactions (as studied by imaging and by other methods) of implants and bone.

J. H. Dobyns, MD

Seventeen-Year Survivorship Analysis of Silastic Metacarpophalangeal Joint Replacement
Trail IA, Martin JA, Nuttall D, et al (Wrightington Hosp, Wigan, England)
J Bone Joint Surg Br 86-B:1002-1006, 2004   19–9

We reviewed the records and radiographs of 381 patients with rheumatoid arthritis who had undergone silastic metacarpophalangeal joint replacement during the past 17 years. The number of implants was 1336 in the course of 404 operations. Implant failure was defined as either revision or fracture of the implant as seen on radiography. At 17 years, the survivorship was 63%, although on radiographs two-thirds of the implants were seen to be broken. Factors which improved survival included soft-tissue balancing, crossed intrinsic transfer and realignment of the wrist. Surgery to the thumb and proximal interphalangeal joint had a deleterious effect and the use of grommets did not protect the implant from fracture.

▶ Silicone metacarpophalangeal joint arthroplasty has been performed for rheumatoid hand for the past 40 years. Although short-term results are quite satisfactory, long-term outcome studies revealed a number of problems, such as implant fracture and recurrent ulnar deviation. This article presented an interesting retrospective analysis on 381 patients who had 1336 implants placed over a course of 17 years. Regression analysis and survival curves were performed to determine factors associated with implant breakage.

The implication of this article is that despite Swanson silicone implants' worldwide popularity, implant breakage occurs at an unacceptably high rate. Most surgeons accept this problem because the Swanson implant is easy to place and is relatively inexpensive. This article, along with other long-term series, has shown a lack of durability of the Swanson design. After many years of field trials documenting a high breakage rate, surgeons should demand from the manufacturer investment of greater research effort in developing new silicone materials that will be less prone to breakage.

The Swanson implant does not simulate a joint but rather is a spacer. Many anatomical implants are on the market now, and long-term follow-up will determine whether other implant designs will replace the Swanson implant for joint replacement in the rheumatoid hand. Until then, the silicone implant will continue to be used. The findings in this article should be a stimulus to improving existing implant materials and designs and maintaining the alignment of the metacarpophalangeal joints.

K. C. Chung, MD, MS

Metacarpophalangeal Joint Mechanics After 3 Different Silicone Arthroplasties
Weiss A-PC, Moore DC, Infantolino C, et al (Brown Med School, Providence, RI)
J Hand Surg [Am] 29A:796-803, 2004   19–10

Background.—Patients with rheumatoid arthritis frequently have involvement of the metacarpophalangeal (MCP) joints. Silicone implants are the most commonly used types of implant for surgical arthroplasty of significant MCP joint pathology in patients with rheumatoid arthritis. A number of silicone MCP joint replacements are available for clinical use, and each has unique design features. MCP joint mechanics after arthroplasty was compared with 3 currently available silicone implants (Fig 3) and how postarthroplasty mechanics compares with the mechanics of the intact joint was investigated.

Methods.—Planar 2-dimensional kinematic analysis was performed with digitized radiographs of 10 isolated fingers harvested from 5 fresh-frozen human cadavers. Radiopaque markers were affixed to the metacarpals and proximal phalanges, the flexor and extensor tendons, and the stems and hinges of the implants. Each finger was tested intact and after MCP joint replacement. Lateral radiographs were taken at approximately 10° intervals and digitized on a high-resolution scanner.

The instantaneous center of rotation (ICR), tendon excursion, and tendon moment arm were calculated. Statistical analysis was performed by repeated measures 1-way analysis of variance and Dunnett post tests.

Results.—The ICRs of the intact and implanted MCPs did not follow a smooth path. The variability of the ICRs of the intact MCP joints was 2.1 ±

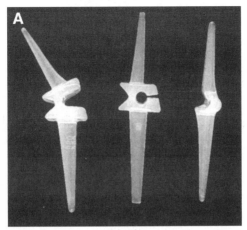

FIGURE 3.—A, Implants tested (top to bottom: Swanson, Avanta, NeuFlex). (Reprinted from Weiss A-PC, Moore DC, Infantolino C, et al: Metacarpophalangeal joint mechanics after 3 different silicone arthroplasties. *J Hand Surg [Am]* 29A:796-803. Copyright 2004, with permission from The American Society for Surgery of the Hand.)

0.8 mm. The variations in the Avanta and DePuy implants were similar (3.1 ± 1.0 mm and 3.5 ± 1.5 mm, respectively), whereas the Swanson implant was higher (4.9 ± 1.7 mm). Implant pistoning was most pronounced with the Swanson implant; the Avanta and DePuy implants pistoned significantly less than the Swanson implant.

Flexor tendon excursion was similar for all implants. The flexor tendon moment arm was similar for the intact joint and the Avanta and NeuFlex implants but was reduced significantly with the Swanson implant. Extensor tendon moment arms were similar for all implants.

Conclusion.—Overall, the NeuFlex implant most closely matched the instantaneous center of rotation, tendon excursion, and moment arm of the intact native metacarpophalangeal joint.

▶ Complications of MCP joint arthroplasties include subluxation, bone erosion, loosening, and implant abrasion. These are all related to implant mechanics. After arthroplasty, the finger kinematics should approximate those of the intact finger. The implant center of rotation should approximate that of the intact joint to balance the flexor and extensor tendon forces. This study evaluated tendon excursion and moment arms and also compared the ICR for 3 implants (NeuFlex, Avanta, and Swanson in Fig 3A).

In this study's evaluation of implant ICR, the proximal shift with the NeuFlex implant was significantly less than with the Swanson implant. None of the implants functioned as a pure hinge, although the NeuFlex implant was closest. The total motions of the Avanta and NeuFlex implants were significantly less than those of the Swanson implant, in both directions. Motions of the Avanta and NeuFlex implants were not significantly different from each other.

This study demonstrated significant reductions in flexor tendon excursion with all 3 implants, and significant reduction in flexion for the Swanson compared to the other 2. No significant change in extensor tendon excursion or moment arm for any of the 3 implants was found. This study confirms previous reports of improved flexion with the NeuFlex over Swanson implant. The most common complication of MCP arthroplasties is fracture, which has been shown to be decreased with the use of grommets for Swanson implants.

The weakness of the study is that the authors do not evaluate the reduction of the greatest complication risk, which is fracture, and the potential for the use of grommets with the NeuFlex implant. Additionally, there is potential bias of the authors toward their implant.

B. Wilhelmi, MD

Long-term Assessment of Swanson Implant Arthroplasty in the Proximal Interphalangeal Joint of the Hand
Takigawa S, Meletiou S, Sauerbier M, et al (Mayo Clinic, Rochester, Minn)
J Hand Surg [Am] 29A:785-795, 2004   19–11

Purpose.—The purpose of this study was to evaluate the clinical results of Swanson silicone implant arthroplasty of the proximal interphalangeal (PIP) joint, specifically evaluating clinical results with long-term assessment.

Methods.—A retrospective review of 70 silicone implants of the PIP joint in 48 patients was performed with an average follow-up period of 6.5 years (range, 3–20 y). Clinical assessment included motion, stability, and alignment. Radiographic assessment included implant fracture, deformity, and cystic bone resorption. The pathology consisted of degenerative joint disease in 14, posttraumatic arthritis (TA) in 11, rheumatoid arthritis (RA) in 13, and idiopathic arthritis (IA) associated with collagen disease in 12 patients. Swan neck and boutonniere deformities were assessed separately. Statistical analysis of preoperative risk factors was compared with the postoperative assessment of pain, motion, and function (return to work).

Results.—There was no significant change in the active range of motion (ROM) before and after PIP arthroplasty (26° vs 30°). Correction of swan neck and boutonniere deformities was difficult, usually leading to poor results. There was improvement in maximum active extension before surgery lacking 32° to after surgery lacking 18°. From a statistical standpoint rheumatoid joint involvement with PIP arthroplasty had poorer results than degenerative or posttraumatic arthritis with respect to pain relief and ROM. Pain relief was present in 70% of replaced PIP joints with residual pain and loss of strength in 30%. Radiographic analysis showed abnormal bone formation (cystic changes) in 45%. There were 11 implant fractures and 9 joints that required revision surgery.

Conclusions.—Silicone replacement of the PIP joint is effective in providing relief of pain from arthritis but does not provide improvement in motion or correction of deformity. It provided a poorer outcome in rheumatoid disease in comparison with degenerative, posttraumatic, or idiopathic arthritis.

▶ This retrospective study reports outcomes from multiple surgeons for PIP joint arthritis treated with a Swanson silicone implant arthroplasty. Seventy implants were studied with an average follow-up of 6.5 years. Although 70% of patients reported pain relief, there was not a significant change in motion before and after the replacement (26° vs 30°). Correction of deformity could not be achieved with use of this implant. Results were also poorer in the rheumatoid population when contrasted with the degenerative, traumatic, or idiopathic forms of arthritis of the PIP joint. This editor questions the use of the Swanson silicone implant based on these and other historical results. Having said that though, I still wonder whether we have found the optimal technique for reconstruction of the PIP joint in the face of arthritis and deformity of this difficult joint.

C. Carroll IV, MD

Comparing the AUSCAN Osteoarthritis Hand Index, Michigan Hand Outcomes Questionnaire, and Sequential Occupational Dexterity Assessment for Patients With Rheumatoid Arthritis

Massy-Westropp N, Krishnan J, Ahern M (Flinders Univ, Daw Park, Australia; Flinders Med Ctr, Daw Park, Australia; Repatriation Gen Hosp, Daw Park, Australia)
J Rheumatol 31:1996-2001, 2004   19–12

Objective.—The Australian Canadian Osteoarthritis Hand Index (AUSCAN), Michigan Hand Outcomes Questionnaire (MHQ), and the Sequential Occupational Dexterity Assessment (SODA) are assessments of hand function. Investigation of psychometric properties, administration, acceptability, and content of an assessment add strength to the findings of research and treatment. We evaluated the validity and reliability of the AUSCAN, MHQ, and the SODA for assessing disability in patients with rheumatoid arthritis (RA).

Methods.—Sixty-two patients with RA completed the AUSCAN (visual analog scale version), the MHQ, and the SODA. Seventeen patients repeated the assessments within one week.

Results.—The assessments recorded high variability within the sample of 62 patients with RA. The AUSCAN and MHQ provided patient and context-specific information, while the SODA provided more impairment information that could be readily compared between patients. Seventeen patients were tested twice within 5 days, showing good reliability of all assessments. Unlike the MHQ, AUSCAN and SODA do not provide information about individual hands or hand dominance. The physical function scales of the AUSCAN and the SODA were related (r = 0.81), and the AUSCAN and MHQ pain scales were related (r = 0.68).

Conclusion.—Clinicians and researchers should decide whether impairment, ability, or handicap outcome is the goal of assessment, and whether bilateral function or the function of one hand is of interest before choosing a hand assessment. The AUSCAN and MHQ are valid and reliable for assessment of hand disability in patients with RA, and they allow the patients to answer questions about their home environment. The SODA is also valid and reliable for assessing disability in a clinical situation that cannot be generalized to the home.

▶ The field of hand surgery has enjoyed an intensive effort to measure outcomes. Many outcome tools are currently available for the hand and the upper extremity. Associated with the luxury of having many choices is the difficulty in choosing the best outcome tool for ones practice or research projects.

The AUSCAN is yet another questionnaire that is designed to measure outcomes in the rheumatoid patient. The MHQ, which was developed in 1998, was used as a comparison questionnaire for validity testing. Overall, the AUSCAN appeared to have good reliability and validity for the rheumatoid hand. The current status of hand outcome questionnaires is analogous to the car industry.

With so many available car designs in the market, the consumer must be aware of the quality of each car model to make an informed choice. Ultimately, the outcome questionnaire that is superior in field testing and has withstood the test of time will be adopted as the dominant tool in the hand surgery field.

K. C. Chung, MD, MS

20 Hand: Microsurgery & Flaps

The International Registry on Hand and Composite Tissue Transplantation

Lanzetta M, Petruzzo P, Margreiter R, et al (Milano-Bicocca Univ, Italy; Hopital Edouard Herriot, Lyon, France; Universitatsklinik fur Chirurgie, Innsbruch, Austria; et al)

Transplantation 79:1210-1214, 2005   20–1

Background.—Since May 2002 all groups performing hand transplantations have supplied detailed information to the International Registry on Hand and Composite Tissue Transplantation. This inaugural report provides a review of all hand transplants performed to date.

Methods.—Between September 1998 and September 2004, 18 male patients underwent 24 hand/forearm/digit transplantations (11 monolateral and 4 bilateral hand transplantations, 2 bilateral forearm transplantations, and 1 thumb transplantation). The level of amputation was mostly at the distal forearm or wrist. The average age of the patient was 32 years. Time since hand loss ranged from 2 months to 22 years. Immunosuppressive therapy included tacrolimus, mycophenolate mofetil, rapamycin, and steroids; polyclonal or monoclonal antibodies were used for induction. Topical immunosuppression was administered in some patients. Follow-up period ranged from 17 to 70 months.

Results.—Patient survival was 100%. Graft survival was 100% at 1 and 2 years. Two cases of graft failure at a later date were caused by severe inflammation and progressive rejection in a noncompliant patient. Acute rejection episodes occurred in 12 patients within the first year. Rejection was reversible in all compliant patients. Side effects included opportunistic infections and metabolic complications. No life-threatening complications or malignancies were reported. All patients had achieved protective sensation, and 17 patients also achieved discriminative sensation. Extrinsic and intrinsic muscle recovery enabled patients to perform most daily activities.

Conclusions.—Despite the enormous antigen load associated with composite tissue allograft, hand transplantation became a clinical reality with immunosuppression comparable to transplantation of solid organs.

▶ Despite considerable controversy, hand transplantation has moved forward and, over the last 7 years, has become a reality. The authors of this article review the 18 cases to date and note the importance of establishing an international registry. The results of hand transplantation have been encouraging in that only 2 failures have occurred. Functionality improved in all patients. I am in complete agreement with the need for a registry. Because these patients receive immunosuppression, it is important that they be followed up through a registry so that the short- and long-term outcomes can ultimately determine the value of this extraordinary development of our specialty.

M. Rizzo, MD

Functional and Cosmetic Results of Fingertip Replantation: Anastomosing Only the Digital Artery
Matsuzaki H, Yoshizu T, Maki Y, et al (Akita Red Cross Hosp, Japan; Niigata Hand Surgery Found, Akita, Japan)
Ann Plast Surg 53:353-359, 2004   20–2

Abstract.—In fingertip amputations, conventional stump plasty provides an almost acceptable functional result. However, replanting fingertips can preserve the nail and minimize loss of function. We investigated the functional and cosmetic results of fingertip replantation at the terminal branch of the digital artery. Outcomes were nailbed width and distal-segment length; sensory recovery; and range of motion (ROM) of thumb-interphalangeal (IP) or finger–distal interphalangeal (DIP) joints, and total active motion (TAM) of the replanted finger. Of 15 fingertips replanted after only arterial anastomosis, 13 were successful, and 12 were studied. After a median of 1.3 years, mean nailbed widths and distal-segment lengths were 95.4% and 93.0%, respectively, of the contralateral finger. Average TAM and ROM of the thumb-IP or finger-DIP joints were 92.0% and 83.0% of normal, respectively. Semmes-Weinstein results were blue (3.22 to 3.61) in 4 fingers and purple (3.84 to 4.31) in 8; the mean result from the 2-point discrimination test was 5.9 mm (range, 3 to 11 mm). Thus, amputated fingertips should be aggressively replanted.

▶ The authors present beautiful results for replantation of distal amputations within Tamai zone I. At such a level, arterial anastomosis is only possible. In this study, blood letting was required for a period of 7 days to prevent venous congestion and fingertip loss. The average follow-up was at a median of 1.3 years, and excellent preservation of the nail bed width and distal segment length was seen. Two-point discrimination was 5.9 mm. Although the results are encouraging, these patients required the additional use of IV urokinase and heparin. No comment is made about the transfusion requirements or overall hospital length of stay. In addition, all fingers experienced cold intolerance. For the benefits of this procedure to be truly evaluated, in light of the additional economic costs and risks to the patient (in terms of transfusion reactions and viral transmission), a prospective study should be performed comparing simple amputation closure to replantation for injuries at this level.

S. L. Moran, MD

Restoration of Function and Sensitivity Utilizing a Homodigital Neurovascular Island Flap After Amputation Injuries of the Fingertip
Varitimidis SE, Dailiana ZH, Zibis AH, et al (Univ of Thessaly, Larissa, Greece)
J Hand Surg [Br] 30B:338-342, 2005   20–3

Background.—The pulp of the fingertip has the richest vasculature and the highest density of nerve ends of any region of the finger. A normal digital pulp is vital to the interaction between the brain and the upper extremity required in the finest activities of daily living. Unfortunately, injury of the fingertip is the most common injury to the hand, and fingertip amputation is the most common amputation in the upper extremity.

Surgical repair should aim at preservation of adequate and functional length of the digits, immediate coverage of the wound, preservation of sensibility at the distal pulp, adequate distal interphalangeal joint motion, a painless scar, short hospital stay and minimum morbidity, and early return to work and other daily activities. However, management of these injuries is controversial. Presented were the results of a large series of patients who were treated with homodigital neurovascular island flaps based on a single neurovascular pedicle for reconstruction of amputated fingertips.

Methods.—From 1995 to 2002, there were 77 reconstructions of fingertip amputations in 62 patients. All were reconstructed in the first 24 hours after injury with the use of a homodigital neurovascular island flap technique based on a single neurovascular pedicle without further shortening of the distal phalanx. The procedure was performed with the patient under regional anesthesia and with the use of a tourniquet and 2 magnifying loupes. Follow-up ranged from 14 to 94 months, with a mean of 46 months.

Results.—All of the flaps survived and achieved normal or adequate 2-point discrimination without any painful scar or hypersensitivity to cold. However, 15 patients reported some loss of distal interphalangeal joint extension.

Conclusion.—The outcome of treatment of fingertip injuries with homodigital neurovascular island flaps based on a single neurovascular bundle is predictable and satisfactory for patient and surgeon. However, careful preoperative planning is required, particularly in the design of the flap. Caution is needed at all stages of the procedure to avoid problems with the flap. A functional digit with normal sensitivity of the pulp is attainable and should be expected.

▶ This large clinical case series provides evidence of the safety and versatility of the homodigital island flap following acute fingertip injuries. The authors show full flap survival in all cases and good acceptance of the clinical outcome by the patients. Higher ratings were seen in patients with the less severe Allen II type injuries versus Allen III and IV type injuries. The authors also document good retention of 2-point discrimination and only mild loss of distal interphalangeal joint motion in the average case.

A variety of treatment modalities have been described for the treatment of fingertip injuries. The main advantage of this flap is that it limits morbidity to the affected finger (discounting the skin graft for the donor site), and there is no period of immobilization involved, unlike distant flaps like a cross-finger or thenar flap. It is most useful for small to moderate-size defects. However, some degree of microsurgical expertise is required for these small island flaps and venous congestion, particularly, can be a problem. To prevent this, the authors recommend taking a cuff of fibrofatty tissue with the neurovascular bundle.

In their experience, the authors report that final sensation is achieved within 12 weeks. This flap and its variations are a useful tool in the hand surgeon's armamentarium to cover moderate-size defects of the fingertip.

A. Chong, MD

Antebrachial Reverse Island Flap With Pedicle of Posterior Interosseous Artery: A Report of 90 Cases
Lu LJ, Gong X, Liu ZG, et al (The First Clinical College Affiliated to Jilin Univ, Chang chun, People's Republic of China)
BJPS 57:645-652, 2004   20–4

Background.—For several decades, antebrachial reverse island flaps have been used to repair soft tissue defects or for thumb reconstruction. Difficulties stemming from the necessary sacrifice of either the radial or ulnar artery have included impaired hand vascularity, causing cold intolerance. After a consistent anastomosis was noted between the posterior interosseous artery and anterior interosseous artery on the dorsal aspect of the wrist, a new antebrachial reverse island flap based on the posterior interosseous artery was developed. Between 1985 and 2000, 90 patients had soft tissue repair or thumb reconstruction with this flap. The results were reported.

Methods.—Patients ranged in age from 6 to 58 years and included 26 female and 64 male subjects. The largest flap was 16 × 10 cm with a pedicle of 7.0 cm, and the smallest was 7 × 6 cm with a pedicle of 8.0 cm. Bone grafts varied from 3 to 6 × 1 to 2 cm, and tendon grafts measured between 4 and 7 cm. The flaps were used for repairing the first web space, palmar skin defects of the hand, dorsal skin defects of the hand, and dorsal skin defects of the finger; for thumb reconstruction; and for repairing volar and dorsal skin with tendon defects.

Results.—The flap survival rate was 98.89%, with only one failing because of vascular insufficiency. Eight cases had venous stasis that led to epidermal necrosis at the distal end. Six cases required lipectomy or modification 3 to 6 months postoperatively. After 3 months, the sensation over the repaired area was similar to that of normal hand areas. Flaps not involving nerve repair recovered within 2 years of the surgery. None of the tendon graft cases required tendon release. All bone grafts healed within 3 months. Neither hand function nor forearm function was adversely affected by the repair or donor site morbidity.

Conclusions.—The advantages of using the antebrachial reverse island flap based on the posterior interosseous artery pedicle include good texture and color and thickness appropriate to the hand. Soft tissue defects with or without nerve, tendon, and bone defects can be reliably repaired. The flap is also suitable for reconstruction of the first web space and thumb. The series reported included a flap survival rate of nearly 99%. Donor site morbidity was acceptable, with minimal interference with mobilization.

▶ In a retrospective review, the authors evaluated a series of 90 cases of antebrachial reverse island flap with pedicle of the posterior interosseous artery. In 1985, the authors found a consistent artery anastomosis between the posterior interosseous artery and the anterior interosseous artery on the dorsal side of the wrist. Based on this finding, they designed a new antebrachial reverse island flap based on the posterior interosseous artery and reported their initial 6 cases in the *Chinese Association of Hand Surgery* in 1986. Two years later, the posterior interosseous flap was published by Costa. Only one of their cases failed. The authors present 4 cases to demonstrate their indications and the characteristics of the flap. Essentially, this is a case series without a significant detailed statistical evaluation.

A. Y. Shin, MD

Delayed Microsurgical Reconstruction of the Extremities for Complex Soft-Tissue Injuries
Riccio M, Pangrazi PP, Campodonico A, et al (Univ of Ancona, Italy)
Microsurgery 25:272-283, 2005   20–5

Background.—The treatment of severe wounds of the extremities caused by crush injuries is characterized by large posttraumatic tissue loss and can present difficult clinical problems. These problems are particularly difficult when the lesion is surrounded by large areas of ischemic dystrophic tissue that progressively aggravates and extends the initial lesion. The result is often exposure of the bone and joint structure, making amputation of the limb inevitable.

In severe and wide lesions of the limbs, microsurgery procedures can successfully be combined, after debridement, with hyperbaric oxygen (HBO), vacuum-assisted closure therapy (VAC), and selective antibiotic therapies to limit the extension of the area to be repaired, improve the trophism of the chronically inflamed tissue around the ulcer, and create the conditions most suitable for implantation of free flaps. Experience with this approach was presented.

Methods.—From 1999 to 2003, 8 patients were treated for large, severe lesions of the skin and soft tissue of the limbs, with exposure of the bone and joint structures after serious crush injuries. Treatment consisted of debridement surgical procedures, medical support methods (HBO or VAC), and definitive surgery by microsurgical free-tissue transfer. The average age of the 6 men and 2 women was 23.25 years, with a range of 8 to 58 years. The follow-up ranged from 6 to 36 months.

Results.—All of the patients tolerated the therapy well, with no problems in any of its phases. In 2 cases of HBO therapy, the presence of sequelae of otitis media in 1 patient and chronic sinusitis in another caused difficult pressure compensation between the environment and the middle ear. However, these problems did not diminish the effectiveness of HBO treatment and had no consequences for the patients. The combination of medical support methods and microsurgery allowed complete and quick resolution of the clinical problem.

Conclusion.—A protocol based on medical support methods such as HBO and VAC in combination with microsurgical reconstruction has allowed successful treatment of severe posttraumatic sequelae of the limbs and provided satisfactory morphofunctional restoration with reduced duration of hospitalization.

▶ This clinical case series describes the use of adjunctive HBO therapy and VAC dressings prior to microsurgical reconstruction of complex contaminated or infected extremity wounds. In 7 of 8 cases, the subsequent flap reconstruction was successful. In the final case of a degloved foot injury, another free flap had to be performed for a decubitus ulcer over the flap that developed 6 months later.

The authors deserve much credit for successful reconstruction of defects where the alternative would have been amputation. They suggest that the use of HBO and VAC combined with repeated surgical debridement and delayed microsurgical flap reconstruction in selected cases can reduce the risk of complications associated with microsurgical flap reconstruction. These modalities help to prepare the tissue bed for flap coverage and contribute to combating infection. These do not replace surgical debridement or antimicrobial therapy, but act as adjunctive therapies.

The approach taken for the cases presented is logical. However, given the small numbers presented and the lack of controls, it is not possible to assess the actual contributions of HBO and VAC to the final outcome. A larger body of data with appropriate controls would be needed before this treatment algorithm can be more widely applied.

A. Chong, MD

Free Muscle Flap Transfer as a Lymphatic Bridge for Upper Extremity Lymphedema

Classen DA, Irvine L (Royal Univ, Saskatoon, SK, Canada; Univ of Saskatchewan, Canada)
J Reconstr Microsurg 21:93-99, 2005   20–6

Background.—There have been limited reports of the use of a pedicle muscle or skin flap as a lymphatic bridge for the treatment of obstructive lymphoma. Spontaneous regeneration or reconnection of lymphatic vessels has been documented when a part is replanted. Studies of patients with free-flap reconstruction have documented the reestablishment of lymphatic pathways after free-tissue transfer. These studies have also documented lymphatic drainage from the free flap by direct intraflap injection of radionucleotide. A case of the successful regeneration of lymphatics across a free muscle flap was presented.

Case Report.—Girl, 17, was seen with complaints of recurrent cellulitis in her hand. She had a history of excision of a circumferential congenital nevus of the left forearm at 1 year of age. The defect had been skin grafted. During childhood the patient would have occasional bouts of cellulitis in the distal hand, which were treated with antibiotics. However, prior to surgical treatment, the patient had experienced 3 episodes of cellulitis over a 2-year period despite chronic suppressive antibiotic treatment.

Preoperative examination showed a circumferential skin graft scar with mild distal swelling caused by obstructive lymphedema. The patient had decreased range of motion of her wrist and fingers because of the tight skin graft scar. The circumferential skin graft was excised in combination with extensor tenolysis. The right latissimus and lower 4 slips of the serratus anterior muscle were transferred as a combined free flap for coverage of the circumferential wound. The flap pedicle was anastomosed to the ulnar vessels, and a split-thickness skin graft was applied to the muscle surface. Postoperatively, the patient had improved range of motion with complete resolution of the distal edema in the hands and digits.

The patient has had no bouts of cellulitis in the 3 years since the surgical treatment. Comparison of preoperative and postoperative lymphoscintigrams showed significant improvement, with axillary lymph nodes imaged on the 30-minute postinjection view. Follow-up lymphoscintigrams have shown maintenance of normal lymphatic flow in the left upper extremity matching that of the right upper extremity.

Conclusion.—This is the first report of the use of a free flap to reestablish lymphatic flow in a limb. Lymphatic drainage may be restored across areas in which lymphatic flow is lacking, because of a loss of lymphatic pathways, by transfer of a muscle flap to act as a lymphatic bridge.

▶ Extremity lymphedema represents a clinical phenomenon without a clear surgical solution. Lymphatic channels appear to reform approximately 3 weeks after disruption, but only if the segmental disruption is small (eg, after replantation). Lymphedema reduction after free-tissue transplant—muscle or fasciocutaneous—is not a new phenomenon. However, the literature is relatively sparse as to its exact science and role in treatment. The authors present a case report of successful treatment of lymphedema in a 17-year-old female with a large, chronic, circumferential scar bed in the forearm, using a latissimus-serratus muscle transplant. Preoperative and postoperative lymphoscintigrams were done to demonstrate improved lymphatic flow.

We have seen lymphatic reduction after free-tissue transplants as a consequence of procedures for soft tissue coverage. On occasion, free-tissue transplants have been used to treat lymphedema, with variable success. It is very likely that there is some creation of lymphovascular channels with a healthy, vascularized flap. The role of bacterial involvement, nature of the scar bed, radiation, age, and other causative factors need to be investigated prior to establishing free-tissue transplantation as a definite modality in treating this difficult problem.

C. Lee, MD

Successful Correction of Severe Contracture of the Palm Using Arterialized Venous Flaps
Nakazawa H, Nozaki M, Kikuchi Y, et al (Tokyo Women's Med Univ)
J Reconstr Microsurg 20:527-531, 2004   20–7

Background.—Mild or moderate contractures of the palm after trauma can be treated effectively by resurfacing with skin grafts or local flaps. However, patients with severe contracture will have great difficulty performing activities of daily living. There have been many reports of the use of arterialized venous flaps for reconstruction of the hands and fingers. However, there have been no previous reports of palm reconstruction with arterialized venous flaps. Four cases of successful improvement of severe and extensive contracture of the palm using large arterialized venous flaps were presented.

Methods.—Four large arterialized venous flaps were used to resurface the palm and for release of severe contracture. After release, the recipient vessels were identified in all 4 cases. The flap was harvested from the anteromedial lower leg, which was selected as the donor site because it was wide enough to allow harvesting of a large flap and the donor site would be hidden by trousers.

The flaps were elevated off the fascia and contained the greater saphenous vein and the subdermal vein of the lower leg. The subdermal veins of the flap were anastomosed to the recipient arteries, and the greater saphenous veins were anastomosed to the recipient veins. Thus, blood flow in these venous flaps was antegrade through the venous valves. Donor sites were covered with split-thickness skin grafts.

Results.—All flaps showed complete survival with uneventful clinical courses and without any need for postoperative anticoagulant therapy. None of the flaps required defatting after the operation.

Conclusion.—The use of arterialized venous flaps may be a useful method for reconstruction of the palm of the hand.

▶ Severe palmar contractures in the hand may require microvascular free-tissue transfers to adequately resurface the palm for sensate, pliable, and durable reconstruction. This can be accomplished by sensate fasciocutaneous flaps such as the anterolateral thigh, thoracodorsal artery perforator, and lateral arm flaps with minimal donor site morbidity.

The authors describe the use of large venous flow-through flaps for subtotal palmar resurfacing in a series of 4 patients. The aesthetic and functional results are good; however, the donor site morbidity using large, saphenous venous flow-through flaps is not addressed. The orientation of the flap as a flow-through flap can lead to complicated designs for anastomotic setup (such as a radial artery to an ulnar-sided dorsal vein), but this would disregard the useful cephalic vein.

The Buncke Clinic experience with venous flow through flaps has been mainly for small defects with harvest from the volar forearm. These postage stamp–sized flaps have minimal donor site morbidity. Use of the large venous flow-through flaps described in this article is another reconstructive option for subtotal palmar resurfacing, despite my concerns with donor site morbidity.

C. Lee, MD

Long-term Results of Replantation of the Proximal Forearm Following Avulsion Amputation
Atzei A, Pignatti M, Baldrighi CM, et al (Azienda Ospedaliera Universitaria di Verona, Italy)
Microsurgery 25:293-298, 2005   20–8

Abstract.—This study reports on the long-term functional outcomes of a homogeneous series of 10 cases of successful replantation of an avulsed proximal forearm and its acceptance on the part of patients. After a minimum follow-up of 3 years (average, 4.7 years), muscular and sensory recovery was evaluated with the Medical Research Council scale, and global function according to the demerit score system of Chen (China Med 5:392-397, 1967). Subjective evaluation and patient satisfaction were investigated by means of a questionnaire. One patient was classified as grade 2, 4 patients as grade 3, and 5 patients as grade 4 according to Chen (China Med 5:392-397, 1967). However, in spite of the poor objective results, patient satisfaction was obtained in 90% of cases, and the replanted extremity was considered of help for common activities of daily living. In conclusion, replantation of an avulsed proximal forearm should be considered only in patients who are strongly motivated to maintain body integrity, and who are aware of the expected functional limitations.

▶ Hand amputations at the level of the mid forearm are extremely destructive by virtue of mechanism and anatomy. These injuries typically involve an avulsive mechanism with severe proximal muscle and nerve injury. Good functional outcomes are difficult to achieve.

The authors present a series of 10 patients with a mean follow-up of 4.7 years. Results are variable, with half of the patients having moderate to good outcomes and the other half having poor functional outcomes. During replantation, the bone was shortened an average of 4 cm to obtain primary repair of nerves and vessels. Vein grafts for the artery or vein were used in several patients, which would indicate significant gap or zone of injury. No primary nerve grafts were performed, and secondary operations did not include free functional muscle transplants or aggressive nerve reconstruction despite poor sensory and motor recovery.

Our experience at the Buncke Clinic includes aggressive primary nerve grafting, additional soft tissue reconstruction with free tissue transplants, and free functional muscle transplants for severe motor deficits. These procedures can lead to improved function for these devastating injuries. Our conclusion is the same, however: patient selection and realistic expectations are important before embarking on this complex course of reconstruction.

C. Lee, MD

Reverse Dorsal Digital and Intercommissural Flaps Used for Digital Reconstruction
Keramidas E, Rodopoulou S, Metaxotos N, et al (Gen State Hosp of Athens, Greece)
Br J Plast Surg 57:61-65, 2004   20–9

Summary.—Reverse dorsal digital and intercommissural flaps offer a simple and versatile option for skin cover of distal finger defects, especially when other local flaps are not available. Twenty-one reverse dorsal digital flaps were used, on an outpatient basis, to cover dorsal soft tissue defects over or beyond the PIP joint. All the flaps were transposed as reverse island flaps. The average size of the defects was 2.5 cm² and they were all used to cover exposed tendon, bone, joint or a combination. Twenty flaps survived completely and did not present any feature of circulatory difficulty. Marginal necrosis of one flap was noticed, while two patients complained of swollen finger 6 months later. No morbidity was reported and the patients maintained good range of motion. Various other types of flaps that have been used to reconstruct distal digital skin defects are reviewed and compared with the reverse dorsal digital and metacarpal flaps.

▶ A common complication of reverse flow flaps is venous congestion. The authors describe use of flaps based on the reliable arterial system on the dorsum of the finger as reported by Strauch and de Moura.[1] This flap was originally described by Pelissier et al.[2] These authors have used the reverse dorsal finger flap for 21 wounds with only 1 case of venous congestion. They describe using a pedicle base that is as wide as the flap, which most likely contributes to their low complication rate of venous compromise. Another advantage of this flap exists when the donor site does not require a skin graft and the donor can be closed primarily. This allows early motion to be started. When harvested from the dorsum of the proximal phalanx, this flap can be innervated by dorsal branches from the proper digital nerves, which could be coapted to a digital nerve in the wound.

B. Wilhelmi, MD

References

1. Strauch B, de Moura W: Arterial system of the fingers. *J Hand Surg* 15A(1):148, 1990.
2. Pelissier P, Casoli V, Bakhach J, et al: Reverse dorsal digital and metacarpal flaps: A review of 27 cases. *Plast Reconstr Surg* 103:159, 1999.

Sensate First Dorsal Metacarpal Artery Flap for Resurfacing Extensive Pulp Defects of the Thumb
Chang S-C, Chen S-L, Chen T-M, et al (Tri-Service Gen Hosp, Taipei, Taiwan)
Ann Plast Surg 53:449-454, 2004   20–10

Abstract.—Finding an appropriate soft-tissue grafting material to close a wound located over the distal phalanx of the thumb, especially the pulp region, can be a difficult task. A sensate first dorsal metacarpal artery flap, mobilized from the dorsum of the adjacent index finger and used as an island pedicle skin flap, can be useful for this purpose. The pedicle includes the ulnar branch of the first dorsal metacarpal artery, the dorsal veins, and the cutaneous branch of the radial nerve. Although this tiny artery is anatomically variable, safe dissection can be achieved by including the radial shaft periosteum of the secondary metacarpal bone and the ulnar head fascia of the first interosseous muscle.

This approach has been used for 8 individuals with extensive pulp defects of the thumb over the past 3 years. Skin defects in all patients were combined with bone, joint, or tendon exposure. All flaps survived completely. This 1-stage procedure is reliable and technically simple. It provides sensate coverage to the pulp of the thumb but also avoids nerve repair or more complicated microsurgery.

▶ This is a small case series of 8 patients treated with the first dorsal metacarpal artery island flap for thumb defects. The authors obtained very good results for return of static 2-point discrimination, which are better than those previously reported in the literature. Previous results reported in the literature note 2-point discrimination averaging about 10 mm.

The authors also report reorientation of sensation in all patients, and the earliest was seen at 4 months. I have found reorientation to be difficult in patients older than 50 years. To improve on reorientation, I anastomose the dorsal radial sensory nerve directly to one of the intact digital nerves of the thumb; however, a previously published study by Germann's group[1] found no significant difference in reorientation between patients younger than and greater than 50 years. I have noted difficulty in reaching the tip of the thumb with this flap, which the authors do not note in this article.

S. L. Moran, MD

Reference

1. Trankle M, Sauerbier M, Heitmann C, et al: Restoration of thumb sensibility with the innervated first dorsal metacarpal artery island flap. *J Hand Surg* 28:758-766, 2003.

'Distally Based Dorsal Hand Flaps': Clinical Experience, Cadaveric Studies and an Update
Vuppalapati G, Oberlin C, Balakrishnan G (Broomfield Hosp, Essex, England; Inst D'Anatomie de Paris; Stanley Med College, Chennai, India)
Br J Plast Surg 57:653-667, 2004   20–11

Summary.—Many developments have taken place in the area of distally based dorsal hand flaps since 1988. This paper reported these developments as well as our clinical experience and cadaveric studies. Thirty-three reverse dorsal metacarpal artery (RDMA) flaps, 11 reverse dorsal digital artery (RDDA) flaps and five extended RDMA flaps done in the Institute for Research and Rehabilitation of Hand, Stanley Hospital, Chennai, India during the period between 1996 and 2002 are reviewed. In our series, we used simple, composite, fasciocutaneous and adipofascial flaps, encountered 4% total loss and 6% partial loss. A series of injected cadaveric hands were studied in the Institute D'Anatomie de Paris. An important anatomical finding in this cadaveric study is the dorsal metacarpal artery terminating at the confluence of common digital artery branching into digital arteries proper to the neighbouring digits in all the eight hands dissected. We undertake a critical review of the literature, highlighting the sequence of developments in the knowledge of relevant anatomy and various flap designs as distally based dorsal hand flaps since their first popular report in 1990.

▶ This article presents the combined series of the 2 senior authors for a total of 46 distally based dorsal hand flaps. The flap loss was low, and functional results were good. The article presents some beautiful figure drawings of the arterial anatomy of the fingers, as well as some cadaveric injection studies, which help one to better visualize the course of the dorsal metacarpal arteries.

S. L. Moran, MD

Extending the Reach of the Heterodigital Arterialized Flap by Vein Division and Repair

Tay S-C, Teoh L-C, Tan S-H, et al (Singapore Gen Hosp)
Plast Reconstr Surg 114:1450-1456, 2004

20–12

Abstract.—The heterodigital arterialized flap is ideal for nonsensory reconstruction of sizable soft-tissue defects in the proximal fingers, web spaces, and the hand. The inclusion of a dorsal vein augments the venous drainage of this digital island flap and avoids the problem of postoperative venous congestion, which is a common problem in digital island flaps. However, the presence of a dorsal vein pedicle inhibits flap mobility somewhat, and the reach of the flap is mainly limited to adjacent fingers. In situations that demand a transfer from a nonadjacent donor finger or when the reach from the adjacent donor finger is inadequate, the dorsal vein pedicle can be temporarily divided and then anastomosed microsurgically after flap transfer is performed. This enables the reach of the flap to be extended up to two fingers from the donor finger. The authors performed this "partially free" heterodigital arterialized flap in 11 consecutive patients between 1991 and 2001. The average size of the defects was 4.4 × 2.3 cm. All of the flaps survived completely, without any evidence of postoperative flap congestion. Healing of all of the flaps was primary and did not result in any scarring. All of the donor fingers had "normal" two-point discrimination of 3 to 5 mm. All of the donor fingers retained excellent or good total active motion, as graded by the criteria of Strickland and Glogovac.

▶ The authors describe a variation of the Littler neurovascular island flap where finger defects are reconstructed with a heterodigital arterialized flap based on the proper digital artery of another finger. In this article, they perform microanastomosis of a dorsal vein to extend the reach of the flap.

The disadvantage of this flap is the donor finger requirement for skin graft and the risk for consequent contracture. Also, it is critical to perform an intraoperative digital artery Allen's test with a microclamp before sacrificing the arterial supply to the donor finger. Continuing the dissection of the proper digital artery proximally lengthens the pedicle by inclusion of the common digital artery. This permits the pivot point of the flap to be the superficial palmar arch, as described by Littler. The venae comitantes that travel with the digital artery can be used to provide venous outflow for this flap, obviating the need for dorsal venous microanastomosis.

The authors reported on 3- to 5-mm 2-point discrimination of the flap, but did not discuss whether the proper digital nerve to the flap was harvested from the donor finger, or whether a nerve was coapted to the flap. The donor finger proper digital nerve can be preserved to maintain sensation to the donor finger. A dorsal nerve branch to the flap can be coapted to make this a sensate flap. The advantage of coapting a nerve to the flap is 2-fold: donor sensation is preserved, and there is no need for cortical reorientation. The main contribution of this report is that a dorsal vein can be repaired if the Littler flap appears to be venous congested.

B. Wilhelmi, MD

Tendofascial Island Flap Based on Distal Perforators of the Radial Artery: Anatomical and Clinical Approach
El-Khatib HA (Rumailah Hosp, Cairo)
Plast Reconstr Surg 113:545-549, 2004   20–13

Background.—The possibility of the transfer of vascularized tissue for restoration of function and resurfacing of large defects, in conjunction with the use of composite flaps, has resulted in advances in "one-stage" reconstructive surgical procedures. A previous study reported that the tendofascial flap is supplied with blood by 5 to 7 of the most distal fascial perforators of the radial artery. In the present study, the blood supply of the flexor carpi radialis tendon was further studied in 5 fresh adult cadavers. Dissection under low magnification showed that 2 networks arising from the radial artery provide the main blood supply to the tendon. From 4 to 10 transfascial branches were seen to penetrate the paratenon anteriorly and the surrounding loose areolar connective tissue. The confirmation that the arterial supply to the flexor carpi radialis tendon arises from the radial artery made it possible to develop an alternative for a vascularized tendon graft, which is described in this article.

Methods.—The tendofascial island flap was used to treat 4 male patients, 2 of whom demonstrated loss of soft tissue on the dorsum of the hand, with segmental losses of the extensor digitorum communis to the index and middle fingers. The other 2 patients had been referred from the orthopedic department 7 days after intramedullary nail fixation of the distal ulna and had secondary raw areas on the dorsum of the hand, with segmental losses of the extensor digitorum communis to the middle fingers and exposed metacarpal bones.

Results.—Stable wound closure was obtained in all 4 patients. The total active range of motion of the repaired digits ranged from 245° to 260°. The range of motion for the wrist was normal in all 4 patients, the aesthetic results for the hand and donor sites were acceptable, and donor-site morbidity was minimal. The only adverse effects at the donor site were temporary hair loss and impaired sensation over the scar.

Conclusions.—The tendofascial island flap is a completely vascularized, single-stage, composite flap. The use of this flap in 4 patients was accomplished without sacrifice of the radial artery. It resulted in good functional and aesthetic outcomes and minimal donor-site morbidity.

▶ Interest has been growing in alternatives to microsurgery for limb reconstruction. Microsurgery remains an excellent tool (and often is the gold standard by which other methods are measured), but it is time- and labor-intensive, requires specialized equipment, and carries with it variable donor morbidity.

Alternative techniques may be faster and easier to perform, providing the surgeon additional reconstructive options.

The distally based adipofascial flap has long been described as a reconstructive option for the lower extremity, and a similar procedure for hand reconstruction has been available for almost a decade. In this article, the author adds the harvest of the flexor carpi radialis to this adipofascial forearm flap to allow immediate tendon reconstruction.

Several other reconstructive options exist for the defects shown in the article:

1. Coverage with free-tissue transfer (temporal parietal fascia flap, serratus flap, or free omental flap) and immediate tendon reconstruction
2. Coverage with free-tissue transfer and delayed tendon reconstruction (placement of Hunter rods)
3. Coverage with free-tissue transfer and donor tendon (dorsalis pedis flap)
4. Coverage with meshed Integra + VAC dressing over Hunter rods (delayed tendon reconstruction)
5. Pedicled groin flap coverage with delayed tendon reconstruction
6. Reversed radial forearm flap with palmaris longus tendon
7. Reversed adipofascial flap (as described in this article)

In my experience, the reversed adipofascial flaps are not as robust as some of the other flap options. When I use this flap, I defer skin grafting for 1 week not only to ensure that the entire flap will survive but also to allow the flap time to develop adequate granulation tissue, which further augments the likelihood of skin graft survival. Nevertheless, the flap modification described in this article offers a useful 1-stage alternative.

M. Concannon, MD

Ulnar Recurrent Adipofascial Flap for Reconstruction of Massive Defects Around the Elbow and Forearm

Hayashi A, Maruyama Y, Saze M, et al (Toho Univ, Chiba, Japan; Toho Univ, Tokyo)
Br J Plast Surg 57:632-637, 2004   20–14

Background.—The ulnar recurrent fasciocutaneous flap is a versatile option for coverage of soft tissue defects around the elbow. This flap can facilitate 1-stage reconstruction, and its use negates the need for long-term immobilization of the involved elbow. However, 2 major disadvantages of these flaps are their bulky appearance and limitations in the dimensions of skin paddle for primary closure of the donor site. These complications were addressed with the development of an ulnar recurrent adipofascial turnover flap based on the ulnar recurrent vessels (Fig 1). This graft should cover massive and complicated defects around the elbow and provide a vascularized bed for skin grafts. The use of this graft in 2 patients is described.

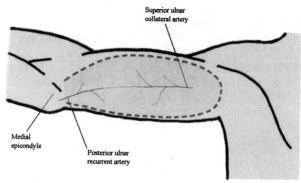

FIGURE 1.—Schematic representation of the pattern of the posterior ulnar recurrent artery, and planning of the ulnar recurrent adipofascial flap. (Reprinted by permission of the publisher from Hayashi A, Maruyama Y, Saze M, et al: Ulnar recurrent adipofascial flap for reconstruction of massive defects around the elbow and forearm. *Br J Plast Surg* 57:632-637. Copyright 2004 by Elsevier.)

Case 1.—Man, 63, had a large soft tissue tumor in the radiodorsal aspect of the proximal half of his left forearm. The tumor, the brachioradialis, supinator, the extensors, the radial nerve, and periosteum of the radius and ulna were resected en bloc and left a massive skin and soft tissue defect measuring 20 × 11 cm. An ulnar recurrent adipofascial flap was raised and turned over to cover the proximal two thirds of this defect and sutured to stumps of the remaining extensors. A split-thickness skin graft was placed over the flap and muscles. The flap survived completely, and the graft healed without problems.

Case 2.—Man, 59, had a localized recurrence of a malignant fibrous histiocytoma in the posteroradial aspect of his left elbow. Wide resection of the lesion was performed with partial resection of the triceps, brachioradialis, extensor carpi radialis longus, the musculocutaneous nerve, and the distal portion of the humerus measuring 2 × 1 × 8 cm³. The adipofascial flap was turned over and transferred through a subcutaneous tunnel to cover the defect, and a split-thickness skin graft was placed over the flap. The donor site was closed completely, and the graft healed uneventfully.

Conclusions.—The ulnar recurrent adipofascial flap is an easy, dependable option for single-stage reconstruction of massive defects around the elbow.

▶ This article provides additional clinical examples of the use of adipofascial flaps for soft tissue coverage at the elbow. Advantages of this type of flap include relatively little donor morbidity and the ease of harvesting. It does not require costly equipment or materials and does not sacrifice a major arterial supply in an already injured extremity. Disadvantages include the fact that these flaps are not particularly robust in their vascular supply, and survival (particularly the distal portion of the flap) is not assured. For this reason, I prefer to delay skin grafting of these flaps for at least 1 week. This flap option is attractive for large defects of this type, which otherwise would likely require either free-tissue transfer or flap substitution with the use of a dermal substitute such as Integra.

M. Concannon, MD

Functional Biceps Brachii Reconstruction Using the Free Tensor Fasciae Latae

Kobayashi MR, Brenner KA, Gupta R, et al (Univ of California, Irvine)
Plast Reconstr Surg 114:1208-1214, 2004   20–15

Background.—Injuries to the upper extremity nerve and muscles can result in severe morbidity, with limited options for reconstruction. The ability to place the hand in a functional position is further impaired by a loss of elbow flexion and supination. Both acute and chronic tendon injuries of the biceps can be repaired surgically, either by direct tendinoplasty or with the use of free tendon grafting. A loss of muscle bulk or innervation is more difficult to treat surgically. Surgical muscle transfers can improve elbow mobility but provide only partial range of motion and suboptimal postoperative strength.

The tensor fasciae latae musculocutaneous flap was first described by Nahai et al in 1978. The first use of delayed functional reconstruction of the biceps using the tensor fasciae latae was described.

Methods.—From September 1998 to May 2001, 3 patients underwent upper extremity reconstruction using innervated free tensor fasciae latae. The patients ranged in age from 18 to 41 years. Two patients had complete loss of biceps muscle function as a result of trauma, and the third patient lost his biceps from tumor ablation. The tensor fasciae latae was inset at the fascial origin of the biceps muscle.

Tension was placed on the flap until previously marked 5-cm intervals were reestablished. The distal inset was then initially placed with the elbow at 90° of flexion. In all 3 cases, the tensor fasciae latae was sewn directly to the remaining native tendon or tendon cuff. After completion of the inset and anastomosis, routine Doppler signal markings were placed for postoperative monitoring, and the arm was dressed with a bulky Robert Jones dressing and placed in a posterior long-arm splint with 90° of elbow flexion. The patients' arms were immobilized in supination for 3 to 4 weeks, after which passive range-of-motion exercises were begun.

Results.—The overall outcome was excellent for all 3 patients. There were no flap losses, infections, or other complications. In 1 patient, a seroma developed at the tensor fasciae latae donor site and required aspiration drainage. The seroma eventually resolved. None of the patients had donor-site lateral thigh bulging after absorption of the Vicryl mesh used during repair. In all 3 patients, 5/5 strength developed. Two patients had flexion from 0° to 135°, and the third had flexion of 15° to 120°. The third patient returned 1 year after the initial procedure for a biceps tendon shortening procedure to increase proximal flexion excursion.

Conclusion.—Free-flap reconstruction with tensor fasciae latae is the best choice for reconstruction of severe biceps injuries.

▶ Loss of elbow flexion results in severe functional arm disability. The biceps brachii, brachialis, and brachioradialis muscles provide elbow flexion, but the biceps is the major elbow flexor and contributes to supination of the forearm. The biceps can be repaired when directly lacerated, but loss of biceps from nerve injury or direct tissue loss is more difficult to repair.

The authors describe a technique of functional biceps reconstruction using the tensor fascia latae muscle as a functional microvascular transplant. The flaps were harvested with a 10 × 15-centimeter skin paddle and on the lateral femoral circumflex pedicle and a branch of the superior gluteal nerve. The flaps were inset by Pulvertaft weave into the distal biceps and after vessel repair, it was coapted to the musculocutaneous nerve in 2 cases. In the other case, it was repaired to the thoracodorsal nerve powering the previous latissimus transfer.

All 3 patients obtained 5/5 strength postoperatively and had from 135° to 120° of elbow flexion. In the cases presented, functional loss before reconstruction was severe.

Although the muscle length of the tensor fascia latae is shorter than the gracilis, the gracilis is somewhat long and deficient in cross-sectional area. The area of cross section of a muscle is proportional to the force it can generate. Therefore, the larger cross section and large distal fascial insertion make the tensor fascia latae a good choice for elbow reconstruction. The shorter length does not seem to limit excursion enough to affect elbow flexion. The donor defect is prone to herniation and more conspicuous than the gracilis donor scar, and this should be discussed with the patient preoperatively. Conversely, the gracilis donor site is relatively inconspicuous.

R. Buntic, MD

The Multiple Monoblock Toe-to-Hand Transfer in Digital Reconstruction: A Report of Ten Cases

Julve GG, Villén GM (Regional Centre for Surgery of the Hand, Zaragoza, Spain)
J Hand Surg [Br] 29B:222-229, 2004   20–16

Background.—Multiple finger amputations or congenital absences represent difficult problems for surgical reconstruction. The single toe-to-hand transfer has been widely accepted as a reconstructive option in these cases, but this approach is insufficient when multiple fingers are absent. Many authors have used multiple toe-to-hand transfers. Most often, simultaneous or delayed transfers of the second toe of each foot are used. Most reports of monoblock transfer have involved the second and third toes. Experience with double monoblock transfer of the great and second toes and triple monoblock transfer from the great, second, and third toes was described.

Methods.—Of the 56 toe-to-hand transfers performed from 1991 to 2002, 10 were monoblock transfers. In 8 cases, the monoblock transfer included the great and second toes. In 1 case, the transfer included the great toe and the vascularized metatarsophalangeal joint of the second toe; in the last patient, the transfer included the great, second, and third toes. The mean age of the patients was 24 years, with a range of 3 to 49 years. Seven of the 10 patients were men.

The monoblock technique allowed multiple toes to be transferred as a single anatomical structure with a common vascular axis. Only part of the great toe was ever taken. Taken in 8 cases was the distal phalanx and in 2 cases the head of the proximal phalanx to incorporate the interphalangeal joint. The great toe was always used for reconstruction of the thumb. The second toe was transferred totally or partially, depending on need.

Results.—In 9 hands, there were no vascular problems. In the remaining hand there were alternate phases of poor and good perfusion, which were treated by irrigation with normal saline and sulmetin papaverine at 38°C. Signs of ischemia appeared in this hand 3 hours later, and an arterial occlusion was discovered at reexploration. The occlusion was treated by removal of a thrombus and re-anastomosis. However, skin necrosis was present 24 hours later.

Soft tissues were removed from the transferred toes, and their bones were covered with an abdominal wrap-around flap. The mean follow-up was 6 years (range, 2 months to 12 years). The functional results were much better in the traumatic cases than in the congenital cases in which radial deviation of the transferred toes occurred. Postoperative re-innervation allowed development of 2-point discrimination sensitivity sufficient for protective sensation in 8 of 10 hands.

The cosmetic results were secondary to the functional outcomes, but 3 cases, including a triple transfer, were considered to have good cosmetic results. Complications requiring revision surgery included commissurotomy of the web space in 5 cases, excision of the index metacarpal in 6 cases, tenolysis in 3 cases, and an abdominal wrap-around flap for skin necrosis in 1 case.

Conclusion.—Monoblock transfers are recommended for treatment of multiple digital loss but not for single-toe transplants.

▶ Multiple finger loss or congenital absence is difficult to reconstruct. Typically great-toe transplants are used for the thumb and second toe transplants are used individually (sometimes bilaterally) for finger reconstruction. The authors present monoblock transfers of the great and second toe in a single contiguous flap and 1 case of a triple toe monoblock transfer. Nine hands had a history of trauma, 1 had congenital absence. The authors had 1 case of vascular arterial insufficiency resulting in partial necrosis requiring an abdominal wrap-around flap for salvage. Significant details of joint range of motion, pinch strength, and grasp size are reported. Eight of 10 patients had protective sensation.

The authors recommend monoblock transfer for multiple digital loss and also recommend 3 venous anastomoses per transplant but present no data to support this latter recommendation. The data presented do not support monoblock transfer preferentially to single-toe transplants.

R. Buntic, MD

Free Vascularized Fibula Grafting for Reconstruction of the Wrist Following Wide Tumor Excision
Muramatsu K, Ihara K, Azuma E, et al (Yamaguchi Univ, Japan; Ogori Daiichi Gen Hosp, Japan)
Microsurgery 25:101-106, 2005   20–17

Background.—Some reconstructive procedures have been reported for defects of the distal radius after wide resection of a malignant tumor. Radial carpal joint reconstruction using the free vascularized proximal fibula graft is an attractive procedure because of its similarity in shape to the distal radius. However, some major postoperative complications have been reported, including progressive degenerative changes, bony collapse caused by poor vascularity of the fibular head, and volar subluxation as a result of incongruity between the fibular head and the proximal carpal row. Three cases of distal radius reconstruction following wide tumor resection were presented.

Case 1.—Woman, 35, noted pain and swelling in her right wrist. Radiographs revealed an extensive lytic lesion on the distal radius with partial invasion of the cortex on the radial side. An open biopsy and histologic examination confirmed the diagnosis of a typical giant cell tumor. After en bloc resection of the distal radius, the resulting defect was repaired with fibular head transfer along with the shaft to replace the radial joint surface.

Case 2.—Boy, 16, noticed pain in his left wrist. A radiograph at initial presentation showed an osteoblastic periosteal reaction at the distal radius. The diagnosis of an osteosarcoma was confirmed by an incisional biopsy. Wide tumor resection was performed after 4 months of preoperative chemotherapy. The subsequent defect was reconstructed with fibulo-scapho-lunate fusion.

Case 3.—Boy, 14, had a painful lump in his left forearm. He underwent initial treatment at a hospital other than the study hospital, and marginal tumor resection was performed. Local recurrence occurred at 3 months postoperatively. Radiographic examination showed that the tumor had expanded widely to the distal half of the radius and ulna. Wide tumor resection was performed 8 months after the initial operation. The bony and soft tissue defects were reconstructed with a free vascularized fibula graft combined with a peroneal skin flap. The wrist was totally stabilized by a reconstruction plate.

Discussion.—The therapeutic goal in bone tumor reconstruction is a 1-stage procedure that provides secure bony consolidation, early physical therapy, and additional adjuvant treatment. Reconstruction of massive radial and ulnar defects is often accomplished with a complete wrist arthrodesis using a free vascularized fibula graft.

This procedure can provide stability for the wrist, but the loss of wrist motion can impair activities of daily living. Radial carpal joint reconstruction using a free vascularized fibula is recommended for patients engaged in nonheavy manual work. Fibulo-scapho-lunate fusion is recommended for young patients with high activity in daily living if the carpal bones can be preserved.

▶ Vascularized fibula transplantation has become less common for long-bone reconstruction with increasing use of Ilizarov techniques. However, vascularized fibula remains an excellent choice in long defect radius and ulna reconstruction and avoids prolonged use of an external frame and percutaneous pins. The authors report 3 cases of fibula flaps for defects of the radius at the level of wrist due to tumor extirpation with wide resection (giant cell, osteosarcoma, and desmoplastic fibroma).

All fibula transplants were successful. The first case is notable for the incorporation of the fibular head in the transplant to reconstruct a radiocarpal composite joint with fibula. The second patient had limited wrist fusion of the radioscapho-lunate joint to preserve mid carpal motion, while the third patient had complete wrist fusion. Although the authors did not note degenerative changes 10 years later in the reconstructed radiocarpal joint after fibular head transplantation, this technique is very technically demanding and potentially can harm the peroneal nerve as it travels around the neck of the fibula. Under most circumstances, wrist fusion or limited wrist fusion would be advisable with vascularized fibula when the radial head must be excised.

R. Buntic, MD

21 Hand: Soft Tissue

Surgery for Dupuytren's Disease in Japanese Patients and a New Preoperative Classification
Abe Y, Rokkaku T, Ofuchi S, et al (Chiba Univ, Japan; Chiba Municipal Hosp, Japan; Awa-Ishikai Hosp, Japan)
J Hand Surg [Br] 29B:235-239, 2004   21–1

Abstract.—The surgical outcome of Dupuytren's disease was evaluated in 73 hands of 57 patients in a Japanese population. Subtotal fasciectomy was performed in all cases. Surgical results were evaluated using the percentage improvement of extension in each finger joint. Statistical analyses were performed on the risk factors associated with recurrence and extension.

The surgical outcome depended on the degree of contracture of the proximal interphalangeal joint. Recurrence of disease occurred in eight patients (14%) and extension occurred in nine (16%). Recurrence and extension frequently occurred in those who had ectopic lesions or involvement of the radial side of the hand. The present results suggested that the Dupuytren's diathesis had an influence on recurrence and extension.

We proposed a new classification of Dupuytren's disease that might help to predict the surgical outcome and facilitate surgical planning.

▶ Dupuytren's disease is considered a rare disease in the non-Caucasian population and has been poorly documented in the Asian literature. The authors describe a large series in Japan over a 15-year period on 57 patients. Subtotal fasciectomies were performed, and various parameters were characterized about these patients. Results were good with nonspecific follow-up time. Ectopic lesions and radial-sided involvement were statistically significant factors in recurrence.

This article adds significantly to the literature on Dupuytren's disease as it dispels the myth that Dupuytren's disease is either different or nonexistent in the Asian population. Management principles are also similar, due to phenotypic homogeneity across races.

C. Lee, MD

Expression of Bone Morphogenetic Proteins by Dupuytren's Fibroblasts

Shin SS, Liu, C, Chang EY, et al (New York Univ; Univ of Minnesota, St Paul)
J Hand Surg [Am] 29A:809-814, 2004   21–2

Purpose.—Dupuytren's fibroblasts, or myofibroblasts, are the primary cell type in Dupuytren's disease. Growth factors play a role in the differentiation of fibroblasts to myofibroblasts. Myofibroblasts are specialized fibroblasts that display morphologic and biochemical features similar to smooth muscle cells. Cytokines, adhesion molecules, and extracellular matrix components are all thought to play a role in myofibroblast transdifferentiation. Recent research has shown that specific cytokines, such as transforming growth factor β_1 (TGF-β_1), can modulate myofibroblast expression. We hypothesize that bone morphogenetic proteins (BMPs) play a role in the modulation of Dupuytren's fibroblasts.

Methods.—Dupuytren's fibroblasts and normal palmar fascia fibroblasts (control) were analyzed for messenger RNA expression of BMPs (BMP-1, -2, -3, -4, -5, -6, -7, -8, -9, -10 and -11), their receptors (BMPR-IA, BMPR-IB, and BMPR-II), and their antagonists (follistatin and noggin) by reverse-transcription polymerase chain reaction (PCR). Western blot analysis and immunostaining also were used to confirm the differential expression of BMP-4.

Results.—With reverse-transcription PCR the expression profile for normal palmar fascia fibroblasts versus Dupuytren's fibroblasts was found to show similar expression of BMP-1 and -11; qualitatively decreased expression of BMP-6, BMP-8, BMPR-IA, BMPR-IB, and BMPR-II in Dupuytren's fibroblasts; and no expression of BMP-4 in Dupuytren's fibroblasts. There was no expression of BMP-2, -3, -5, -7, -9, and -10 in both the control fibroblasts and Dupuytren's fibroblasts. In line with the messenger RNA expression pattern BMP-4 was detected in only the control fibroblasts and not in the Dupuytren's fibroblasts, whereas BMP-8 (chosen for comparison purposes) was detectable in both cell populations. Immunostaining for BMP-8 and BMP-4 confirmed our findings with reverse-transcription PCR and Western blot analysis.

Conclusions.—This study reports on the expression of BMPs in Dupuytren's fibroblasts. We characterized the expression of BMPs in both normal palmar fascia fibroblasts and in Dupuytren's fibroblasts through reverse-transcription PCR, Western blot analysis, and immunostaining. The most significant difference in expression profiles was in the expression of BMP-4; that is, BMP-4 was expressed in the normal fibroblasts but not in the Dupuytren's fibroblasts. Whether BMP-4 is necessary and/or sufficient for maintaining a normal palmar fascia fibroblast phenotype is not yet known. Further studies are needed to elucidate the exact role of BMPs, and especially BMP-4, in Dupuytren's fibroblasts.

▶ The authors show evidence of differential BMP expression in Dupuytren's fibroblasts compared with control fibroblasts obtained from carpal tunnel release. Most marked is the absence of BMP-4 expression in Dupuytren's fibroblasts. BMPs have been shown to be important in musculoskeletal development and healing, and it would be consistent that derangements in their expression could be involved in the pathogenesis of Dupuytren's disease. This study provides support for BMPs as candidates in the pathogenesis of Dupuytren's disease. The number of samples for each group is not stated, so it is unclear whether the findings are truly generalizable. Confounding factors such as age differences between samples were not discussed. One weakness in studies involving tissue analysis from Dupuytren's disease is that the findings only present a snapshot of the disease in time. Dupuytren's disease is known to have histologic phases, and plausibly, gene expression may differ early in the disease compared with later phases of the disease, when surgery is usually performed. More research will be required to establish whether changes in BMP expression are causative for the development of Dupuytren's disease. Ultimately, the relevance for the practicing hand surgeon is whether modulation of these factors can reverse or retard disease.

A. Chong, MD

The Surgical Treatment of Dupuytren's Contracture: A Synthesis of Techniques
Skoff HD (Harvard Med School, Boston)
Plast Reconstr Surg 113:540-544, 2004   21–3

Dupuytren's disease is an affliction of the palmar fascia. Selective fasciectomy is recommended once contracture has occurred. Alternatives for wound closure include tissue rearrangement, the open palm technique, and full-thickness skin grafting. In this prospective study, a new "synthesis" technique was used to treat a cohort of patients with advanced Dupuytren's disease. The results were then compared with those of a second cohort of patients who underwent the open palm technique. Thirty consecutive patients were selected. Ten patients (nine men and one woman; average age, 67 years) underwent the open palm technique, and 20 patients (18 men and two women; average age, 70 years) underwent the synthesis method. Follow-up was 3.5 years for the open palm group and 2.7 years for the synthesis group. All patients in both groups improved with respect to motion, function, appearance, and satisfaction. Objectively, for the open palm technique, metacarpophalangeal joint contracture decreased from 50 degrees to 0 degrees, and proximal interphalangeal joint contracture decreased from 40 degrees to 6 degrees. Using the synthesis method, metacarpophalangeal joint contracture decreased from 57 degrees to 0 degrees, and proximal interphalangeal joint contracture decreased from 58 degrees to 10 degrees. The Disabilities of the Arm, Shoulder, and Hand Test scores decreased from 37 to 30 in both groups. There were no significant differences between groups in these parameters. The two significant intergroup differences were healing time (40 days for the open palm technique versus 28 days for the synthesis method) and recurrence rate (50 percent for open palm versus 0 percent for synthesis). The synthesis technique combines with success the best features of current methods for the surgical treatment of advanced Dupuytren's disease.

▶ The authors compare results of patients treated with the open palm technique (McCash) with a group combining the open palm technique but adding a full-thickness skin graft at 4 days postoperatively. Both groups regained excellent range of motion (ROM). Two concerns are the need for possibly one necessary return to the operating room in the first week (at least this is my understanding from the paper) and the use of a nontraditional incision. The ROM and Disabilities of the Arm, Shoulder, and Hand scores postoperatively were similar and reasonable in both groups. A more relevant comparison might be immediate versus delayed full-thickness skin graft.

J. A. Katarincic, MD

The Effect of Cellular Proliferative Activity on Recurrence and Local Tumour Extent of Localized Giant Cell Tumour of Tendon Sheath
Kitagawa Y, Ito H, Yokoyama M, et al (Nippon Med School, Tokyo)
J Hand Surg [Br] 29B:604-607, 2004   21–4

Background.—Localized giant cell tumor of tendon sheath (GCTTS) is one of the most common soft tissue tumors of the hand. However, the etiology of GCTTS has not been discerned. The recurrence rate for GCTTS after surgery has been reported to range from 9% to 44%, and occasionally, spreading of the tumor circumferentially around the phalanx and involvement of adjacent structures make complete surgical excision difficult. Some clinical risk factors for the recurrence of localized GCTTS have been reported. The cellularity and mitotic activity of GCTTS have been reported to be related to recurrence, but this is a controversial view. Whether the proliferative activity of GCTTS is related to its recurrence rate and local aggressiveness was investigated.

Methods.—The clinicopathological and immunohistochemical features of localized GCTTS of the fingers, including the area around the metacarpophalangeal joint, were studied in 30 patients (21 men, 9 women) 9 to 63 years of age. All had undergone excision of a GCTTS between 1993 and 2001 at one institution. Four of the 30 patients had undergone surgery for recurrent GCTTS, which had originally been performed at another institution. Immunohistochemical staining with the MIB-1 monoclonal antibody was performed on formalin-fixed paraffin-embedded tissue sections. Correlations between the MIB-1 staining index of nonrecurrent lesions and that of recurrent lesions and between that of lesions with no bone involvement and that of those with bone involvement were analyzed with the use of the Mann-Whitney U test.

Results.—No significant difference in the MIB-1 staining index was found between the lesions that recurred and those that did not recur. In addition, no significant association was found between local aggressiveness and the MIB-1 staining index.

Conclusions.—The proliferative activity of localized GCTTS does not seem to be related to its high recurrence rate and local aggressiveness.

▶ This study proposed to use a histologic marker to predict the aggressiveness (and, ultimately, the risk of a recurrence) of GCTTS. Unfortunately, the particular marker tested (MIB-1 staining index) was not clearly effective in making any distinctions between aggressiveness or the lack thereof and the rate of recurrence of these tumors. Without such a tool, the hand surgeon must continue to focus on meticulous dissection and complete resection.

M. Concannon, MD

Tuberculosis of the Metacarpals and Phalanges of the Hand
Subasi M, Bukte Y, Kapukaya A, et al (Univ of Dicle, Diyarbakir, Turkey)
Ann Plast Surg 53:469-472, 2004   21–5

Abstract.—Skeletal tuberculosis (TB) is less common than the pulmonary form. Involvements of the metacarpals and phalanges of the hand are infrequent. The authors report their experience with treatment and outcome of TB of the metacarpals and phalanges of the hand in 7 patients. There were 4 women and 3 men in the study who ranged in age from 3 to 60 years (average age, 22.7 years). The duration of complaints at presentation ranged from 4 to 17 months (average, 9 months). The most common presentation was pain and swelling. The presumptive preoperative diagnoses were bone tumor in 4 patients, spina ventosa in 2, and chronic pyogenic osteomyelitis in 1 patients. The results of the laboratory examination showed a mild increase in the erythrocyte sedimentation rate. No patient had an active tubercular lesion or history of pulmonary disease. The diagnosis was based on the clinical picture and radiographic features, and was confirmed by open biopsy. No patient had bony debridement or arthrodesis to control the infection. The treatment of all patients began with a 4-drug regimen for 2 months, followed by a 2-drug regimen for 10 months. The mean follow-up was 30.28 months (range, 16–52 months). At the time of the last follow-up, all lesions had healed with no recurrence. The functional results were satisfactory in all patients. One patient with thumb metacarpophalangeal TB had joint irregularity and thumb metacarpal shortening. Arthrodesis was not needed in any patient. TB of the metacarpals and phalanges of the hand can be difficult to diagnose during the early stages. TB should be suspected in cases of long-standing pain and swelling in the metacarpals and phalanges. It is necessary to keep TB in mind when making the differential diagnosis of several osseous pathologies.

▶ The authors report their experience with 7 patients with TB of the metacarpals and phalanges of the hand. All patients had pain and swelling of the affected regions and radiographic evidence of osseous involvement. Of the 7 patients, only 3 had a positive Mantoux test, and the diagnosis of osteoarticular TB was confirmed by culture or histologic findings, or both. Treatment consisted of 12 months of antituberculosis drugs without the need for surgical debridement or arthrodesis. In the last few decades, the incidence of extrapulmonary TB has increased. Therefore, tuberculosis should be included in the differential diagnosis of patients with long-standing pain in metacarpal and phalangeal joints and radiographic evidence of osseous pathology.

K. Azari, MD

Epithelioid Sarcoma of the Hand

Herr MJ, Harmsen WS, Amadio PC, et al (Mayo Clinic, Rochester, Minn)
Clin Orthop 431:193-200, 2005   21–6

Twenty-eight patients were treated for a primary epithelioid sarcoma of the hand. Twenty-seven patients (96%) had excisions before evaluation, including 11 (39%) with multiple prior excisions with varying diagnoses before epithelioid sarcoma, and all had surgical treatment after referral. The patients' surgical management included three patients with amputation at the forearm, three patients with wide excision, and 21 patients with a partial amputation of the hand. The follow-up period averaged 120 months (range, 24–276 months). Eighteen patients have no evidence of disease at last follow-up. Treatment failures included one local recurrence, four regional metastases, and five distant metastases. Five patients died secondary to disease. Two patients are alive with disease, and three are alive with no evidence of disease after additional treatment. After aggressive surgical management with negative margins, 71% of the patients were alive without evidence of disease at the last follow-up, with a 5- and 10-year survivorship of 85%. Our goal is to review: (1) the effectiveness of preoperative imaging, (2) the role of adjuvant therapy, (3) survival after alternative resections, and (4) function after resection.

▶ This article examining a single institution's retrospective experience with epithelioid sarcoma of the hand is a helpful and important contribution to the literature. As with previous studies, wide excision (whenever possible) is the treatment of choice and leads to improved functionality compared with partial amputation. MRI is very useful and demonstrates an excellent positive predictive value. Although not statistically significant, negative outcome variables include male gender, advanced age, larger tumor size, prior biopsy or surgery, and a residual neoplasm at the time of surgery. An interesting point made in the article is that many of these tumors present without pain and are slow growing, which makes differentiation from more common benign lesions difficult.

M. Rizzo, MD

Human Orf (Ecthyma contagiosum)

Georgiades G, Katsarou A, Dimitroglou K (Limnos Gen Hosp, Greece)
J Hand Surg [Br] 30B:409-411, 2005   21–7

Background.—Orf, or ecthyma contagiosum, is a cutaneous lesion caused by an epitheliotropic DNA parapoxvirus that is especially adapted to epidermal cells. It has been recognized since 1934 as a common occupational disease among persons in contact with infected animals or contaminated meat, such as farmers, butchers, and veterinarians. The true prevalence of human orf infection is likely underestimated because orf is a self-limiting condition that is easily recognized by persons at risk who do not always seek medical care. This report described 31 cases of orf and considered its pathology, characteristic appearance, diagnosis, treatment, and complications.

Case Reports.—From 1988 to 2003, 31 cases of human orf were diagnosed in 21 men and 10 women at one hospital. The mean age of the patients was 51 years (range 17-70 years). All but one of the patients were farmers who had been exposed to infected animals. Ten patients had an animal bite in the vicinity of the lesion. The lesions typically were 1 to 3 cm in diameter and were located on the extensor surface of the digits in 20 cases, the dorsum of the hand in 6 cases, and the palm in 5 cases. Twenty-two patients presented with the typical lesion-a painless, itchy macule that developed into a papule. After 1 to 2 weeks the lesion developed a red center surrounded by a white ring and a red halo. In the following 2 weeks the lesion changed to a nodular shape with central umbilication and then took on a papillomatous shape. Two patients experienced systemic symptoms such as fever and malaise. In all patients, the only specific local treatment was local wound care. The lesion was kept clean with local antiseptic under a moist and later a dry dressing. Misdiagnosis as a pyogenic granuloma led to incision of the lesion in three patients. Symptomatic therapy, including local steroids and oral antihistamines, was administered to the four patients who developed erythema multiforme. In 19 patients with a typical lesion, complete regression occurred in 4 to 7 weeks without residual scarring with no treatment other than local wound care. In the other 12 patients, who developed superimposed infection or erythema multiforme, or had the lesion incised, healing occurred in 4 to 9 weeks, also without residual scarring.

Conclusions.—The diagnosis of human orf is based on the history of contact with infected animals and the clinical features of papular skin lesions. Differential diagnosis should include "milker's nodules," pyogenic granuloma, skin anthracosis, keratoacanthoma, and malignant tumors. The use of gloves and isolation of infected animals are effective preventive measures. There have been no reports of human-to-human spread of orf. Orthopaedic, hand, and plastic surgeons not experienced with orf lesions should be aware of the disease and should include it in the differential diagnosis of hand infections.

▶ Human orf is a viral infection that is more common in rural areas and in patients who handle sheep and goats. The authors provide an excellent review of the disease process and remind us that no specific treatment, other than local wound care, is usually necessary. It is important to consider human orf in patients who have had contact with animals in the differential diagnosis. Only cases with large or persistent lesions, or patients who are immunosuppressed may require more aggressive management. Many of us who rarely see (or consider) this lesion need to keep it in mind.

M. Rizzo, MD

22 Hand: Miscellaneous

Forearm Compartment Syndrome: Anatomical Analysis of Surgical Approaches to the Deep Space
Ronel DN, Mtui E, Nolan WB III (Cornell Univ, New York)
Plast Reconstr Surg 114:697-705, 2004   22–1

Abstract.—Forearm compartment syndrome is a surgical emergency that usually requires release of the superficial muscle compartments. In some clinical situations it is imperative to also explore the deep muscle compartments. There are no anatomical guides for surgical exploration of the deep compartments that would minimize collateral damage to surrounding vessels, nerves, and muscles. Surgical injury in the setting of ischemia, especially vascular injury, compounds the tissue damage that has already occurred. The authors evaluated four surgical approaches (three volar and one dorsal) to the deep forearm by performing detailed anatomical dissections on 10 embalmed and plastinated cadavers. They used a scoring system to rate the approaches for their ability to visualize the deep space without causing iatrogenic injury to superficial muscles, arteries, and nerves. In the volar forearm, an ulnar approach to the deep space is simple, causes the least iatrogenic surgical injury, and provides access to the deep volar forearm structures. The plane of dissection is between the flexor carpi ulnaris and the flexor digitorum superficialis. Dividing one or two distal segmental branches of the ulnar artery to the distal flexor digitorum superficialis exposes the pronator quadratus. Lifting the ulnar neurovascular bundle with the flexor digitorum superficialis in the middle third of the forearm exposes the flexor digitorum profundus and the flexor pollicis longus. This approach to the deep space requires no sharp dissection. In the dorsal forearm, a midline approach between the extensor digitorum communis and the extensor carpi radialis brevis is simple and safe.

▶ This study investigated the ability of 4 surgical approaches (radial, central, ulnar, and dorsal) to visualize the deep musculature of the forearm without iatrogenic harm to the muscles, nerves, and arteries. A detailed anatomic study of the forearm was performed in 10 embalmed and plastinated cadavers, and a scoring system was devised to rate the degree of harm to the muscles, nerves, and arteries with each surgical approach. The ulnar approach accessed the deep space between the flexor carpi ulnaris and flexor digitorum superficialis muscles and appeared to be least damaging to the musculature and blood supply in each of the forearm compartments.

In most cases, release of the superficial volar compartments is sufficient treatment for forearm compartment syndrome. However, there are instances such as high-voltage electrical injury, severe crush injuries, and ongoing myonecrosis despite superficial fasciotomy, that mandate the exploration and release of the deep volar or dorsal compartments. In these situations, this ulnar approach to the deep volar forearm compartment should be considered.

K. Azari, MD

Surgical Management of Hypothenar and Thenar Hammer Syndromes: A Retrospective Study of 31 Instances in 28 Patients
Dethmers RSM, Houpt P (Centre for Plastic, Reconstructive and Handsurgery, Zwolle, The Netherlands)
J Hand Surg [Br] 30B:419-423, 2005   22–2

This retrospective study assessed the results of treatment of 29 cases of hypothenar hammer syndrome and two cases of thenar hammer syndrome. Three hands were symptom free, 15 were improved, 11 were unchanged and two were worse at a mean follow-up of 43 (range 4–60) months. Follow-up colour-coded Duplex sonography of revascularizations ($n = 27$) revealed 13 patent, five occluded and one partially thrombosed grafts, seven grafts with aneurysmal dilatations and one coiled graft. Colour-coded Duplex sonography results after venous interposition graft combined with endoscopic thoracic sympathectomy were no better than venous interposition graft alone. All three arterial interposition grafts and two end-to-end-reconstructions were patent. The Duplex outcomes of the revascularizations did not correspond well with the clinical outcomes. Endoscopic thoracic sympathectomy was associated with a high rate of inconvenient side effects.

▶ This is a study reviewing 29 cases of hypothenar hammer syndrome and 2 cases of thenar hammer syndrome with a long-term follow-up averaging 43 months. Debate exists within the literature as to whether patients with reconstructed vascular arches have improved outcomes in comparison with simple ligation and resection of the diseased segment. Unfortunately, this article does not clearly answer that question. The major difficulty with the article is the varied treatment methods that existed for the 31 cases. Primary end-to-end repair of the diseased arterial segment was used in 2 patients. Arterial interposition grafting was used in 3 patients. Twenty-four cases were reconstructed with volar forearm veins. Endoscopic thoracotomy was also used in almost half of the patients. Results were somewhat discouraging: only 3 of 31 patients were symptom free at a 4-year follow-up. However, 15 of 31 were improved, 11 of 31 were no better, and 2 of 31 were worse. Endoscopic sympathectomy produced no significant improvement in overall symptomatology. In addition, endoscopic sympathectomy in this study produced a high rate of objectionable hand dryness and compensatory sweating in the contralateral extremity.

Arterial grafts did appear to do better than venous grafts in terms of long-term patency. We favor the use of saphenous vein grafts. Volar forearm veins are thin-walled and tend to coil and become aneurysmal with time, which was certainly confirmed in this study. The work done by Ferris et al[1] with saphenous vein grafts showed excellent patency rates, in contrast to the almost 50% occlusion rate seen with the use of volar venous grafts in this article. The best treatment for hypothenar hammer syndrome still remains to be determined. Further prospective studies will need to be carried out to determine the true benefits of ligation versus vascular reconstruction alone. Until then, we still recommend the use of either arterial grafts or saphenous vein grafts to avoid the problems seen with thinner upper arm veins. We also still believe it is very important to have patients refrain from smoking during the postoperative period, as this contributes to early graft thrombosis.

S. L. Moran, MD

Reference

1. Ferris BL, Taylor LM Jr, Oyama K, et al: Hypothenar hammer syndrome: Proposed etiology. *J Vasc Surg* 31:104-113, 2000.

A Controlled Clinical Trial of Postoperative Hand Elevation at Home Following Day-Case Surgery
Fagan DJ, Evans A, Ghandour A, et al (Univ Hosp of Wales, Cardiff, England; Glan Clwyd Hosp, Denbighshire, North Wales, England)
J Hand Surg [Br] 29B:458-460, 2004   22–3

Although elevation of the upper limb is considered valuable for the prevention of and the reduction of swelling following major surgery or severe injuries to the hand, it is not clear how much elevation, if any, is required following minor surgery such as carpal tunnel decompression. We investigated this by randomizing patients undergoing carpal tunnel decompression into two groups - one having high elevation at home and one being treated with a simple sling. Volumetric analysis of the swelling of the hand 5 days postoperatively showed no significant difference between the two groups. In the trial group, the mean increase in volume of the operated hand was 11 ml (95% CI +4 to +17) or 2.7%. In the control group, the mean swelling was 13 ml (95% CI +4 to +21) or 3.6%. The findings of this study do not support the use of routine high arm elevation following day-case surgery of the hand.

▶ In upper extremity surgery, postoperative edema is one of the main barriers to surgical success. Edema may contribute to stiffness, poor wound healing, and increased chance of infection. It may also increase the chance of complex regional pain syndrome. Therefore, an aggressive approach to postoperative edema is the highest priority of physicians and therapists who treat patients after upper extremity surgery.

As such, one should welcome any attempt at studying the effects of treating edema in the postoperative setting. This study isolates the effect of elevation alone on the presence of edema in a series of patients who underwent open carpal tunnel release. The conclusion of the study is that elevation alone does not significantly affect the amount of postoperative swelling at the fifth day after surgery. Unfortunately, it is quite difficult to show meaningful results of intervention when the measured variable is quite small in both the control and the intervention groups. In this case, the amount of increase in upper extremity volume was 11 mL and 13 mL in the intervention and control groups, respectively. In other words, carpal tunnel release surgery does not routinely result in much postoperative edema. Therefore, it is difficult to study postoperative edema in this group of patients.

I hope that this study does not lead surgeons and therapists to think that postoperative elevation is completely unhelpful. Yes, in a very limited sense one could rightly conclude that elevation is a bit superfluous in treating patients after an uncomplicated carpal tunnel release procedure. However, there is quite likely an important role for elevation after upper extremity trauma such as a wrist fracture and in more extensive surgeries. Moreover, elevation is just one component of a postoperative anti-edema program. Elevation should be combined with compression, decongestive massage, and active range of motion of the arm. The simplest anti-edema program is to instruct the patient as follows: "Put your hand over your head and open and close your fist 10 times. Perform this exercise every hour, or as often as you think about it, until your first postoperative appointment."

K. Bengtson, MD

Mechanical Load on the Upper Extremity During Wheelchair Activities
van Drongelen S, van der Woude LH, Janssen TW, et al (Vrije Universiteit, Amsterdam; Delft Univ of Technology, The Netherlands; Rehabilitation Ctr Amsterdam; et al)
Arch Phys Med Rehabil 86:1214-1220, 2005   22–4

Objective.—To determine the net moments on the glenohumeral joint and elbow joint during wheelchair activities.

Design.—Kinematics and external forces were measured during wheelchair activities of daily living (level propulsion, riding on a slope, weight-relief lifting, reaching, negotiating a curb) and processed in an inverse dynamics biomechanic model.

Setting.—Biomechanics laboratory.

Participants.—Five able-bodied subjects, 8 subjects with paraplegia, and 4 subjects with tetraplegia.

Interventions.—Not applicable.

Main Outcome Measure.—Net moments on the glenohumeral joint and elbow joint.

Results.—Peak shoulder and elbow moments were significantly higher for negotiating a curb and weight-relief lifting than for reaching, level propulsion, and riding on a slope. Overall, the elbow extension moments were significantly lower for subjects with tetraplegia than for those with paraplegia.

Conclusions.—The net moments during weight-relief lifting and negotiating a curb were high when compared with wheelchair propulsion tasks. Taking the effect of frequency and duration into account, these loads might imply a considerable risk for joint damage in the long term.

▶ The upper extremities of individuals of paraplegia and tetraplegia perform all the tasks required of both the arms and legs in able-bodied individuals. Since the arms perform double duty, they are subject to extra forces and are, therefore, at higher risk for various overuse injuries compared to ambulating individuals. This article attempts to quantify these forces based on biomechanical monitoring of the elbows and glenohumeral joints during various tasks that are unique to individuals who function from a wheelchair base. The authors also attempt to show a difference between individuals with high spinal cord injuries (SCIs) compared with those with lower SCIs. One might expect in a person with injury to the C6-7 level of the spinal cord—where there is paralysis of many of the muscles that normally move the shoulder and elbow as well as stabilize the shoulder—that the biomechanical forces on these joints would be different than in those individuals with all the upper-extremity muscles intact. Therefore, the authors compare those with C6-7 level of injury with those who have T3-12 SCIs, as well as with normal subjects.

Surprisingly, the tasks of wheelchair propulsion, weight relief lifting, and reaching showed only a small significant difference among the groups. The authors conclude that the increased incidence of upper-extremity injury is due to the repetitive nature of these tasks rather than an increase in joint forces.

From this study one may draw the correlation that operative procedures on the shoulder and elbow in tetraplegic individuals require no significant modification to allow for differing biomechanical properties of either joint. However, one should not ignore the significant difference in the postoperative rehabilitation phase for these individuals. The wheelchair-based patient will require additional support for mobility and activities of daily living while recovering from upper extremity surgery. Often this involves a nursing home stay until they are completely recovered. Additionally, one must account for increased reconditioning time to reach the higher level of strength and function required in the patient functioning from a wheelchair base.

K. Bengtson, MD

Providing Care for Hand Disorders a Re-Appraisal of Need
Burke FD, Dias JJ, Palou CH, et al (Pulvertaft Hand Ctr, Derby, England)
J Hand Surg [Br] 29B:575-579, 2004   22–5

An audit of hand surgery activity in Derby during the period 1989–1990 produced manpower and resource recommendations for the speciality per

100,000 of population per year for the United Kingdom. The decade that
followed the audit has seen major changes in health care provision, including reduced service activity by trainee doctors through restricted hours of
work and less unsupervised surgery. A further audit of hand surgery activity
was performed during 2000–2001 to assess the effects of these and other
changes. This showed that there has been a 2% rise in trauma attendances,
though trauma bed utilization had reduced by 12% and surgery time by
38%. Trauma out-patient visits had also reduced by 11%. Day-case trauma
surgery rates were virtually unchanged at 63%. Women attend more frequently with traumatic hand injuries than they did 10 years ago and there is
a rising incidence of hand injuries in the home, with a falling incidence at
work. Elective referrals have risen by 36% and operations by 34%. The top
ten diagnoses relate to the same conditions although their rankings have
changed. Elective day-case surgery rates have risen from 64% to 94% over
the decade. The 34% increase in elective operations has been absorbed
within a 5% reduction in elective bed use and a 23% reduction in surgery
time. Elective out-patient visits have also dropped 14% overall. This audit
indicates that in 2000–2001 one whole time equivalent hand surgeon can
service a population of 125,000. The national requirement for a 56 million
population would be 448 whole time equivalent hand surgeons.

▶ The authors report their audit of hand surgery activity in one area of the
United Kingdom where there has existed a well-known hand surgery unit for
many decades. They analyze a number of parameters that have changed over
the interval between this and a preceding study (1989-1990). They make conclusions related to hand surgeon requirements per 100,000 of population.

The numbers are what they are. Conclusions may differ. Relevance to other
regions of the United Kingdom—much less to other countries with differing
populations, industries, health care systems, etc—may be less clear. Nonetheless, these data are absolutely necessary for a health system in which care
is based on a 1-payor, universal coverage paradigm.

V. R. Hentz, MD

**The Patient Outcomes of Surgery-Hand/Arm (POS-Hand/Arm): A New
Patient-Based Outcome Measure**
Cano SJ, Browne JP, Lamping DL, et al (London School of Hygiene & Tropical
Medicine)
J Hand Surg [Br] 29B:477-485, 2004   22–6

The purpose of this study was to develop and validate a new patient-based
outcome measure for hand/arm disorders for use in audit, clinical trials and
effectiveness studies. There were three stages. First, we carried out inter-
views with 40 patients with hand/arm disorders to develop and pilot questionnaire content. Second, in a postal survey with 165 pre- and 181 post-
surgery patients, we reduced the number of items and identified scales.

Third, in a postal survey with 132 pre- and 204 post-surgery patients we evaluated the psychometric properties of the measure.

Findings confirmed the acceptability, reliability, validity and responsiveness to clinical change of the questionnaire. The Patient Outcomes of Surgery-Hand/Arm (POS-Hand/Arm) is a new surgical outcome measure that can be used before and after surgery (29 and 33 items, respectively) to evaluate and compare new techniques, surgical teams and units.

▶ This is yet another questionnaire that was reported to be suitable to measure outcomes after hand surgery. The questions in this questionnaire overlapped with the questions in the DASH and the Michigan Hand Outcomes Questionnaire.

There are descriptive nouns added to this questionnaire—such as cramp, stiffness, joint locking, and tightness—that attempt to measure how much these symptoms bother the patients. There are questions in the functional domain that include using a remote control and pouring from a teapot. Some of these functional questions are suitable for the British patients but may not be applicable to patients in the United States or in other countries. It appears that this questionnaire is a variation of questionnaires that are currently used in the United States, but the questions are adapted for British subjects.

More testing is necessary to evaluate whether this questionnaire is responsive for a variety of hand surgery conditions and whether this questionnaire is suitable for international use. Additionally, psychometric testing is necessary to assess whether additional descriptive terms will enhance the applicability of this questionnaire.

K. C. Chung, MD, MS

Telemedicine Consultation for Patients With Upper Extremity Disorders Is Reliable
Abboud JA, Bozentka DJ, Beredjiklian PK (Univ of Pennsylvania, Philadelphia)
Clin Orthop 435:250-257, 2005   22–7

Abstract.—Telemedicine is a valuable resource for the delivery of health care to patients in underserved areas. The purpose of this study was to assess the reliability of asynchronous teleconsultation in the diagnosis and establishment of treatment plans for patients with disorders of the upper extremity. One hundred patients with disorders of the upper extremity were prospectively evaluated. Initial patient evaluations, done by an independent evaluator, involved a medical history, physical examination, digital images of the patient, and digitized radiographic studies. This patient information was presented electronically to two hand surgeons 6 months after one surgeon independently evaluated the patients in the outpatient clinic. The physicians formulated diagnosis and treatment plans for the patients based on the blinded electronic information. These findings then were compared with the treatment plans made by the physicians at the time of the patients' visits. Telemedicine consultation resulted in excellent agreement within observers

($\kappa = .92$) and between observers ($\kappa = .86$). Telemedicine consultation seems to be a reliable method for diagnosis and establishment of treatment plans in the management of upper extremity disorders.

▶ The authors compared the reliability of noninteractive (asynchronous) teleconsultation with face-to-face consultations for the diagnosis and treatment of 100 consecutive patients with upper extremity disorders. The asynchronous format was chosen because it is less costly and more readily available than the live, interactive telemedicine format. The results showed excellent agreement between the face-to-face and telemedicine consultations.

The major limitation of this study and asynchronous teleconsultation is the quality of the examiner. Here, a senior orthopedic surgery resident served as the examiner. However, one can easily imagine that an examiner with less orthopedic experience may lead to decreased teleconsultation reliability. Another shortcoming of this study is the electronic format reevaluation of the same patient by the same surgeon 6 months after the face-to-face consultation. This relatively short period to repeat evaluation may have introduced recall bias in the present study.

Despite these limitations, telemedicine holds great potential for delivery of health care to underserved areas. As technologies improve and become less costly, the live, interactive format may become more prevalent and may help improve reliability with less experienced examiners.

K. Azari, MD

Subject Index

position of crossing branches of the
medial antebrachial cutaneous
nerve in, 109
posttraumatic stiffness, surgical
treatment of, 89
reconstruction of soft tissue defects,
ulnar recurrent adipofascial flap
for, 257
ulnar neuropathy, follow-up and
prognostic factors determining
outcome, 111
valgus laxity of, effects of elbow flexion
and forearm rotation on, 92
Elderly, distal humerus fractures in
fixation with and without
Kirschner-wire augmentation, 73
noncustom total elbow replacement for,
75
treatment considerations, 74
Epicondylectomy
frontal partial medial, for cubital tunnel
syndrome, 113
Epithelioid sarcoma
of the hand, 270
Essex-Lopresti injury
failure of fresh-frozen radial head
allografts in treatment of, 83

F

Fat pad sign
following elbow trauma in adults,
usefulness and reliability in
diagnosis of occult fracture, 93
Fingers
(*see also* Thumb)
arthroplasty
long-term assessment of Swanson
implant in, 240
mechanics after 3 different silicone
implants, 238
osteolysis following use of Swanson
and Sutter prostheses, 236
with Swanson prosthesis, 17-year
survivorship analysis, 237
bioabsorbable osteofixation devices in,
217
chronic joint instability,
bone-ligament-bone graft from the
iliac crest for reconstruction, 224
fractures
base of distal phalanx in children,
218
extra-articular metacarpal, 3 cast
techniques for, 215
management principles, 219
nerve repair
end-to-side neurorrhaphy for, 195

limited, protected postsurgical motion
and results of, 198
reconstruction
distally based dorsal flaps for, clinical
experience and cadaveric studies,
254
heterodigital arterial flap for,
extension of reach by vein division
and repair, 255
reverse dorsal digital and
intercommissural flaps for, 252
surgical results in severe scleroderma,
234
tendon repair
A1 pulley release of locked trigger
digit by percutaneous technique,
206
comparative analysis of
biomechanical behavior of 5 flexor
tendon core sutures, 210
dental rolls as model for practicing
techniques, 208
early active mobilization with 2
Kessler 2-strand core sutures and a
strengthened circumferential suture,
212
partial A2 pulley excision, effect on
gliding resistance and pulley
strength in vitro, 205
Seprafilm for prevention of
peritendinous adhesions following,
211
terminal tendon of the digital extensor
mechanism
anatomy, 203
kinematic analysis, 204
tip amputation
homodigital neurovascular island flap
for restoration of function and
sensitivity, 245
replantation, functional and cosmetic
results, 244
toe-to-hand transfer
multiple monoblock, report of 10
cases, 260
total foot-to-hand transfer for
monodactyly, 178
transthecal vs. traditional digital block
for anesthesia of, 191
tuberculosis of the metacarpals and
phalanges, 269
Flexor pollicis longus tendon
early active mobilization of primary
repairs with 2 Kessler 2-strand core
sutures and a strengthened
circumferential suture, 212

Author Index

A

Abboud JA, 279
Abe Y, 265
Acland RD, 49
Adamczyk MJ, 144
Adams R, 100, 104
Adams RA, 101
Agel J, 137
Agrawal V, 27
Ahern M, 241
Akuthota V, 192
Aldridge JM III, 90
Al-Harran H, 126
Ali A, 76
Al-Qattan MM, 178
Amadio PC, 205, 213, 270
Ameur N, 60
Ashammakhi N, 217
Athwal GS, 230
Atkins TA, 90
Atzei A, 251
Aydin A, 169
Azuma E, 262
Azzopardi T, 130

B

Bach PB, 33
Backman C, 229
Bain GI, 121
Bajhau A, 121
Balakrishnan G, 254
Baldrighi CM, 251
Barron OA, 198
Beaupre LA, 127
Bednar DA, 126
Beekman R, 111
Bell MJ, 91
Bellaïche L, 24
Belt EA, 232, 236
Bennett WF, 54
Beredjiklian PK, 279
Berger RA, 156
Bergman GJD, 21
Bhat M, 165
Bicknell RT, 26
Björkenheim J-M, 1
Bogdanske J, 14
Bohnsack M, 63
Boll T, 131
Boyer MI, 200
Bozentka DJ, 279
Brady O, 233
Brenner KA, 259
Browne JP, 278

B

Bryant D, 36
Bukte Y, 269
Burge P, 151
Burkart A, 17
Burke FD, 277
Burke MS, 171
Burkhart BG, 73

C

Campodonico A, 247
Candal-Couto JJ, 81
Candido KD, 72
Cano SJ, 278
Catalano LW III, 198
Chammas M, 59
Chang EY, 266
Chang S-C, 253
Charousset C, 24
Chassery C, 71
Chen S-L, 253
Chen T-M, 253
Chenkin J, 230
Chennagiri R, 151
Chiang AS, 44
Choi B-H, 195
Chuang DC-C, 69
Classen DA, 249
Cofield RH, 28
Cohen MS, 97
Collins DN, 34
Cooney WP, 83, 156
Coulet B, 59
Coulton T, 130
Court-Brown CM, 2
Culp RW, 188

D

Dailiana ZH, 245
Daluiski A, 117
Dao KD, 116
David TRC, 233
Davila S, 6
Davis TRC, 165
DeFranco MJ, 20
de la Cerda J, 77
de las Heras J, 77
Dellon AL, 65, 110
Dethmers RSM, 274
Devnani AS, 77
Dias JJ, 233, 277
Dimitroglou K, 271
Dines JS, 7
Doi K, 61, 68

D

Doornberg J, 80
Doty R Jr, 72
Douglas H, 76
Draganich LF, 223
Dubberley JH, 95
Dubert Th, 113
Ducic I, 65, 110
Dunham RC, 103
Dunn WR, 23
Dunning CE, 193
Durán D, 77
Duranthon LD, 24

E

Ebaugh DD, 31
Eckstein F, 11
Edelson G, 218
Ehrendorfer S, 130
El-Khatib HA, 256
Elliot D, 187, 212
Elsaidi GA, 151
Evans A, 275

F

Faber KJ, 95
Fagan DJ, 275
Ferreira L, 26
Ferri M, 25
Finlay K, 25
Fitzgerald BT, 116
Fitzgerald D, 94
Frankle M, 41
Franzblau A, 182
Freeland AE, 5
Fujita S, 227

G

Galarza M, 112
Ganayem M, 218
Gardner MJ, 7
Geissler WB, 5
Gelberman RH, 200
Gell N, 182
Georgiades G, 271
Gerber C, 3
Getz CL, 16
Ghandour A, 275
Gilbart MK, 234
Gilbert A, 68
Ginn TA, 133
Givissis PK, 98

293